Success in Medical School and Beyond

MNEMONICS AND PEARLS

Success in Medical School and Beyond

MNEMONICS AND PEARLS

Steve C. Christos, MS, DO, FACEP, FAAEM
Chairman, Department of Emergency Medicine
Clinical Assistant Professor
Vituity | At the heart of better care - Vituity Partner
AMITA Health Resurrection Medical Center – Chicago

William G. Gossman MD, FAAEM
Chairman, Department of Emergency Medicine
Medical Director, Physician Assistants Program
Creighton University Medical School

2021 Ed.

Success in Medical School and Beyond Mnemonics and Pearls
By Dr. Steve C. Christos, FACEP, FAAEM and William G. Gossman, MD, FAAEM

Layout and Cover Design - Sherry Gossman, RN, BSN
Cover Photo by Luis Melendez on Unsplash

SPECIAL THANKS TO OUR FRIENDS AND REVIEWERS:

Karl Ambroz, MD, FACEP
Clinical Assistant Professor
Department of Emergency Medicine
AMITA Health Resurrection Medical Center

Amy Archer, MD, FACEP
Attending Physician
Department of Emergency Medicine
Advocate Lutheran General Hospital

George Chiampas, DO, FACEP
Clinical Assistant Professor
Department of Emergency Medicine
Northwestern University Feinberg School of Medicine

Nicole Colucci, DO, FACEP, FAAP
Clinical Assistant Professor
Department of Emergency Medicine
Vituity | At the heart of better care Vituity Partner
AMITA Health Resurrection Medical Center

Brian Donahue, MD, FACEP
Clinical Assistant Professor
Department of Emergency Medicine
Vituity | At the heart of better care Vituity Partner
AMITA Health Resurrection Medical Center

Marc Dorfman, MD, FACEP
Director, Emergency Medicine Residency
Clinical Assistant Professor
Department of Emergency Medicine
Vituity | At the heart of better care Vituity Partner
AMITA Health Resurrection Medical Center

Brett Hanson, MD
Emergency Medicine Resident Physician
AMITA Health Resurrection Medical Center
Department of Emergency Medicine

Matthew Jordan, MD, FACEP
Clinical Assistant Professor
Department of Emergency Medicine
Vituity | At the heart of better care Vituity Partner
AMITA Health Resurrection Medical Center

Jason Langenfeld, MD, FACEP
Assistant Professor of Emergency Medicine
University of Nebraska Medical Center

Procopio M. LoDuca, MD
Northwest Infectious Disease Consultants
AMITA Health Resurrection Medical Center

Tony Macasaet, MD, FACEP
Medical Director, Emergency Services
Vernon Memorial Healthcare, Viroqua, WI

Ruba S. Odeh, DO
Northwest Infectious Disease Consultants
AMITA Health Resurrection Medical Center

Robert Oelhaf, MD, FAAEM
Attending Physician
Department of Emergency Medicine
Penn Highland Healthcare
Elk Regional Health Center, St. Marys, PA

William Parente, MD
Emergency Medicine Resident Physician
AMITA Health Resurrection Medical Center
Department of Emergency Medicine

Kristin Peterson, MD, FACEP
Clinical Assistant Professor
Department of Emergency Medicine
Vituity | At the heart of better care Vituity Partner
AMITA Health Resurrection Medical Center

Scott Plantz, MD, FAAEM
Associate Professor of Emergency Medicine
University of Louisville Emergency Medicine

Mark Postel, DO
Emergency Medicine Resident Physician
AMITA Health Resurrection Medical Center
Department of Emergency Medicine

Thomas Topalis, DO
Emergency Medicine Resident Physician
AMITA Health Resurrection Medical Center
Department of Emergency Medicine

Leo L. Viray, MD
Emergency Medicine Resident Physician
AMITA Health Resurrection Medical Center
Department of Emergency Medicine

Special thanks to Sherry Gossman, Kelly Delaney, Catherine Deregla, Denise Toriani, Sally Lorentz, Ellie Barberis, Christina, Peter, Sam and Demetra Christos for their efforts.

CONTENTS

CONTENTS

CONTENTS

CONTENTS

CONTENTS

CONTENTS

CONTENTS

CONTENTS

CONTENTS

CONTENTS

CONTENTS

CONTENTS

CONTENTS

GENERAL

HISTORY OF PRESENT ILLNESS

Mnemonic - (O P_3 Q R S_3 T)

O	**O**nset - What time did the symptoms start - What activity caused the symptoms
P3	**P**ain location **P**alliative (what makes the pain better) **P**rovocactive factors (what makes the pain worse)
Q	**Q**uality (sharp, dull, heavy, burning, squeezing, etc.
R	**R**adiation (arms, jay, back, groin, etc.
S3	**S**everity (use pain scale 1 to 10, ten being the most severe pain) **S**ymptoms associated (nausea, vomiting, diaphoresis, SOB, F/C) **S**imilar episodes in past
T	**T**iming (how long, constant vs. intermittent)

DETERMINING THE ETIOLOGY OF DISEASE PROCESSES

Mnemonic - (AN INDICATIVE DIFFERENTIAL DIAGNOSIS DD)

A	**A**llergy
N	**N**eoplasm

I	**I**nfection
N	**N**osocomial
D	**D**rugs
I	**I**ntoxication
C	**C**ongenital
A	**A**utoimmune
T	**T**rauma
I	**I**nflammation
V	**V**ascular
E	**E**ndocrine

D	**D**eficiency
D	**D**egenerative

If you come up empty with all the above consider PSYCH

MORE HISTORY

Mnemonic - **(AMPLE FAMILY)**

A	**A**llergies
M	**M**eds
P	**P**revious medical history / **P**revious surgical history
L	**L**ast meal in/ **L**MP
E	**E**vents
FAMILY	**FAMILY** History

SYMPTOM / SIGN

Symptom: Patient's presenting complaint (dyspnea, chest pain, etc.)
Sign: Physical exam finding (hypoxia, hypotension, etc.)

CAUSES OF CHEST PAIN

Mnemonic - (MAPLE)3 (PCP$_2$)

M	**M**yocardial Infarction (*33% of patients with AMI do not have chest pain at presentation)* **M**usculoskelatal (Costochondritis, Tietze Syndrome) **M**yocarditis
A	**A**ortic dissection **A**ngina (40% of patients with UA progress to AMI) **A**nxiety
P	**P**E **P**neumothorax **P**neumonia
L	**L**ow H/H **L**ung CA **L**esions, Skin (Herpes Zoster)
E	**E**sophageal rupture **E**sophagitis G**E**RD

P	**P**yelonephritis
C	**C**holecystitis
P	**P**ancreatitis
P	**P**ericarditis

TIETZE SYNDROME

- Painful, non-suppurative localized swelling of the costosternal, sternoclavicular, or costochondral joints
- Differentiated from costochondritis based on the finding of swelling
- Usually involves the 2cd and 3rd ribs
- Cause = unknown; there is a relationship with a recent respiratory illness and coughing

MAJOR RISK FACTORS ASSOCIATED WITH ISCHEMIC HEART DISEASE

- Age > 40
- Male sex
- Family history
- Cigarette smoking
- HTN
- DM
- Hypercholesterolemia
- Obesity
- Known CAD

HEART SCORE

Predicts 6-week risk of **Major Adverse Cardiac Event (MACE)**

HISTORY	ECG	AGE
Highly suspicious +2	Significant ST-depression +2	≥ 65 +2
Moderately suspicious +1	Non specific repolarisation disturbance +1	45-65 +1
Slightly suspicious 0	Normal 0	≤ 45 0

RISK FACTORS		TROPONIN
Hypercholesterolemia, Hypertension, Diabetes, Smoking, + Family history, Obesity	≥ 3 risk factors or history of atherosclerotic disease +2	≥ 3× normal limit +2
	1-2 risk factors +1	1-3× normal limit +1
	No risk factors known 0	≤ normal limit 0

The HEART Score is a propspectively studied scoring system to help emergency departments risk-stratifiy chest pain patients: who will have a MACE within in the next 6 weeks and who will not?

- It involves only a 1-time troponin, at admission.
- The rest of the score is based on age, history, risk factors, and ECG.
- Low risk patients have a score 0-3 and have a less than 2% risk of MACE at 6 weeks.
- MACE is defined as: all-cause mortality, myocardial infarction, or coronary revascularization.
- All other scores are high risk (risk increasing exponentially) and require further management and admission.

CAUSES OF ST SEGMENT ELEVATION

Mnemonic (ELEVATION) 2 [Acad Emerg Med, 1999;6:930, with modifications]

E	**E**lectrolyte abnormalities (↑ K+) **E**xcitation (WPW→ Delta wave)
L	**L**eft bundle branch block **L**eft ventricular hypertrophy
E	**E**arly repolarization **E**mbolism
V	**V**entricular paced rhythms **V**ariant angina (Prinzmetal's angina)
A	**A**neurysm (left ventricular) **A**MI
T	**T**rauma (contusion) **T**reatment (pericardiocentesis)
I	**I**ntracranial hemorrhage **I**nflammation (pericarditis/myocarditis)
O	**O**sborn J waves (hypothermia) **O**verdose-cocaine
N	**N**SSTT – wave change **N**onocclusive vasospasm - (Prinzmetal's angina, cocaine)

ECG FINDINGS IN AMI

ECG diagnosis of AMI: > 1 mm (0.1 mV) of STE in limb leads, and at least 2 mm elevation in the precordial leads

	ECG Findings	Coronary Artery Involvement
Septal	V1-V2	LCA → LAD → septal branch
Anterior	V3-V4	LCA → LAD → diagonal branch
Lateral	I, aVL plus V5, V6	LCA → Circumflex branch
Inferior wall	II, III, aVF	RCA (90%)
Posterior	V8-V9	LCA → Circumflex or RCA → PDA
	STD w/upright T V1	
	R/S ratio > 1 V1-V2	
Right Ventricle	V4R (II, III, aVF)	RCA → proximal branches

QUICK ECG INTERPRETATION OF STEMI V1-V6

Mnemonic - (SSAALL)

S	S	A	A	L	L
V1 **S**EPTAL	V2 **S**EPTAL	V3 **A**NTERIOR	V4 **A**NTERIOR	V5 **L**ATERAL	V6 **L**ATERAL

AMI IN LBBB (SGARBOSSA CRITERIA)

- STE > 1mm concordant with QRS — 5 points
- ST depression > 1mm in V1, V2, V3 — 3 points (STD in V1-V3 concurrently = 3 points)
- STE > 5mm discordant with QRS — 2 points
- Score > 3 suggest MI (90% specific, however 36% sensitive)

Clinical utility of criteria are insensitive and probably have relatively low utility

SGARBOSSA CRITERIA / LBBB PACED RHYTHM

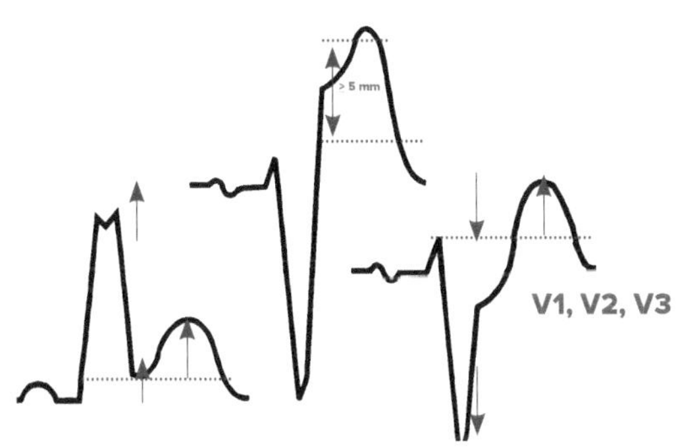

WELLEN'S SYNDROME

T-waves

1. Biphasic T wave (Type A)
2. Deeply inverted T wave (Type B) = most common, 75% of cases

- High-grade critical STENOSIS (not occlusion) of the proximal LAD
- Usually have anterior wall STEMI 30-90 days later
- Patient's are usually asymptomatic at time of ED presentation
- ECG findings present when patient is pain free
- Cardiac enzymes: usually normal or slightly elevated
- Correct disposition: admit, obtain cardiology consult for cardiac catheterization;
  If the patient does not have CP, cardiac catheterization can be done on admission; if the patient has CP, then emergent cardiac catheterization must be performed.

BRUGADA SYNDROME

- Transmembrane ion channelopathy
- Inherited disorder of transmembrane Na, Ca, or K channels that affects myocardial depolarization
- Predisposes young individuals to malignant ventricular dysrhythmias and sudden death
- Family History of Sudden Death or Cardiac Syncope without structural heart disease
- Sudden cardiac arrest (usually young patients <30 years old) may be the initial presentation in approximately 30% of patients; however, SYNCOPE = most common presentation
- Death resulting from Brugada syndrome is related to subsequent Polymorphic VT or VF
- Disposition: cardiac monitoring, admit and cardiology consult
- Treatment: placement of an automatic implanted cardiac cardioverter-defibrillator (AICD)

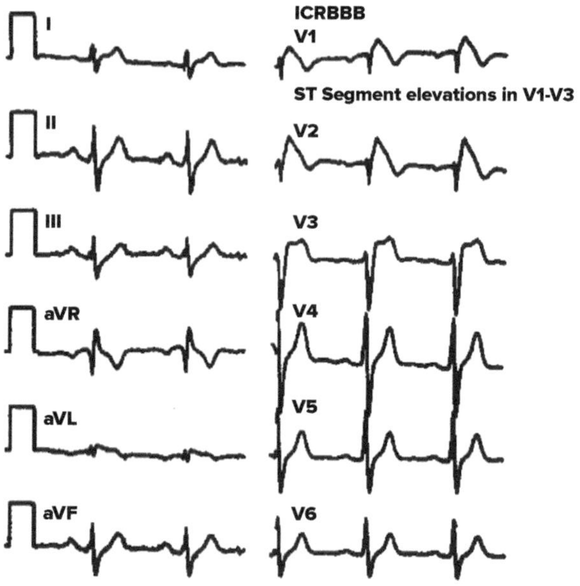

ST segment elevation V1-V3 and/or "saddle deformity" of ST– T segment, with RBBB with or without the terminal S waves in the lateral leads that are associated with typical RBBB. For ECGs of Brugada Types 1-3 go to litfl.com/brugada-syndrome-ecg-library/

ACUTE CORONARY SYNDROMES

- **Stable angina**: activity induced discomfort; predictable and reproducible; relieved by rest or nitroglycerin
- **Unstable angina (UA)**: angina new in onset that occurs at rest or with minimal exertion, OR a worsening change in a previously diagnosed stable angina
- **AMI:** now defined mainly by an increase in serum troponin (involves myocardial cell death and necrosis)
- **Vasospastic angina**, was previously referred to as Prinzmetal or variant angina = Coronary Artery Spasm
- Incompletely occlusive **White Thrombus** = thought to cause UA/NSTEMI
- Completely occlusive **Red Thrombus** = cause of AMI
- **White Thrombus**: platelet rich, gradual onset, partially occlusive; like rings of tree
- **Red Thrombus**: fibrin rich plaque ruptures, sudden, complete occlusion, clotting factors involved

TREATMENT OPTIONS IN ACUTE CORONARY SYNDROME

Mnemonic - (HE BE MOAN) uptodate.com/contents/image?imageKey=CARD%2F75032&topicKey=CARD%2F68&source=see_link

HE	**HEparin**
	
	UFH
	#1 Activates Antithrombin
	➔ inhibits activity of Factor Xa
	➔ Thrombin (IIa)formation from prothrombin inhibited
	
	#2 Activates Antithrombin
	➔ inactivates Thrombin(IIa) directly
	
	LMWHs also activate antithrombin however: Primarily inhibit Factor Xa
	Minimal affect Thrombin (Factor IIa)
		UNFRACTIONATED HEPARIN (UFH) IV
		STEMI and NSTEMI
		• 60 U/kg IV bolus
		  • Max 4,000 U if using Thrombolytic for STEMI
		  • Max 5,000 U if STEMI (PCI) or NSTEMI invasive approach
		• Followed with 12 U/kg/hr infusion (max 1,000 U/hr)
		
		ENOXAPARIN (LOVENOX) DOSAGES - STEMI FIBRINOLYSIS
		• **Dose for patients age < 75 years with normal CrCl**
		  • Lovenox 30mg IV bolus
		  • First SQ dose administered with IV dose 1mg/kg SQ q12hrs. The first two SQ doses maximum = 100mg
		• **CrCl < 30ml/min:** loading dose of 30mg IV followed by 1 mg/kg SQ every 24 hrs
		
		• **Dose for patients ≥ 75 y/o with normal CrCl**
		  • No Lovenox bolus
		  • Lovenox dose: 0.75 mg/kg SQ q 12 hr Max 75 mg/dose for first 2 doses
		
		• **CrCl < 30 mL/min:** 1mg/kg SQ q 24 hours
		No IV loading dose
		
		PERCUTANEOUS CORONARY INTERVENTION (PCI)
		• If last SQ dose of Lovenox was < 8 hours before PCI ➔ no additional dosing needed
		• If > 8 hours bolus with Enoxaparin (Lovenox) 0.3 mg/kg IV
		
		ENOXAPARIN (LOVENOX) DOSAGES - NSTEMI
		• 1mg/kg SQ q 12 hours
		• Reduce dose if creatinine clearance < 30 mL/min: 1mg/kg SQ daily

BE	**BE**ta Blocker *Decrease myocardial oxygen demand, Catecholamine-induced tachycardia and contractility*	**NSTEMI** Oral beta-blocker within 24 h; Metoprolol 50 mg po or Lopressor 5 mg IV at 5 min intervals x 3 = total 15 mg in the absence of contraindications (Severe COPD/Asthma, CHF, bradycardia, ED meds, hypotension)
M	**M**orphine *Theoretically decrease in myocardial oxygen demand by decreasing pain and anxiety; some vasodilatory effects; Never proven in trials; no mortality benefit.*	**NSTEMI patients:** potentially adverse effects of morphine in patients with UA/NSTEMI **STEMI patients:** *Avoided if possible and reserved for patients with an unacceptable level of pain since a large but retrospective study suggests its use is associated with an adverse effect on outcome.*

O	**O**xygen Oxygen saturation > 90%	The usefulness of supplementary oxygen therapy has not been established in normoxic patients. In the prehospital, ED, and hospital settings, the withholding of supplementary oxygen therapy in normoxic patients with suspected or confirmed acute coronary syndrome may be considered
A	**A**ntiplatelet **Aspirin** inhibits the synthesis of thromboxane A2 (TxA2), a potent stimulator of platelet aggregation **P2Y12 Adenosine Diphosphate (ADP) platelet receptor antagonists** Inhibition of P2Y12 receptor on platelet cell membranes → blocks activation / transformation of glycoprotein IIb/IIIa receptors → decreased platelet aggregation **Thienopyridines** (prodrugs that need to converted to an active metabolite) IRREVERSIBLE Inhibition **Prasugrel (Efient)** **Clopidogrel (Plavix)** **Non-Thienopyridines** (act directly on receptor and do not need metabolic activation and therefore have faster, greater and more consistent ADP receptor inhibition then Thienopyridines) REVERSIBLE inhibition of P2Y12 receptor **Ticagrelor (Brilinta)**	**ASA** 162-325 mg po/crushed/chewed; vomiting: 300mg rectal; ASA alone provided a 23% reduction in 30-day mortality If ASA contraindicated: clopidogrel (Plavix) 300 mg po **NSTEMI Conservative Therapy** ASA + add **Ticagrelor (Brilinta), loading dose 180mg** **NSTEMI Invasive Strategy** Angiography within 4 to 48 hours < 75 years old Give ASA + Ticagrelor (Brilinta), loading dose 180mg GB IIb/IIIa inhibitor prior to diagnostic angiography (either eptifibatide or triofiban) **STEMI** < 75 years old treated with primary PCI ASA + add Ticagrelor (Brilinta), loading dose 180mg Patients at high risk of bleeding or for whom prasugrel or ticagrelor cannot be used - give clopidogrel 600mg **Fibrinolytic therapy:** ASA + add clopidogrel 300 mg po (If age > 75 years give loading dose of 75mg)
N	**N**itroglycerin	**NTG** 0.4 mg sublingual or spray every 5 minutes; if no improvement after 3 tablets/sprays, start IV NTG at 10mcg/min continuous infusion, ↑ 10 mcg /min every 3 to 5 min until relief or hypotension Hold if patients have recently taken ED meds sildenafil (Viagra) or vardenafil (Levitra), tadalafil (Cialis) Hold if extreme bradycardia (<50 bpm) or tachycardia (>100 bpm) in absence of heart failure Hold in patients with RV infarct

TREATMENT OPTIONS IN ACS

- Nonsteroidal anti-inflammatory drugs (except aspirin) should be discontinued immediately due to an increased risk of cardiovascular events associated with their use.
- If CABG planned → Hold Clopidogrel (Plavix) for 5 days; Prasugrel (Efient) and Ticagrelor (Brilinta) for 7 days
- Prasugrel (Effient) is contraindicated in patients with history of TIA, CVA; use with caution in patients > 75 years old or < 60 kg due to risk of fatal bleeding, ICH and uncertain benefit; Not recommended in STEMI patients managed with fibrinolysis.
- Start statin, atorvastatin, as early as possible and preferably before PCI in patients not on statin
- Correct any electrolyte abnormalities, especially hypokalemia and hypomagnesemia, which often occur together.
- No clinical trials documenting the benefits of electrolyte replacement in acute MI.
- However most recommend maintaining K above 4.0 meq/L and a serum magnesium concentration above 2.0 meq/L

GLYCOPROTEIN IIB/IIIA INHIBITORS

Prevent fibrinogen/vWF crosslinking → ↓ platelet aggregation

Abciximab (ReoPro)

- **STEMI with emergent PCI**
    - 0.25 mg/kg IV bolus 10 to 60 minutes before PCI followed by
    - 0.125 mcg/kg/minute (max of 10 mcg/minute) IV infusion for 12 hours
- **NSTEMI Invasive Strategy** (PCI planned within 24 hours)
    - 0.25 mg/kg IV bolus, then
    - 10 mcg per minute IV infusion for 18 to 24 hours, end 1 hour after PCI
- Must use with heparin

Eptifibatide (Integrilin) – NSTEMI Invasive Strategy

- 180 mcg/kg IV bolus over 2 minutes then begin 2 mcg/kg/min IV infusion repeat 180 mcg/kg IV bolus over 2 minutes in 10 minute
- Maximum dose (121-kg patient) for PCI: 22.6 mg bolus; 15 mg per hour infusion
- Infusion duration 18 to 24 hours after PCI
- Reduce infusion rate by 50% if CrCl < 50 mL/min

Tirofiban (Aggrastat) – NSTEMI Invasive Strategy

- 0.4 mcg/kg/min IV for 30 minutes and then continued at 0.1 mcg/kg/min IV infusion for 18 to 24 hours after PCI
- Reduce infusion rate by 50% if CrCl < 30 mL/min

MANAGEMENT OF COCAINE-INDUCED ACS

- SL NTG and a CCB (e.g., diltiazem 20 mg IV); avoid B-blockers
- If **ST-segment elevation** is present and the patient is unresponsive to initial treatment, immediate coronary angiography is preferred over fibrinolytic therapy.

- UA/NSTEMI → observed and managed medically for 9 to 24 h. If ECG and biomarkers are normal and the patient is stable, the patient can be discharged.

PERCUTANEOUS CORONARY INTERVENTION (PCI) - STEMI

- Duration of STEMI < 2 hours: PCI should be initiated within 60 minutes
- Duration of STEMI 2 to 3 hours: PCI should be initiated within 120 minutes
- Cardiogenic shock + STEMI: PCI; fibrinolysis has little outcome benefit
- No shock, symptoms < 12 hours, PCI can be done in <120 minutes: transfer to PCI capable hospital
- "Door to balloon" time for percutaneous coronary intervention (PCI): 90 minutes

DIAGNOSTIC ANGIOGRAPHY IN NSTEMI PATIENTS

- Hemodynamic instability or cardiogenic shock
- Severe left ventricular dysfunction / CHF
- Recurrent or persistent rest angina despite intensive medical therapy
- New or worsening mitral regurgitation or new ventricular septal defect
- Sustained ventricular arrhythmias

THROMBOLYTIC AGENTS RECOMMENDED (AMI)

Presentation < 12 hours in context of signs and symptoms of AMI

- ST-segment elevation (> 1 mm in > 2 contiguous leads)
- Posterior-wall MI
- New or presumably new left bundle-branch block
- No exclusion criteria

Altepase (tPA) – Accelerated infusion regimen is given over 1.5 hours
Give 15mg IV Bolus
Then 0.75 mg/kg (max 50 mg) over next 30 minutes
Then 0.50 mg/kg (max 35 mg) over next 60 minutes

Reteplase (Retavase)
10 U IV over 2 min
30 minutes later give second 10 U IV bolus over 2 minutes

Tenecteplase (TNKase)
Bolus: 30 to 50 mg, weight adjusted (not to exceed 50 mg)

IV bolus over 5-10 seconds
< 60 kg: 30 mg
≥ 60 to < 70 kg - 35 mg
≥ 70 to < 80 kg - 40 mg
≥ 80 to < 90 kg - 45 mg
≥ 90: 50 mg

Heparin in AMI

- Begin heparin with fibrin-specific lytics (tPA, Retavase and TNKase)
- Unfractionated Heparin (UFH) or LMWH

THROMBOLYTIC AND HEPARIN DOSING IN CVA AND PULMONARY EMBOLISM

Acute Ischemic Stroke (AIS)
Tissue Plasminogen Activator (tPA) (Alteplase, Activase®)

- Dose: 0.9 mg/kg, max 90mg
- First 10% bolus over 1 min, remaining infused over next **60 minutes**
- Do not administer **heparin** or ASA during the first 24 hrs of fibrinolytic therapy

Tenecteplase (TNKase)

- 0.25 mg/kg (rounded to the nearest 0.2 mL) IV Bolus over 5 to 10 seconds
- Max 25 mg

Pulmonary Embolism - You will find three different protocols for tPA

- 100 mg over 2 hours (FDA approved regimen, most textbooks) *or*
- 15 mg bolus, then 85 mg continuous infusion over 2 hours *or*
- Accelerated infusion regimen used in AMI

Hold heparin during fibrinolytic infusion. At the conclusion of alteplase infusion begin heparin infusion without a bolus when aPTT has decreased to less than < 80 seconds

tPA for PE Associated with Cardiac Arrest

- 50 mg bolus over 1 minute
- If no response to initial bolus or if patient continues to deteriorate 15 minutes after initial bolus →
- Bolus #2 = 50 mg bolus over 1 minute

Pulmonary Embolism - Tenecteplase (TNKase)

- Bolus: 30 to 50 mg, weight adjusted (not to exceed 50 mg)
- IV bolus over 5-10 seconds
- < 60 kg: 30 mg
- ≥ 60 to < 70 kg - 35 mg
- ≥ 70 to < 80 kg - 40 mg
- ≥ 80 to < 90 kg - 45 mg
- ≥ 90: 50 mg

CONTRAINDICATIONS AND CAUTIONS FOR FIBRINOLYSIS USE

Absolute contraindications

- Any prior ICH
- Known structural cerebral vascular lesion (neoplasm, AVM, aneurysm)
- Known malignant intracranial neoplasm (primary or metastatic)
- Contraindicated if CVA < 1 year ago
- Suspected aortic dissection
- Active bleeding or bleeding diathesis (excluding menses)
- Significant closed head or facial trauma within 3 months
- Suspected pericarditits

Relative contraindications

- History of chronic severe, poorly controlled hypertension
- Severe uncontrolled hypertension on presentation (SBP > 180 mm Hg or DBP > 110 mm Hg)
- History of prior ischemic stroke greater than 3 months, dementia, or known intracranial pathology not covered in contraindications
- Traumatic or prolonged (> 10 minutes) CPR or major surgery (< 3 weeks)
- Recent internal bleeding (within 2 to 4 weeks)
- Noncompressible vascular punctures
- For streptokinase/anistreplase: prior exposure (> 5 days) or prior allergic reaction to these agents
- Pregnancy
- Active peptic ulcer
- Current use of anticoagulants: the higher the INR, the higher the risk of bleeding

ADULT CARDIOPULMONARY RESUSCITATION

- Compression position: lower half of sternum
- Compression depth: 2 inches
- Compression rate: 100-120/min
- 30 compressions: 2 breaths
- High quality chest compressions: 10-20 mm Hg CO2
- Factors that worsen CPR: Compression interruption, excessive ventilation, poor technique

VENTRICULAR FIBRILLATION/PULSELESS VENTRICULAR TACHYCARDIA (VT)

Definition

- > 3PVCs = VT
- < 30 seconds = non-sustained VT
- > 30 seconds = sustained VT
- Start CPR, provide maximum oxygen, attach monitor/defibrillator →
- Unsynchronized Cardioversion: Biphasic preferred, manufacturer recommendation (120 to 200J); if unknown use max available →
- Resume CPR immediately – 2 minutes → check rhythm → shockable rhythm →
- 200J Biphasic or → Resume CPR immediately
- When IV available →
  Epinephrine 1 mg IVP repeat every 3 to 5 minutes
- CPR 2 minutes → check rhythm → shockable rhythm →
- 200J Biphasic →
  Amiodarone 300 mg once IVP; second dose (if needed) 150mg IVP
- Most common cause of Monomorphic VT = re-entrant mechanism through scarred myocardium (chronic forms of ischemic heart disease - patient had MI in the past); can also be seen in the setting of myocardial ischemia, however more often from re-entrant mechanism
- Most common cause of Polymorphic VT = myocardial ishchemia

CARDIOPULMONARY ARREST - IMPROVED OUTCOMES

- AED use
- Early bystander CPR
- Presenting rhythm: v-tach/v-fib
- CPR prior to defibrillation
- Amiodarone use in shock resistant v-tach/v-fib
- Therapeutic hypothermia

THERAPEUTIC HYPOTHERMIA (TARGETED TEMPERATURE MANAGEMENT (TTM)

- 32 to 36°C
- 89.6 to 96.8°F
- PaCO2: 40 to 45 mm Hg
- Oxygen saturation: 94-96%
- MAP: 65 to 100 mmHG
- Strict avoidance of hypo- or hyperglycemia
- Glucose: 108 to 144 mg/dL
- Best chance for good neurologic outcome following cardiac arrest:
  a) Patients treated with therapeutic hypothermia early
  b) Initial rhythm of ventricular tachycardia (VT) or ventricular fibrillation (VF)
- Cooling should be maintained for at least 48 hours post-arrest
- Adequate sedation to suppress shivering

COMPLICATIONS FROM COOLING

- Bleeding from coagulopathy
- Cardiac dysrhythmias
- Sepsis
- Hypo-heart rate (bradycardia common)
- Hypo-kalemia
- Hypo-magnesemia
- Hypo-phosphatemia
- Hypo-volemia (cold diuresis)
- Hyper-movement (shivering)
- Hyper-QT: (prolonged QT interval interval)
- Hyper-glycemia (insulin resistance) - need larger amounts of insulin to maintain euglycemic state.
- **PEARL:** Therapeutic hypothermia is recommended for all post-cardiac arrest patients, however best prognosis = VT and VF

MEDICATIONS THAT CAN BE GIVEN DOWN ET TUBE IN ADULTS

Mnemonic (NAVEL)

N	**N**arcan
A	**A**tropine
V	**V**alium & **V**asopressin
E	**E**pinephrine
L	**L**idocaine

Pediatrics: All meds are the same except no V (Valium and Vasopressin)
LANE: **L**idocaine, **A**tropine, **N**arcan and **E**pinephrine are medications that can be given down ETT in kids

ATRIAL FIBRILLATION

Atrial fibrillation = Most common sustained arrhythmia in adults
Rate = irregular
Rhythm = irregular
No defined P waves

CAUSES OF ATRIAL FIBRILLATION

Mnemonic (ME WITH MITCH PhD)

Atrial rate = 350-500, ventricular rate = 100-160; Irregular

M	**M**itral valve disease (MS, MR) in underdeveloped countries, most common cause of AF is Rheumatic Heart Disease.
E	**E**lectrolytes
W	**W**PW
I	**I**ntoxication/ETOH (holiday heart)
T	**T**hyrotoxicosis

H	HTN
M	**M**yocarditis
I	**I**diopathic
T	**T**ox (CO, cocaine, amphetamines, heroin)
C	**C**AD
H	**H**ypoxia (COPD) *although more commonly Multifocal Atrial Tachycardia (MAT)*
P	**P**E
h	**H**ypothermia
D	**D**rugs (see tox above)

ATRIAL FIBRILLATION

If unstable (ie hypotensive) → "Synchronized" Cardioversion
Synchronized cardioversion is shock delivery that is timed (synchronized) with the QRS complex. This synchronization avoids shock delivery during the relative refractory portion of the cardiac cycle, when a shock could produce VF.

- Biphasic 120 to 200 J preferred, if not available then monophasic cardioversion at 200J
- If the initial shock fails, providers should increase the dose in a stepwise fashion
- Electrical cardioversion in Digoxin Toxicity → malignant ventricular arrhythmias
- Avoid electrical cardioversion if patient is on Digoxin unless condition is life-threatening, then use lower dose → 10 to 20 J

Treatment Options

1. **Rate control**
   - Diltiazem (Cardizem 0.25 mg/kg IV bolus over 2 min; 5-15 mg/hr maintenance infusion. If the first dose does not produce the desired response (20% reduction in heart rate from baseline or a HR < 100 bpm) within 15 minutes, then a second bolus of 0.35 mg/kg is given over 2 minutes
   - B-blockers Metoprolol (Lopressor) 5 mg IV every 5" for total of 15 mg
   - Esmolol: very short half-life
     Loading dose (optional): 500 mcg/kg IV over 1 minute
     Follow with 50 mcg/kg/minute infusion for 4 minutes
     If adequate response continue at 50 mcg/kg/minute
     If inadequate response: titrate upward in 50 mcg/kg/minute increments
     Increased no more frequently than every 4 minutes to a maximum of 200 mcg/kg/minute
   - Amiodarone 150 mg IV over 10 min, then 1 mg/min for 6 hrs, than 0.5 mg/min over 18 hours. **Rhythm control strategy is not preferred;** long-term risk of many side effects: limited role in chronic rate control; use second line if 1st line unsuccessful
   - Digoxin 0.25 mg IV each 2 hours, up to 1.5 mg
     1 hour delay before onset of action, peak effect does not develop for up to 6 hours
     Digoxin is not the first line drug unless advanced CHF or significant hypotension; Usually added to CCB or Beta-blocker patients who do not respond to initial therapy
   - Some patients have a greater degree of rate control with a beta blocker than with a CCB, and vice versa. Thus, in patients who have an inadequate response to one of these drugs, switching

to a drug from the other class is an alternative to adding digoxin. If patient is already taking a B-blocker, you can begin management with intravenous B-Blocker
PEARL: There is no mortality benefit of rhythm control vs rate control; therefore, rate control treatment strategy is preferred

2. Catheter ablation
3. Caution with cardioversion in stable patients; if AF > 48 hours - anticoagulate for 21 days prior to cardioversion
4. Determine need for anticoagulation; CHA2DS2-VASc risk stratification score ≥ 2 anticoagulation significantly reduces the incidence stroke

CHA_2DS_2-VASc SCORE

In patients with nonvalvular AF, the CHA_2DS_2-VASc score is recommended for assessment of stroke risk
[http://circ.ahajournals.org/content/early/2014/04/10/CIR.0000000000000041.full.pdf]

Stroke Risk Stratification With CHA_2DS_2 - VASc Scores

CHA_2DS_2-VASc	SCORE
Congestive HF	1
Hypertension	1
Age greater than or = to 75	**2**
Diabetes Mellitus	1
Stroke / TIA / TE Thromboembolism	**2**
Vascular disease (Prior MI, PAD, or aortic plaque)	1
Age 65 - 74 y	1
Sex category (ie female)	1
Maximum Score	9

CHA_2DS_2-VASc	Adjusted stroke rate (% per year)
0	0%
1	1.3%
2	2.2%
3	3.2%
4	4.0%
5	6.7%
6	9.8%
7	9.6%
8	6.7%
9	15.20%

ANTITHROMBOTIC THERAPY FOR ATRIAL FIBRILLATION

- AF and mechanical heart valves: warfarin is recommended
- Nonvalvular AF, prior stroke, TIA or a CHA_2DS_2-VASc score ≥ 2: oral anticoagulants are recommended. Options include: warfarin (INR 2.0 to 3.0), dabigatran, rivaroxaban or apixaban
- For patients with nonvalvular AF unable to maintain a therapeutic INR level with warfarin: use of a direct thrombin or factor Xa inhibitor (dabigatran, rivaroxaban, or apixaban) is recommended.
- Renal function should be evaluated prior to initiation of direct thrombin or factor Xa inhibitors and should be re-evaluated when clinically indicated and at least annually
- For patients with atrial flutter, antithrombotic therapy is recommended according to the same risk profile used for AF
- CHA_2DS_2-VASc score of 1: no antithrombotic therapy or treatment with an oral anticoagulant or aspirin may be considered.

WOLFF-PARKINSON-WHITE (WPW) SYNDROME

- Wolff-Parkinson-White (WPW) syndrome = pre-excitation syndrome
- Accessory electrical conduction pathway directly connects the atria to ventricles, bypassing the AV node
- The clinical hallmark = narrow complex supraventricular tachycardia at a rate of 150 to 300 beats/minute
- The accessory pathway impulse is not subject to the normal conduction delay of the AV node ——> therefore the impulse arrives earlier to the ventricles ——> this results in triad of ECG findings which correspond to the aberrant activation through the accessory pathway

Triad of ECG Findings in WPW

1. Short PR Interval (PR < 120 msec)
2. Wide QRS complex (QRS > 120 msec)
3. Slurred upstroke of QRS complex ("delta wave")

- Most common tachydysrhythmia = atrioventricular reentry tachycardia (AVRT), which can be either:
- Orthodromic or Antidromic

Orthodromic AVRT

- Antegrade conduction via the AV node
- Retrograde conduction via the accessory pathway
- Narrow complex
- Looks like PSVT
- **Treatment:** #1 Adenosine, #2 option verapamil and #3 beta-blocker or procainamide

Antidromic AVRT

- Antegrade conduction via the accessory pathway
- Retrograde conduction via the AV node
- Wide complex
- Looks like VT
- Treat with procainamide (watch for hypotension, prolonged QRS)

Avoid AV nodal blocking agents (adenosine, beta-blockers, calcium-channel blockers, amiodarone) in **antidromic AVRT** because this can paradoxically enhance conduction via the accessory pathway and trigger VF

WPW is associated with Atrial Fibrillation (AF)

- Pre-excited AF with rapid ventricular response (RVR) = fast heart rates and symptoms; the heart rates (> 200 beats/minute) are faster > than typical atrial fibrillation rates
- Do NOT use standard AV nodal blocking medications (ie, beta blockers, calcium channel blockers (verapamil and diltiazem), digoxin, adenosine, and amiodarone
- These medications can paradoxically enhance conduction via the accessory pathway and trigger VF

Treatment

- Stable: Prcainamide or ibutilide
- Unstable: cardioversion

MULTIFOCAL ATRIAL TACHYCARDIA (MAT)

1. > 3 differently shaped P waves
2. Varying PP, PR and RR intervals
3. Atrial rhythm between 100 and 180

- "Irregularly irregular" rhythm, "wandering pacemaker", "chaotic atrial rhythm"
- Most common cause of MAT = COPD. Other causes: CHF, sepsis and theophylline toxicity.
- Treatment of MAT is directed toward underlying disorder

ATRIAL FLUTTER

Atrial Rate = 250 to 350 beats/min

The 2:1 conduction ratio accounts for the classic (although not exclusive) ECG appearance of atrial flutter as a **narrow complex tachycardia** with a regular ventricular rate usually in the high 130's to 140's beats/min

- Cardioversion often responds to lower energy levels then Atrial Fibrillation
- Use 50 to 100 J with either a monophasic or biphasic device

ANTIDYSRHYTHMIC DRUGS

Mnemonic: (SOme Block Potassium Channels) [ANK, provided by Dr. Alan Lazzara]

Class I	**SO**me Fast **SO**dium Channel Blockers	Class IA slow conduction through the atria, AV nodes and His-Purkinje systems. Additionally, conduction through accessory pathways is slowed Class IB slow conduction and depolarization and shorten repolarization → slow phase 0 depolarization in His-Purkinje and ventricular myocytes = slow conduction and membrane-stabilization Class 1C slow conduction and depolarization Class IA (Quinidine, Procainamide, Disopyramide) Class IB (Lidocaine, Phenytoin, Mexiletine (Mexitil) Class IC (Flecanide, Propafenone Rythmol) • Toxicity of Class IA, IC meds → ↑ QT → torsade de pointes. Procanimide may lead to hypotension and QRS widening • Toxicity of Class IB Lidocaine = CNS disturbances (lightheadedness, confusion) CV effects (↓ BP, AV block)

Class II	**BLOCK:** Beta Blockers Beta-adrenergic blockers - indirect Ca channel blockade by attenuation of adrenergic activation.	Metoprolol, Atenolol, Esmolol, Propanolol, Timolol
Class III	**POTASSIUM** Channel Blockers Prolong action potential refractoriness (delay repolarization) by blocking potassium channels	Amiodarone, Dofetilide, Sotalol (non-selective beta-blocker) and Ibutilide also share activity with class II agents. Prolong QT risk.
Class IV	**CHANNELS** Ca2+ (slow) Channel Blockers	Verapamil, Diltiazem Non-dihydropyridines

CAUSES OF PAROXYSMAL SUPRAVENTRICULAR TACHYCARDIA (PVST)

Mnemonic: (MI PhD) 2 (CREW)

Rate = 130-220, usually 160; Regular

MI	**MI** **M**V Disease (MV Prolapse, MV stenosis)
P	**P**neumonia **P**ericarditis
H	**H**ypertension **H**yperthyroidism
D	**D**igitalis toxicity **D**rop volume (hypovolemia)

C	**C**OPD (much more common rhythm for COPD = MAT)
R	**R**heumatic Heart Disease
E	**E**TOH
W	**W**PW (40-80% PSVT, 10-20% A fib, 5% Flutter)

PSVT TREATMENT OPTIONS

If unstable → "synchronized" Cardioversion → 50 to 100J biphasic
Vagal maneuvers → Adenosine (Adenocard) 6 mg IVP → Adenosine 12 mg IVP in proximal vein (short half life); may repeat 12 mg IVP dose once → rhythm does not convert →

Is the QRS Narrow or Wide?
→ Narrow QRS consider → Diltiazem or β-blockers
→ Wide QRS consider → Procainamide

Methylxanthines (Theophylline) and caffeine → antagonize Adenosine
Dipyridamole (Persantine) and Carbamazepine (Tegretol) → potentiate Adenosine

- Adenosine ultra short acting, 20 secs → Atrioventricular nodal blocking agent converts > 90% of reentrant SVT
- Most common pediatric dysrhythmia = PSVT heart rate usually > 220 (in adults it's less)
  Treatment: Adenosine 0.1 mg/kg (max 6 mg) → 0.2 mg/kg (max 12 mg), (may repeat x1)
- Verapamil is contraindicated in infants
- Carotid massage is not recommended in infants or children. Hemodynamically stable child in SVT = Application of ice to the face = effective method of converting a to NSR; do not occlude the nose or mouth → apply ice only over the patient's forehead, eyes, and bridge of the nose for 10–15 seconds

CAUSES OF PULSELESS ELECTRICAL ACTIVITY

Mnemonic: (MI OD PATCH$_6$)

MI	**MI**
OD	**O**ver**d**ose (Toxins)

P	**P**E
A	**A**cidosis
T	**T**ension Pneumothorax
C	**C**ardiac tamponade
H6	**H**ypo-xia **H**ypo-thermia **H**ypo-glycemia **H**ypo-volemia **H**ypo-kalemia **H**yper-kalemia

FIRST-DEGREE HEART BLOCK

- Prolonged and constant PR interval without any dropped beats

SECOND-DEGREE HEART BLOCK

- Type I second-degree heart block = progressive PR interval lengthening until a QRS complex is dropped
- Type II second-degree heart block = random dropped QRS complexes without changes in PR interval

THIRD DEGREE HEART BLOCK (COMPLETE HEART BLOCK)

- Rhythm is regular
- P-P regular
- R-R regular
- Independent regular beats from the atria and ventricles
- Treatment
- Atropine or isoproterenol, transcutaneous pacing
- Permanent - pacemaker

TREATMENT OPTIONS: ASYSTOLE / PEA

- Epinephrine 1 mg IVP repeat every 3-5 minutes
- Vasopressin was removed from cardiac arrest algorithm in 2015
- Atropine was removed from the cardiac arrest algorithm in 2010

TRANSCUTANEOUS CARDIAC PACING

Used for unstable AV blocks, bradycardia, and for overdrive pacing of tachydysrhythmias (not for asystole)

- Medicate with anxiolytics or narcotics prior to pacing
- Anterior pacing pad (black) placed over the right superior chest
- Posterior pad (red) placed inferior to the left scapula
- Unstable: set HR between 60 to 80 and amperage to maximum (80 mA)
- Stable: set mA between 40 to 60
- Decreased until threshold for pacing is reached
- Then increase by 5–10 mA to ensure continued capture
- Capture is confirmed when a QRS follows the pacing spike and a corresponding pulse is felt
- Initial pacing should be set to demand pacing (avoid R on T phenomenon and decompensation into dangerous dysrhythmias)
- If transcutaneous pacing fails, transvenous (TV) pacing should follow. TV pacing is temporary until pacemaker placed

Transvenous Pacemakers: Right internal jugular vein (IJ) #1 or LEFT subclavian option #2 if RIJ cannnot be accessed
Transcutaneous: 40 to 60 mA to capture
Transvenous: capture at 5 mA then decrease

Electrical capture without a palpable pulse = PEA

CAUSES OF PROLONGED QT ON ECG

Normal duration (interval) of QRS complex 0.08 to 0.1 seconds, 80 to 100 milliseconds (ms)
Normal QT interval - 0.4 to 0.44 seconds, 400 to 440ms

- Hypo-calcemia
- Hypo-magnesemia
- Hypo-kalemia
- Hypo-thyroidism
- Hypo-thermia (also, see mnemonics: causes of ST segment elevation and Afib)
- Hereditary
- Drugs
  - TCA's
  - Methadone
  - Droperidol (Inapsine)
  - Haloperidol (Haldol)
  - Lithium
  - Phenothiazine
  - Diphenhydramine
  - Cocaine
  - Class IA Antiarrhythmics - Procanimide, Quinidine
  - Class IC Antiarrhythmics - Propafenone, Flecanide
  - Class III Antiarrhythmics - Amiodarone, Ibutilide, Sotalol

    - Erythromycin IV
    - Fluroquinalones
    - Zofran (ondansetron)
- Miscellaneous
    - AMI
    - ↑ICP
    - SAH (also, diffuse deep T-wave inversion with SAH)
    - MVP
    - Targeted temperature management (TTM)

PEARL: Amiodarone can cause chemical epididymitis, hypothyroidism, interstitial lung disease (pulmonary fibrosis), blue-grey skin discoloration, corneal microdeposits : bradycardia, heart blocks, dysrhythmias, hypotention, prolonged QT

CAUSES OF LOW VOLTAGE ECG

Mnemonic: (ME BIRP)

M	**M**yxedema
E	**E**ffusion, pericardial

B	**B**arrel chest/obese
I	**I**mproper lead placement
R	**R**estrictive cardiomyopathy
P	**P**ericarditis / Myocarditis

PERICARDITIS

Men > Women
Elevated WBC, ESR
Fever, myagias, anorexia
CP that improves with leaning forward
ECHO most useful in confirming the diagnosis

FOUR PHASES OF PERICARDITIS

Phase 1	ST-Segment ↑ I, V5, V6 → subepicardial ventricular injury ST segment in concave upward, in AMI = convex upward PR Depression II, aVF and V4 to V6 → subepicardial atrial injury Low voltage PR elevation in aVR with ST depression
Phase 2	ST-Segment returns to isoelectric line, and T-wave amplitude decreases (flattens)
Phase 3	T-wave ↓ inversion in leads which were previously ST ↑ Begins at the end of the second or third week and lasts several weeks
Phase 4	Resolution of repolarization abnormalities

CAUSES OF PERICARDITIS

MNEMONIC: (AMP CARDIAC RIND) [Provided by Dr Mark Postel, with modifications]

A	**A**utoimmune (Dressler's Syndrome - see below)
M	**M**yxedema
P	**P**ost-traumatic (4 to 12 days post-injury)

C	**C**ollagen Vascular Disease (SLE, RA, scleroderma, dermatomyositis, sarcoid, amyloid) Treat with steroids. Most common cardiac manifestation of SLE in 30%
A	**A**ortic dissection
R	**R**adiation (most spontaneously resolve)
D	**D**rug-Induced (procainamide, hydralazine, cromolyn sodium, dantrolene, methysergide)
I	**I**diopathic = Most Common; viral #2 most common cause of pericarditis
A	**A**cute Renal Failure - Uremic pericarditis - do not treat with ANSAIDs. Treatment: Intensive dialysis for 2-6 weeks and steroids 1-2 weeks
C	**C**ardiac Infarction

R	**R**heumatic Fever
I	**I**nfectious: viral (coxsackie B, echovirus, influenza, adenovirus, HIV, EBV, CMV), Staph, Strep pneumo, Strep pyogenes (acute rheumatic fever), Mycoplasma, C. trachomatis, Rickettsia, parasites, TB, Salmonella, Haemophilus influenzae
N	**N**eoplasm, mainly metastatic. Treatment: Chemo; pericardiocentesis; lung worse prognosis
D	**D**ressler syndrome: several weeks after MI Fever, autoimmune, anti-myocardial antibodies Late pericarditis 2-3 weeks post AMI Treatment: NSAIDs; resolution complete/rapid

PERICARDITIS TREATMENT

- NSAIDs
- Adding Colchicine to NSAID treatment can resolve pericarditis symptoms faster AND prevent recurrence
- Corticosteroids reserved if NSAID failure or recurrent pericarditis

PERICARDITIS PEARLS

- **Uremia**: few ECG changes; serous or hemorrhagic effusions; hemorrhagic effusions more common secondary to uremia-induced platelet dysfunction
  - Treatment: hemodialysis, avoid NSAIDs → bleeding
  - Corticosteroids are a second-line treatment for uremic pericarditis, used in patients who do not respond to hemodialysis

- Most common symptom: CP which ↑ when the patient is supine, ↓leaning forward
- Most common physical finding: pericardial friction rub.
- Sternal rub heard best over LSCB 25%; Rub varies with inspiration
- Constrictive pericarditis is long-term, or chronic, inflammation of the pericardium which can lead to dilated cardiomyopathy (DCM) CHF, pulsus paradoxus, Kussmaul's sign, pericardial knock, peripheral edema, ascites, and/or cachexia and pericardial calcifications

HEART FAILURE CAUSES / PRECIPITATIONS FACTORS / PEARLS

Mnemonic: (HEART MISHAPS) 3

Most common cause of heart failure (HF) in the US = Coronary atherosclerosis (50-70%)

Heart Failure

- Systolic dysfunction = impaired cardiac contractility
- Diastolic dysfunction = limitation to diastolic filling and therefore in forward output due to increased ventricular stiffness

H	**H**TN	**H**igh output failure vs low output failure*	**H**IV Infection
E	**E**ndocarditis	**E**ndocrine disorders associated with DCM = hypothyroid or hyperthyroid, DM, Cushings, Pheochromocytoma, Growth hormone excess or deficiency	**E**lectrolyte / renal abnormalities associated with DCM = HYPOcalcemia, HYPOphosphatemia, Uremia, Calcium overload (Paget's Disease)
A	**A**cute Anemia	**A**rrhythmias	**A**V Fistulas
R	**R**heumatic fever	**R**enal failure	**R**educed Vitamins (Nutritional deficiencies as cause of DCM) = Niacin (B3) (pellagra), Carnitine and Thiamine (B1: beriberi)
T	**T**hyroid (hyper or hypo can lead to DCM)	**T**oxins associated with DCM = ETOH, Cocaine, Amphetamines, Lead (Pb), Lithium (Li) and Carbon monoxide (CO)	**T**achycardia

M	**M**R/MS/AR/AS Valvular Heart Disease	**M**yopathies (Dilated / Hypertrophic / Restrictive)**	+ **M**yocarditis
I	**I**schemic Heart Disease	**I**nfiltrative Diseases (Amyloid, Sarcoid, Hemochromatosis)	**I**diopathic Most common cause of DCM and RCM = Idiopathic
S	**S**odium load	**S**tiff ventricles (noncompliant)***	**S**tiff Pericardium (constrictive pericarditis causes = radiation and chronic pericarditis)
H	**H**eat Stroke	**H**ypothermia	++ **H**ypersensitivity myocarditis

A	**A**myloidosis	**A**utoimmune / Inflammatory causes of DCM = SLE, dermatomyositis, RA, scleroderma, Giant cell arteritis or Kawasaki disease	**A**nti-inflammatory (NSAIDS)
P	**P**ulmonary Embolism	**P**regnancy (peripartum cardiomyopathy)	**P**arovirus B19 (most common cause of myocarditis in US)
S	**S**teroids	**S**aline overload	**S**arcoid

***High output failure** examples include: hyperthyroid, Paget's, pregnancy, anemia, AV fistula and beriberi → heart cannot meet elevated circulatory demands. All these conditions lead to dilated cardiomyopathy (DCM)

Low output failure myocardial dysfunction prevents normal metabolic requirements being met.

CARDIOMYOPATHY

a myocardial disorder in which the heart muscle is structurally and functionally abnormal in the ABSENCE of coronary artery disease, hypertension, valvular disease, and congenital heart disease sufficient to explain the observed myocardial abnormality. (Note: cardiology will use terms "ischemic" and HTN cardiomyopathy this term is not supported by the AHA)

****Cardiomyopathies**

1. Dilated cardiomyopathy (DCM)
2. Hypertrophic cardiomyopathy (HCM)
3. Restrictive cardiomyopathy (RCM)

Causes of Dilated Cardiomyopathy (DCM)

- Idiopathic 50%
- Myocarditis 9%
- Ischemic heart disease 7%
- Infiltrative disease 5%
- Peripartum cardiomyopathy 4%
- Hypertension 4%
- HIV infection 4%
- Connective tissue disease 3%
- Substance abuse (ETOH) 3%
- Doxorubicin 1%
- Other 10%

Hypertrophic cardiomyopathy (HCM)

Autosomal dominant inherited disorder that causes LVH; can result in sudden death in young athletes; present with CP, SOB, palpitations or syncope. Amyloid cardiomyopathy may present as a DCM, HCM or RCM

Restrictivecardiomyopathy (RCM)

Reduced compliance is caused by abnormal elastic properties of the myocardium and/or intercellular matrix. RCM is much less common than either DCM or HCM in the US, however is a frequent cause of death in Africa, India, South and Central America, and Asia, primarily because of the high incidence of endomyocardial fibrosis in those regions.

Most common cause of RCM = Idiopathic

- Other causes of RCM: amyloid, sarcoid, hemochromatosis, storage disease (Fabry disease), scleroderma and endomyocardial fibrosis

ECHO: non-dilated, non-hypertrophied ventricles, moderate bilateral atrial enlargement; impaired ventricular filling - need doppler assessment of diastolic transmittal flow velocity to detect filling abnormality

+Infectious causes of DCM = Myocarditis

- Most common cause of myocarditis = Viral
- Most common viral cause of myocarditis = Parovirus B19
- (Coxsackie B was most common in the 1990's); other viruses = Influenza, HH6, HIV, CMV, Hepatitis, Varicella, Mumps; Bacterial causes = Diptheria, Typhoid fever, Brucellosis, Psitticosis, Mycobacterium, Strep - rheumatic fever (RF);
- Rickettsial; Spirochetal: Syphilis, Leptospirosis and Lyme Disease
- Most common cause of Myocarditis worldwide = Trypanosomiasis (Chaga's disease); Other parasites: Toxoplasmosis, Shistosomiasis, Trichinosis
- Fungal: Histoplasmosis and Cryptococcosis

++Hypersensitivity myocarditis (HSM): a form of eosinophilic myocarditis; it is an autoimmune reaction in the heart that is often drug-related and is usually characterized by acute rash, fever, peripheral eosinophilia

***__Stiff ventricles__** /noncompliant - due to hypertrophy or ischemia, requires ↑LVEDP to achieve diastolic filling

Ultrasound Findings in Pulmonary Edema

- B-lines ("Comet-tails") = hyperechoic lines that run perpendicular (vertical) to the pleural line of the lung using high frequency probe;
- Higher number of B-lines within the visualized lung field = more interstitial lung disease and fluid-filled alveoli
- A-lines are horizontal lines created as repetition of the pleural line from air artifact; represent air filled lung tissue (normal lung surface)

PEARL: Hepatization = area of lung tissue looks sonographically like the liver; consolidation (pneumonia) will appear as "hepatization" on ultrasound.

CHF ON CXR

Most common and earliest CXR finding in CHF = Cardiomegaly https://www.med-ed.virginia.edu/courses/rad/cxr/pathology2Bchest.html

Kerley A lines: straight, non-branching lines in the mid and upper lung fields radiate towards the hila, 3 to 4cm long

Kerley B lines: horizontal, non-branching lines seen laterally in lower zones never > 2 cm long

Pulmonary edema, pleural effusions (usually bilateral with right > left, if unilateral almost always right sided), cardiac enlargement without specific chamber enlargement and evidence of ↑pulmonary venous pressure (enlargement of vessel in upper lung zones "**cephalization**")

CHF SIGNS / SYMPTOMS

- CHF occurs if there is acute impairment of at least 25% of the left ventricle
- Most common symptom of left-sided failure = SOB
- LEFT sided failure (reduced flow into aorta and systemic circulation) → fatigue, dyspnea, orthopnea, ↑HR, ↑RR, ↑BP, ↑CO, S3 gallop, diaphoresis, rales/wheezing
- RIGHT sided failure (secondary to elevated systemic venous pressure) → JVD, ↓BP, ↓CO, RUQ pain, peripheral edema, hepatomegaly and hepatojugular reflux
- Don't forget to order Brain Natriuretic Peptide (BNP)

TREATMENT OPTIONS IN CHF

Mnemonic: (L M N O P)

L	**L**asix: 2 mechanisms of action: 1) Vasodilation within few minutes 2) Diuretic response in 10-20" • Dose = equal twice the patient's daily usage, up to a maximum of 180 mg IV • If the patient previously has not been on a loop diuretic, initial dose = 40mg IV • If bumetanide (Bumex) is used, 1 mg of Bumetanide equals 40 mg furosemide • Ethacrynic acid is useful if the patient has a serious ***sulfa*** allergy
M	**M**ilrinone (Primacor); Intravenous inotropic agents such as dobutamine and/or milrinone may be required as a temporizing measure in patients with severe LV systolic dysfunction and low output syndrome
N	**N**itroglycerin 0.4 mg SL q 1-5 min, IV starting dose = 0.2-0.4mcg/kg/min. (Venous > arterial vasodilation, therefore reduces LV filling pressure primarily via venodilation)
O	**O**xygen, CPAP, intubate. Early use of noninvasive positive pressure ventilation (NIPPV) decreases the need for intubation
P	**P**osition – elevate HOB

- Dobutamine acts primarily on beta-1 adrenergic receptors, with minimal effects on beta-2 and alpha-1 receptors
- Milrinone = phosphodiesterase inhibitor that increases myocardial inotropy by inhibiting degradation of cyclic adenosine monophosphate. A potent arterial and venous dilator due to inhibition of vascular smooth muscle phosphodiesterase, leading to decreases in systemic and pulmonary vascular resistance, and right and left heart filling pressures.Together these effects lead to an increase in cardiac index and decreases in LV afterload and filling pressures.
- In patients with heart failure with reduced ejection fraction (HFrEF), chronic blockade of beta adrenergic receptors improves symptoms, reduces hospitalization, and enhances survival

Effects of Beta-blockers in CHF

Reduce detrimental effects of catecholamine stimulation including elevated HR, increased myocardial energy demands, adverse remodeling due to cardiac myocyte hypertrophy and death, interstitial fibrosis, impaired beta-adrenergic receptor responsivenes, arrhythmia promotion, and stimulation of other detrimental systems such as the renin-angiotensin-aldosterone axis

Beta blocker options

(In the absence of contraindications)
for patients with current or prior HF and a LVEF ≤ 40%
Carvedilol (Coreg, Coreg CR)
Metoprolol succinate (Toprol XL)
Bisoprolol (Zebeta)

Bilevel positive airway pressure (BIPAP)

- With each breath BiPap provides
- Inspiratory positive pressure
- End-expiratory positive pressure
- Inspiratory pressure provides for adequate ventilation → reduces the work of breathing
- End-expiratory pressure increases number of recruited alveoli and improves lung edema by shifting fluids from the interstitium of the lungs → back into the vasculature
- The positive pressures → increase intrathoracic pressure Increased intrathoracic pressure → reduces venous return to the heart, thereby lowering LVEDV
- This causes relaxation of the cardiac muscles ——> resulting in a decreased afterload and decreased preload while the cardiac output is maintained.
- Hypoxia can be improved by adding positive end-expiratory pressure (PEEP)

PEARL: For patients with known Systolic heart failure (HF) presenting with signs of acute decompensated heart failure (ADHF) and cardiogenic shock = Discontinue beta blocker therapy. Begin IV inotrope or mechanical support or both

PEARL: For patients with known Diastolic HF presenting with signs of severe acute ADHF & cardiogenic shock

- Treat for possible left ventricular outflow obstruction. Beta blocker. Gentle IV fluid (unless pulmonary edema present). IV vasopressor (phenylephrine or norepinephrine). Do NOT give an inotrope or vasodilator

PEARL: For patients with unknown systolic vs diastolic HF in severe ADHF and cardiogenic shock

- Give an inotrope IV, +/- vasopressor; assess need for mechanical support
- Mechanical support
    - intra-aortic balloon pump (IABP), extracorporeal circulatory membrane oxygenator (ECMO), or extracorporeal ventricular assist devices

PEARL: ECHO - Order stat echocardiogram

AORTOENTERIC FISTULA (AEF)

- **Primary**
    - Erosion of an unrepaired AAA into the duodenum
- **Secondary**
    - More common; the development of a pseudoaneurysm from the AAA repair or by direct mechanical effects of scarring between bowel and the suture line
- Presents years following aortic surgery
- Triad = GI bleed, Abdominal pain & Palpable Mass = 12%
- High mortality; massive hemorrhage = most common presentation
- Some patients present with a "herald bleed", an initial bleed that presents as melena or hematochezia → followed by a catastrophic hemorrhage if not treated
- **Diagnosis:**
    - Hemodynamically unstable → OR
    - Hemodynamically stable → EGD sensitivity 50%
    - CT angiography as a first-line study: if negative → EGD with careful inspection of the distal duodenum
- **Treatment**
    - hemodynamic support, antiboitics, surgical repair or fatal

PEARL: most common intestinal location of fistula formation in an aortoenteric fistula = duodenum

ABDOMINAL AORTIC ANEURYSM (AAA)

- AAA = localized dilation of aorta, involves all three layers of aorta (intima, media and adventitia ... don't confuse with Aortic Dissection
- Aortic Dissection = Separation of the layers of the aortic wall due to an intimal tear. Uncertain whether the initiating event is a primary rupture of the intima with secondary dissection of the media or primary hemorrhage within the media and subsequent rupture of the overlying intima resulting in two channels - true and false lumens
- Men > Female 4:1
- Average age at time of diagnosis = 65 to 70 y/o (75% of AAAs occur in patients > 60 y/o)
- AAAs have traditionally been attributed to Atherosclerosis but other factors probably contribute to their formation → biochemical abnormalities and uncertain genetic basis → Society for Vascular Surgery recommend labeling AAA as "nonspecific" rather than "atherosclerotic"
- Strong risk factor for AAA = Family history → patients with 1st degree relative & AAA have 10-20- fold ↑risk of developing AAA, other risk factors: smoking, HTN, history of CAD or PVD, hyperlipidemia, DM and connective tissue disease, male sex, caucasian race
- Most important risk factor for AAA rupture = size; most ruptures > 5cm
    - Rupture < 4 cm is rare
    - > 4 cm screen every 6 months
    - > 5.5 cm needs surgery
- US: detects and sizes AAA, however does not distinguish intact vs ruptured
- CT: preferred if patient stable, predicts size and extent of AAA and retroperitoneal hemorrhage (not detected by US)
- KUB /cross-table lateral: suggest diagnosis of AAA in > 65% of symptomatic patients (Calcified aorta/loss of renal/psoas shadow)
- Classic TRIAD OF Rupture
    - 1. Hypotension
    - 2. Pulsatile abdominal mass
    - 3. Flank/bak pain
    - Triad may be incomplete in as many as 50%
    - Syncope is common
- Other Findings: abdominal distention, ileus, bruits and "Blue Toe Syndrome"
- Mechanism of pain: 1. Rapid expansion of AAA or 2. Pressure of AAA on surrounding structures like nerves or 3. Presence of free blood in the abdomen or retroperitoneum from leaking or ruptured aneurysm
- Most common site AAA ruptures = Retroperitoneal 75-90% of cases (most common on left)
Most common segment = below renal arteries. 98% are infrarenal
10 to 30% rupture intraperitoneal: if intraperitoneal rupture → rapidly fatal
- Mortality: Elective repair = 4%; after rupture 20-80%
- Increasing use of percutaneous endovascular grafts both for ruptured and unruptured AAA especially in poor surgical candidates

AORTIC DISSECTION

- Thoracic aortic dissection is the most common lethal disease affecting the aorta
- 2-3x more common as ruptured AAA
- Major risk factor for aortic dissection = HTN
  Other: pregnancy, aortic valve disease, connective tissue disease, stimulant use and iatrogenic
- Age > 60 y/o; 3:1 male:female
- Most common locations: 65% ascending > 25% descending > 10% transverse arch
- Type A (proximal): ascending aorta +/- descending aorta = 75% cases; Treatment: surgery
  Type B (distal): confined to descending aorta; Treatment: medical management
- BP difference between upper extremities of > 20 mmHg or a loss/reduction of lower extremity pulses suggests aortic dissection
- Mortality: 25% at 1 hour, 50% at one week and 90% at one year

CXR Findings

- Widened mediastinum (> 8cm) - most common/reliable abnormality occurs 75% of cases
- Tracheal deviation to the RIGHT
- Depressed LEFT mainstem bronchus
- LEFT apical plerual cap
- Loss of aortic arch (Obliterated aortic knob)
- Separation (> 5mm) of intimal calcium from the outer border of the aorta. Calcium “ring” sign
- LEFT pleural effusion (see mnemonic “causes of pleural effusions”)

Cardiovascular

- 90% CP; Migration of pain down back or from chest to back is highly specific for dissection
- Ascending dissections → pain anterior chest
- Arch dissections → neck and jaw pain
- Descending dissections → pain in the interscapular area
- Aortic Insufficiency (diastolic murmur) = common > 50% of patients → Acute CHF
- ECG is abnormal in most patients: varying degrees of heart block, AMI
- Tamponade (blood spreads proximally to open the pericardial space to aortic blood flow)

Neurologic

- 9% syncope (most common cause = tamponade; other: cerebral ischemia)
- Type A→ carotid artery dissection/obstruction → CVA
- Spinal artery of Adamkiewicz blockage → cord ischemia → acute paraplegia
- Horners syndrome = compression of sympathetic chain from enlarged aorta

GI

- Hematemesis
- Accompanied mesenteric ischemia BAD → death rate 88%

Renal

- Hematuria, oliguria
- Decrease blood flow → renin release → refractory ↑BP

CT Chest with IV Contrast

- Reveals true and false lumens
- Reveals other causes of CP (pneumonia, PE)
- Disadvantage: uses IV contrast media

Transesophageal ECHO (TEE)

- Demonstrates involvement of ascending aorta
- Demonstrates aortic insufficiency (AI) and pericardial effusion
- No contrast required
- Disadvantage: availability and technical difficulties

BP management = see HTN Emergencies
Pain management

HYPERTENSIVE EMERGENCY

Severe elevation in BP accompanied by acute target organ damage; treatment = parenteral therapy

MAP = CO x SVR MAP = DBP + 1/3 (SBP – DBP) CPP = MAP - ICP

Normal MAP = 50 to 150mmHg
Normal CCP > 70mmHg
Normal ICP < 20mmHg

Pulse pressure = SBP - DBP (force heart generates each contraction; normal range = 40 to 60 mm Hg)

HYPERTENSIVE EMERGENCIES – TREATMENT OPTIONS

HTN with evidence of acute end-organ dysfunction
Decrease MAP 25% over 1 hour

1. **HTN Encephalopathy**: Nitroprusside or Labetalol or Clevidipine (Cleviprex, new CCB drug, recently approved, may see but will be institution dependent)
2. **Stroke Syndromes:** Labetalol or Nicardapine (Cardene)
   Nimodipine (Nimotop) useful in SAH, 60mg po (Note: Patients with acute ischemic stroke-in-evolution are most often not given antihypertensive drugs unless they are candidates for tissue plasminogen activator and their initial blood pressure is ≥185/110 mmHg. Nitroprusside is NOT a first line agent because of risk of rapid decrease in blood pressure
3. **Acute Coronary Syndromes:** NTG
   Avoid Nitroprusside because of "coronary steal" syndrome
4. **Acute Pulmonary Edema:** NTG and Lasix; Drugs that increase cardiac work (eg, hydralazine) or acutely decrease cardiac contractility (eg, labetalol or other beta blockers) should be avoided
5. **Aortic Dissection:** Nitroprusside + esmolol or labetalol, give β-blocker first to prevent reflex tachycardia. Goal - decrease aortic pressure wave contour (dp/dt); Titrate to a SBP of 110 mmHg
6. **Eclampsia:** Hydralazine (direct arteriolar vasodilator); Magnesium sulfate (MgSO4) for seizures
   Avoid Nipride → fetal cyanide toxicity
7. **Hyperadrenergic States** (MAOI, Pheochromocytoma, Anit-HTN withdrawal)
   Phentolamine + Propranolol; Nitroprusside + Propranolol; Labetalol
   Trimethaphan (ganglion blocker) if Beta Blocker contraindication
8. **Posterior Reversible Encephalopathy Syndrome (PRES)**: seizures (most common presentation), AMS, vision changes and HTN BILATERAL white matter changes in posterior temporal & occipital lobes MRI for diagnosis; Treatment: antiepileptic meds and emergent lowering BP

Do not drop BP too quickly. Ischemic damage can occur in vascular beds that have grown accustomed to the higher level of blood pressure (ie, autoregulation). For most hypertensive emergencies, mean arterial pressure should be reduced by about 10 to 20 percent in the first hour and then gradually during the next 23 hours so that the final pressure is reduced by approximately 25 percent compared with baseline.

Dosing

- Labetalol: 20mg IV over two minutes – repeat or double every 10min to max of 300mg; Infusion rate 1 to 2 mg/min up to 8 mg/min
- Nicardipine (Cardene): 5mg/hr, increase infusion 2.5mg/hr every 10 min to a max of 15mg/hr
- Nitroprusside: start at 0.5 mcg/kg/min IV infusion

Hypertensive Urgency

Severe elevations in BP (SBP > or = 180 mmHg, DBP > or = 120 mmHg), with mild or no acute target organ damage; may reduce BP within hours to days usually with oral medications

HTN without Emergency / Urgency = does not mandate urgent therapy

- Essential HTN = chronic problem and referral to PMD will greatly enhance management of HTN
- Treatment of HTN as an outpatient basis is usually not the responsibility of EM doc.

Rapid lowering of blood pressure in patients with chronic elevated blood pressure can cause organ hypoperfusion brain hypoperfusion) and lead to serious sequelae.

CARDIOLOGY PEARLS - ACUTE CORONARY SYNDROMES / DYSRHYTHMIAS

- Most common complications of Anterior Wall MI = Mobitz type II, ventricular aneurysm, CHB (unlike CHB with IWMI, CHB with AWMI = grave prognosis)
- 33% of patients diagnosed with acute myocardial infarction did not have chest pain on presentation. CP may be pleuritic, postional or even reproduced (5-10%). Elderly and females present with atypical features of ACS; dyspnea = most common atypical symptom
- Diaphoresis is most "suggestive" of ACS other clinical features = CP (most common presenting symptom); mitral regurgitation (MR); hypotension; CHF; dyspnea 30%; nausea / vomiting; syncope; pain in upper extremities; epigastric pain; shoulder, or neck pain ... and of course ... dizziness
- Most common complications of Inferior Wall MI = Acute MR, ↓HR and ↓BP
  First degree AVB, Mobitz type I (Wenckebach, accounts for 90% of 2nd-degree AVB and AMI) and CHB (stable, usually resolves)
- VF occurs in 5% of patients with AMI, 80% present within 12 hours
- Most common cause of VT/VF = AMI / ischemia
- Inverted P's = think Junctional rhythm
- Low magnesium = risk for AICD to fire
- Most common conduction disturbance in AMI = First degree AV block, 15%; more common with IWMI
- Negative Cath - good for 6 to 12 months; negative must truly be negative; 40% lesion could rupture anytime
- Negative Stress test - good for < 6 months; only 60-70% Sn for CAD at time of test! No test is Gold
- Mortality rate with IWMI and CHB = 15%; if RV involved MR rises to > 30%
- Most common rhythm disturbances in AMI = PVC's (>90%), PACs (50%) Sinus tach (33%)
- 50% of patients with AMI have nondiagnostic ECG
- Most common complications of thrombolytic therapy in patients with AMI = Reperfusion arrhythmias; accelerated idioventricular rhythm (AIVR) most common arrhythmia
- AIVR = ventricular rhythm with a rate of between 40 and 120 bpm

- Idioventricular means "relating to or affecting the cardiac ventricle alone" and refers to any ectopic ventricular arrhythmia
  - Treatment = nothing .... stay calm.
  - In addition to reperfusion arrhythmias, AIVR, can also be seen in: RHD, dig toxicity, cocaine toxicity, structural HD, dilated cardiomyopathy
- Earliest ECG findings associated with AMI = hyperacute T → "giant" R wave ("tombstone") → typical ST segment elevation – which is either flat (horizontally or oblique) or convex
- ST-segment elevation in V1, in the absence of ST-segment elevation in the other anteroseptal leads (V2-V3), is suggestive of right-ventricular ischemia/infarction
- Dressler's syndrome: fever, pleuritis, leukocytosis, pericardial friction rub, and evidence of pericarditis or pleural effusion occurring several weeks after MI. Autoimmune. Treatment: NSAIDs or ASA
- LV dysfunction > 40% = Cardiogenic shock
- Cardiogenic shock may not occur immediately post-MI. The median delay from AMI to clinical development of cardiogenic shock may be up to 7 hours
- Most common type of CVA after MI = ischemic thromboembolic
- **AMI 2 Main Complications**
  - Dysrhythmia (early)
  - Pump failure: New CHF, MR = 5%, Mild CHF, MR = 15-20%; Pulmonary Edema, MR = 40% and Cardiogenic Shock, MR 80%
- **Myocardial Rupture**
  - Sudden decompensation of a previously stable patient who recently suffered an AMI = concern for a mechanical complication.
  - Rupture of the ventricular free wall (Myocardial Rupture) is the most common mechanical complication
  - Bimodal: first 24 hours OR 1-2 weeks later
  - Acute onset of tearing CP and signs of pericardial tamponade
  - Another cause of myocardial rupture = trauma
  - Signs & symptoms: Hypotension, elevated CVP, distended neck veins, tachycardia

PACEMAKER DYSFUNCTION

- Most common cause of failure to PACE / pacemaker dysfunction = oversensing
- Oversensing = sensing electrical events NOT associated with atrial or ventricular depolarizations → this suppresses impulse generation in pacemakers in the inhibit mode

Other causes of Failure to Pace

- Wire Fracture
- Battery depletion

Failure to SENSE (undersensing)

- pacemaker spikes occurring at the wrong time
- on the ECG or rhythm strip

Failure to CAPTURE

- Pacemaker impulses fail to trigger myocardial depolarization
- ECG: pacemaker spikes without associated ventricular depolarization

NORMAL DIGOXIN ECG FINDINGS ("DIG EFFECT")

1. Downsloping ST depression (Salvador Dali / sagging / hockey stick appearance)
2. Flattened, inverted, or biphasic T waves
3. Shortened QT interval

Most Common Rhythm Disturbance in Digitalis Toxicity

- PVC 60% > SVT 25% > AV block 20%
- Classic dig toxicity arrhythmia = SVT with a slow ventricular response (atrial tachycardia with block)

CRITERIA FOR DIGIBIND

- Digoxin level > 10 mg/mL
- Cardiovascular instability
- Blocks (Mobitz II, CHB)
- Ventricular dysrhythmia
- K > 5 mEq/L
- AMS attributed to digoxin
- Ingestion
- > 10 mg in adults or
- > 0.3 mg/kg in children

CARDIOLOGY PEARLS - INFECTIVE ENDOCARDITIS (IE)

- Fever is the most common presenting sign of patients with IE
- In patients with rheumatic heart disease, the mitral valve is the most common site of IE involvement
- Most common cause of Native Valve Infective Endocarditis (IE) Staph aureus (no longer Strep Viridans) cover MRSA in IVDA patient
- Treatment: Pen G or AMP + Nafcillin + Gentamycin; Most textbooks: AMP + Gent or Vancomycin + Gentamycin (if MRSA suspected)
  - **PEARL:** Gentamycin addsc synergy; Nafcillin does not cover Enterococci
- Most common cause of Native Valve Right-Sided IE = *Staph aureus* (IVD abusers)
  Most common valve affected = tricuspid; Treatment = Vancomycin
- Culture negative IE = *Haemophilus parainfluenzae, H. aphrophilus, Actinobacillus, Cardiobacterium, Eikenella*, and *Kingella* species (HACEK organisms); Treatment = Ceftriaxone 2gm IV q 24hrs or Amp + Gent
  - Add *Bartonella henselae, B. quinata* = (HABCEK); Treatment = Ceftriaxone + Gentamycin + Doxy
  - Also, *Coxiella burnetii* Treatment = Doxy + Hydroxychloroquine
- Most common cause of Prosthetic Valve IE < 60 days post-op = coagulase negative *Staph. (S. epidermidis)* and *Staph aureus.* Treat = Vancomycin + Gentamycin + Rifampin
- Most common cause of Prosthetic Valve IE > 60 days post-op = similar to Native Valve with Staph aureus now most common etiology
- Association between *Streptococcus bovis* IE and coexisting colon cancer
- Inefective Endocarditis = petechiae, splinter hemorrhages (dark red vertical lesions in nailbeds), Osler nodes (painful, red, raised lesions on distal finger pads), Janeway lesions 35% (flat, red-bluish, painless lesions on palms/soles), fever, murmur, anemia, malaise, Roth spots (retinal hemorrhages with pale center) Fever is the most common presenting symptom

- Most common cause of Acute Aortic Regurgitation (AR) = Infective endocarditis
- In developed countries, the frequency of RHD has declined, and MVP is now the most common underlying condition in patients with endocarditis
- Antibiotic prophylaxis - not recommended GI or GU procedure of active infection

INFECTIVE ENDOCARDITIS

Mnemonic (FROM JANE)

F	**F**ever (most common presenting symptom)
R	**R**oth spots (retinal hemorrhages with pale center)
O	**O**sler nodes (painful, red, raised lesions on distal finger pads)
M	**M**urmur

J	**J**aneway lesions 35% (flat, red-bluish, painless lesions on palms/soles) and petechiae
A	**A**nemia
N	**N**ailbeds - splinter hemorrhages (dark red vertical lesions in nailbeds)
E	**E**mboli

Hallmark of imaging for endocarditis = Echocardiography (transesophageal preferred)

MYOCARDITIS

- Most common cause of myocarditis = Viral
- Most common viral cause of myocarditis = Parovirus B19 (Coxsackie B was most common in the 1990's)
- Other viruses: Influenza, HH6, HIV, CMV, Hepatitis, Varicella, Mumps
- Bacterial causes: Diptheria, Typhoid fever, Brucellosis, Psitticosis, Mycobacterium, Strep - rheumatic fever (RF)
- Rickettsial; Spirochetal: Syphilis, Leptospirosis and Lyme Disease
- Consider CMV and Toxoplasma gondii in Transplant or HIV patient
- Most common cause of Myocarditis worldwide = Trypanosomiasis (Chaga's disease); Other parasites: Toxoplasmosis, Shistosomiasis, Trichinosis
  Chaga's disease: 3/4 of patients have NO symptoms; Spread by reduviid, "kissing" or "assassin" bug
  - Pathognomonic finding in Chaga's = Romana sign (painless unilateral periorbital edema uncommon)
  - Chagoma: painful cutaneous edema at site of skin penetration
  - Treatment: Nifurtimox (Lampit) or Primaquine
- Fungal: Histoplasmosis and Cryptococcosis
- Kawasaki Syndrome (Mucocutaneous Lymph Node Syndrome) = 50% myocarditis; Treat with ASA and IV gammaglobulin
- Chemotherapeutic agent most commonly implicated in causing myocarditis = Doxorubicin
- The most common long-term sequelae of myocarditis = dilated cardiomyopathy

MRI of the heart is becoming the Gold Standard to diagnose Myocarditis

- 78% Accuracy
- Easier then the current Gold Standard (Myocardial Biopsy)

Myocarditis ECG changes: sinus tachycardia; diffuse ST-segment elevation, low voltage, conduction delays, NSST-T wave changes

- Disproportionate tachycardia - tachycardia is out of proportion to fever
- Troponin often elevated
- ECHO: global hypokinesis
- Treatment
  - Usually supportive
  - If patients have a low Ejection Fraction (EF) or new LBBB = may need left ventricular assist device (LVAD) as bridge to cardiac transplantation

CARDIOLOGY PEARLS - VALVULAR HEART DISEASE

- Patent foramen ovale is a risk factor ofr an ischemic stroke from a paradoxial embolus
- Most common cause of Acute AR = Infective endocarditis
- Most common cause of Chronic Aortic Regurgitation (AR) = Rheumatic heart disease (RHD)
- Most common cause of Aortic Stenosis < 65 y/o=Congenital Heart Disease (Bicuspid Valve 50%), 2nd RHD. Crescendo-decrescendo mid-SEM, heard best at the base, radiates to carotids.
- Most common cause of Aortic Stenosis > 65 y/o=Idiopathic calcification/degenerative heart disease
- Most common cause of Acute MR = Rupture of chordae tendineae or papillary muscle (IWMI). Consider in new onset CHF
- Most common cause of Chronic MR = Rheumatic heart disease (RHD)
- Most common cause of Mitral Stenosis (MS) = Rheumatic heart disease (RHD)
- Most common presenting symptom of all cardiac valvular diseases = exertional dyspnea
- Most common symptom of Mitral Stenosis (MS) = Exertional Dyspnea (symptom specific to MS = hemoptysis)
- Most common dysrhythmias associated with MS = Atrial Fibrillation
- Aortic Stenosis (AS) = exertional Syncope, Angina and Dyspnea (mnemonic=SAD)
- AS patients become symptomatic when valve opening decreases to < 1cm
- Avoid vasodilators (NTG) in patients with AS
- Increased risk of sudden death in AS secondary to arrhythmia (25%)
- Most common rapidly lethal complication of Aortic Stenosis (AS) = sudden death
- Most common valvulopathy due to chest trauma = Aortic Regurgitation (AR)
- Aortic Regurgitation (AR) = High Pulse Pressure, head bobbing = prominent ventricular impulse (Musset sign), soft diastolic murmur (Austin-Flint murmur), bounding peripheral pulses (water hammer), pulsations of uvula and nailbed, and SBP of LE > UE (Hill sign); causes: trauma, IE, aortic dissection, Marfan's, syphilis
  - AR: Nailbed pulsations = Quincke's sign
  - AR: To-and-fro murmur over the femoral artery = Duroziez's murmur

- Systolic murmurs = AS (mid-systolic ejection crescendo-decrescendo)
- MS = Rumbling Mid-late diastolic murmur, heard best at the apex, opening snap, does not radite, heart best at apex and in left lateral decubitus position
- Diastolic murmurs = AR (blowing decrescendo) and MS (holodiastolic with opening snap)
- AS = Mid-SEM Crescendo-decrescendo, hard best at the base (Right second intercostal space) radiates to carotids.
- AS, MS, MR, Pulmonary Insufficiency = decrease pulse pressure

MITRAL VALVE PROLAPSE (MVP)

- MVP is billowing of one or both mitral leaflets into the left atrium by increasing pressure in the ventricle during systole
- The murmur is due to the Mitral Regurgitation (MR) that follows the MVP
- Caused by myxomatous degeneration of the valve
- Most common cause of primary valvular disease in industrialized countries
- Most patients are asymptomatic
- Most common symptoms of MVP = CP (sharp, localized) & palpitations; affects 10% of population; majority asymptomatic; ECG abnormal; patients may have pectus excavatum or scoliosis; ↑ migraines, anxiety and CVA. Beta-blocker therapy is indicated if symptoms recur frequently.
  - ↑incidence of sudden death and dysrhythmias. ↑incidence of TIAs under the age of 45;
  - MVP with regurgitation (both leafltets involved; usually affects one – the posterior leaflet) →
  - ↑risk of IE

Auscultation

- Classic mid-systolic click, followed by a late high-pitched systolic crescendo murmur
- Heard best at the apex
- Maneuvers that DECREASE preload (such as valsalva and standing) move the click EARLIER in systole (PEARL: this will make HCM murmur louder)
- Maneuvers that INCREASE preload (such as squatting) or increasing afteroad (such as hand grip) move the click LATER in systole
- Although most patients with MVP are asymptomatic, symptoms can include:
  non-exertional CP, palpitations, SOB, fatigue and anxiety
  Principal determinant of prognosis in mitral valve prolapse = presence and severity of concomitant MR
- **Diagnosis = ECHO**
- The most important use of the Valsalva maneuerer is to distinguish the murmur of AS from HCM. If you decrease the preload (Valsalva or standing from squatting) → the murmur of HCM becomes quite loud.
- Valsalva → ↑intrathoracic pressure → ↓venous return → ↓preload → ↓most murmurs except for Hypertrophic Cardiomyopathy murmur which ↑ because dynamic LV outflow obstruction is accentuated by ↓preload

- **Hypertrophic Cardiomyopathy murmur (HCM)** = harsh mid-SEM crescendo-decrescendo; loud S4; heard best at apex & left sternal border; radiates to the axilla (AS radiates to carotids)

↓ preload (standing, valsalva diuretics or nitrates) or ↓ afterload (vasodilators) →↑gradient → ↑murmur

- HCM = the most common cause of sudden cardiac death in young athletes
- DOE / Syncope
- Murmur worse with valsalva (decrease preload)
- Daggers on ECG
- Treatment = beta blocker

CARDIOLOGY PEARLS

- Amount of fluid in normal pericardial space = 25-50 ml
- Need 250 ml of fluid in pericardial space before cardiac silhouette ↑ on CX
- Beck's Triad: 1) Muffled heart tones 2) ↓BP 3) JVD (↑CVP) = cardiac tamponade
- Most common echocardiographic findings with cardiac tamponade = right ventricular diastolic collapse
- RV diastolic collapse is definitely seen in cardiac tamponade vs Electrical Alternans which is not always seen, however if present is pathognomonic for tamponade
- Most common cause of pericardial tamponade = malignancy 30-60%; uremia 10-15%, idiopathic pericarditis 5-15%, ID 5-10%, anticoagulation 5-10%, connective tissue diseases 2-6%, and Dressler syndrome 1-2%
- Causes of pulsus paradoxus = cardiac tamponade, and obstructive lung disease (asthma, COPD), massive PE, hemorrhagic shock, constrictive pericarditis
- Pulsus Paradoxus = measuring the variation of SBP during expiration and inspiration
- Slowly decrease cuff pressure until systolic sounds are first heard during expiration but not during inspiration, (note this reading)
  - Slowly continue decreasing the cuff pressure until sounds are heard throughout the respiratory cycle, (inspiration and expiration) = note this second reading
  - Drop in SBP > 10mm Hg during normal inspiration = Pulsus Paradoxus

SHOCK

- Shock = imbalance of tissue O2 supply and demand
- No lab test or vital sign can diagnose shock
- Rather, the initial diagnosis is based on clinical recognition of the presence of inadequate tissue perfusion and oxygenation
- Decreased CNS perfusion = agitation and AMS
- **Shock Index (SI)** = HR / SBP
  - Normal range = (0.5 to 0.7)
  - Higher values = occult shock
  - More sensitive (Sn) then vital signs alone to diagnose occult shock
- MAP = DBP + 1/3 (SBP - DBP)
- All patients with shock should receive as the first priority → Supplemental oxygen

- **Four Mechanistic Classifications of Shock**
  1. Hypovolemic (inadequate circulatory volume)
  2. Cardiogenic (inadequate cardiac pump function)
  3. Distributive (peripheral vasodilation and maldistribution of blood flow); examples → neurogenic shock (↓BP and ↓HR), anaphylactic shock, pancreatitis, burns, trauma, adrenal insufficiency, drug or toxin reactions, heavy metal poisoning, hepatic insufficiency
  4. Obstructive (extra-cardiac obstruction to blood flow) cardiac tamponade, PE, tension pneumothorax
- **Shock Treatment Options**
  - Pure alpha adrenergic agent = phenylephrine
  - Mixed alpha and beta adrenergic agents = epinephrine, norepinephrine and dopamine
  - Pure beta or primary beta-agonists = dobutamine and isoproterenol

CARDIAC TUMORS

- Cardiac tumors are a rare and immediately life-threatening finding in any patient regardless of current associated symptoms
- 75% of cardiac tumors are benign, 15% are primary malignant cancers and 10% are metastases
- Cardiac myxomas = the most common cardiac tumor (65%)
- Typically occur in patients in their 40s to 60s
- Symptoms include lightheadedness, dyspnea, palpitations, and chest pain
- Malignant tumors like lymphomas may be accompanied by weight loss, fatigue, night sweats, and cough
- Diagnosis is best assessed by echocardiography, and the presence of thrombus or vegetation should be concurrently assessed
- Computed tomography or magnetic resonance imaging should be secondarily pursued when echocardiography is negative and suspicion persists
- Cardiac tumors place the patient at risk for severe complications: dysrhythmias (e.g., heart block), heart failure, hemorrhagic pericardial effusion (common in malignant tumors), pulmonary embolism, and stroke
- Consequently, immediate surgical treatment is indicated for practically all patients except in the case of lymphomas when radiation and chemotherapy are predominantly used
- Given the rarity and complexity of treatment for these patients, they should be TRANSFERRED to a tertiary care center as they often require interdisciplinary care of oncology, radiation oncology, cardiology, and cardiac surgery

LEFT VENTRICULAR ASSIST DEVICE (LVAD) PEARLS

- Infection is common = 40%
- Most often occurs between 2 weeks and 2 months after implantation
- Driveline (line that exits chest) = most common site for infection

PULMONARY HYPERTENSION

- Mainstay of emergency therapy = adequate intravascular volume
- normal saline recommended
- Maintain right ventricular pressure and ensure adequate CO
- Presentation = exercise intolerance, syncope, near-syncope, DOE
- 50% of patients with Pulmonary HTN experience syncope
- Syncope is typically related to dysrhythmia

FASICULAR BLOCKS

- S1Q3 RAD = Left Posterior Fascicular (LPFB)
- S3Q1 LAD = Left Anterior Fascicular (LAFB)
- LPFB has more serious implications since it implies compromise to both the right and left coronary arteries as well as damage to large areas of myocardial muscle and to the electrical conduction system in the left ventricle [Sensible analysis of the 12-lead ECG By Kathryn Monica Lewis, Kathleen A. Handal, pg. 170]

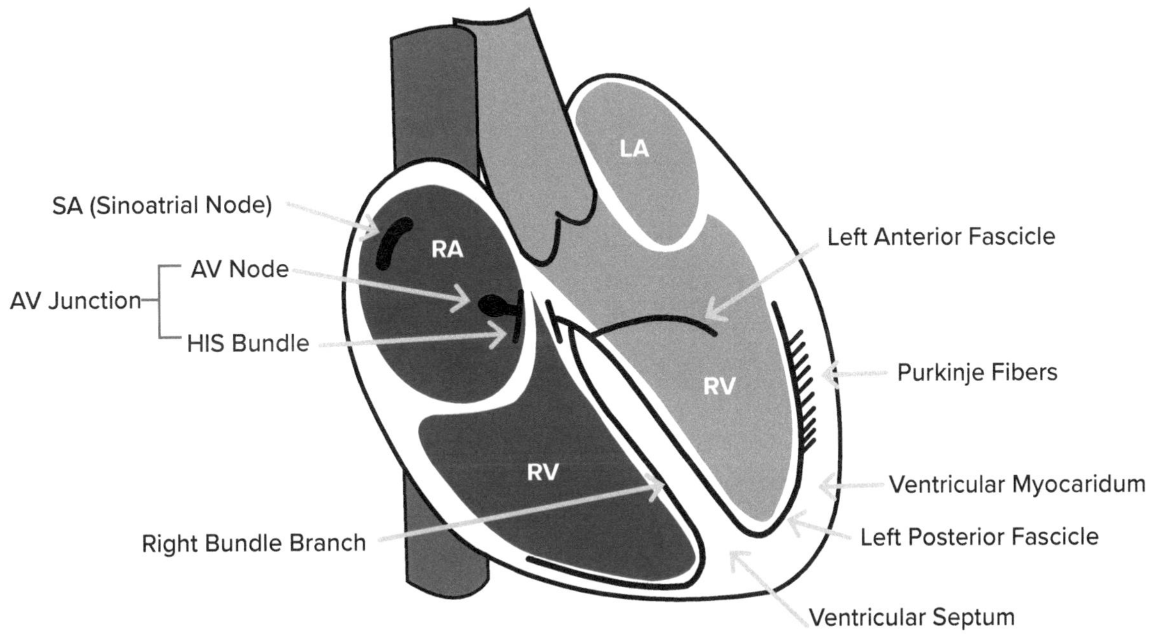

SPECTRUM OF LOWER EXTREMITY THROMBOTIC DISEASE

Simple DVT → phlegmasia alba dolens → phlegmasia cerulea dolens → venous gangrene

PHLEGMASIA ALBA DOLENS

- Painful white inflammation ("milk leg") occurs when venous thrombosis progresses to a massive occlusion of the major deep venous system of the leg compromising arterial flow, but without ischemia.

PHLEGMASIA CERULEA DOLENS

- Massive DVT of the proximal iliofemoral vein
- Most commonly in patient's in their 50–60s, more common in women, history of malignancy
- Sudden, severe unilateral leg pain with significant swelling and edema
- Initially, the leg will appear blanched **(phlegmasia alba dolens),** then will progress to a bluish discoloration due to venous congestion
- Eventually, arterial compromise may occur as the compartment pressure rises above arterial systolic pressure
- **Diagnosis**: Clinical or by duplex ultrasonography (obstructing proximal iliofemoral DVT)
- **Treatment**: Elevate limb, heparin infusion, and vascular surgery consult for thrombectomy or catheter-directed thrombolysis
- **PROVOKED DVT** is caused by a clear inciting factor: recent surgery or trauma, hospitalization with prolonged bed rest, or use of oral contraceptives
- **UNPROVOKED DVT** may be idiopathic or result from inherited or acquired hypercoagulable states such as cancer and pregnancy

RISK FACTORS FOR DVT / PULMONARY EMBOLISM

Mnemonic: (MOIST CAMEL)

M	**M**obility = stasis: prolonged travel, bed rest, paralysis (CVA, spinal cord injury), leg cast
O	**O**besity
I	**I**nflammatory conditions (IBD, SLE, PVD)
S	**S**urgery (especially orthopedic, pelvic & major abdominal surgery)
T	**T**rauma = Intimal damage: trauma, IVDA, surgery, central lines

C	**C**HF / CVA / COPD (respiratory diseases) / Cardiac Disease
A	**A**ntithrombin III, Protein C & S deficiency
M	**M**alignancy / **M**edical patients
E	**E**strogen / pregnancy /postpartum /elective AB or miscarriage
L	**L**ong bone fracture

VIRCHOW'S TRIAD

1) Hypercoagulable state
2) Venous stasis
3) Venous injury

HYPERCOAGULABLE (THROMBOPHILIA) STATES

- Previous DVT/PE
- Nephrotic syndrome (loss of antithrombin)
- Malignancy
- Inflammatory Conditions (IBD, SLE, PVD)
- Sepsis

COAGULATION DISORDERS – INHERITABLE VS ACQUIRED

- Protein C or S deficiency
- Resistance to activated Protein C
- Antithrombin deficiency
- Disorders of Fibrinogen or Plasminogen
- Antiphospholipid antibodies (lupus anticoagulant & anti-cardiolipin)
- Most common inherited hypercoagulable state = Factor V Leiden mutation

INCREASED ESTROGEN (CAUSES URINARY LOSS OF PROTEIN S AND ANTITHROMBIN)

- Pregnancy
- Postpartum status < 3 months
- OCPs
- Elective abortion or miscarriage

D-DIMER

Fibrin fragments found in fresh fibrin clot & in fibrin degradation products. Elevated in many conditions: DVT/PE, CVA, trauma, cancer, surgery, infection/sepsis, sickle cell anemia, postpartum within 1 week and pregnancy (elevated in 75% of patients with a normal pregnancy)

PEARL: AGE-ADJUSTED D-DIMER

In patients older than 50 years deemed to be low or intermediate risk for acute PE, clinicians may use a negative age-adjusted D-dimer* result to exclude the diagnosis of PE
*For highly sensitive D-dimer assays using fibrin equivalent units (FEU) use a cutoff of age10 mg/L
For highly sensitive D-dimer assays using D-dimer units (DDU), use a cutoff of age 5 mg/L

D-DIMER + WELLS CLINICAL SCORE FOR DVT- DIAGNOSTIC STRATEGY

A negative D-dimer result in the *unlikely* group (Wells DVT score < 2) → rules out DVT
All patients with a positive D-dimer result and all patients in the *likely* group (Wells DVT score > 2) → require a diagnostic study (duplex Ultrasonography)

WELLS CLINICAL SCORE FOR DVT

Clinical Parameter	Score
Active cancer (treatment ongoing, or withing 6 mo. or palliative	+1
Paralysis or recent plaster immobilization of the lower extremities	+1
Recently bedridden for >3 days or major surgery < 4wks.	+1
Localized tenderness along the distribution of the deep venous system	+1
Entire leg swelling	+1
Calf swelling >3 cm compared with the asymptomatic leg	+1
Previous DVT documented	+1
Collateral superficial veins (non varicose)	+1
Alternative diagnosis (as likely or greater than that of DVT)	-2
Total of Above Score	
High probability	≥3
Moderate probability	1 or 2
Low probability	0

ANTICOAGULATION TREATMENT OPTIONS FOR VENOTHROMBOEMBOLISM (VTE) - DVT/PE

1. **Injectable indirect factor Xa and IIa (thrombin) inhibitors**
   The effects of indirect inhibitors are mediated through antithrombin (AT)
   a. **Unfractionated heparin (UFH):** Xa and to a lesser extent IIa (thrombin). Also, inhibits factors XIIa, XIa and IXa
   b. **Enoxaparin (Lovenox):** low-molecular-weight-heparin (LMWH); Xa and to a lesser extent IIa (thrombin) inhibitor
   c. **Fondaparinux (Arixtra):** exclusive indirect factor Xa inhibitor

Warfarin

- Overlap Warfarin at the same time as UFH, LMWH or Fondaparinux because early in treatment, warfarin can cause a hypercoaguable state (due to more rapid depletion of protein C and protein S compared to the clotting factors with longer half-lives); Overlap with warfarin for at least 5 days and until INR is in therapeutic (2.0 – 3.0) range for 24 hours.
- **PEARL**: Warfarin is contraindicated in pregnancy

2. **Target-Specific Oral Anticoagulants (TSOACs) or Direct Oral Anticoagulants (DOACs)**
   a. **Direct Thrombin Inhibitors (DTIs) (IIa)**
      i. Dabigatran (Pradaxa)
   b. **Direct Factor Xa Inhibitors ("Xabans")**
      i. Rivaroxaban (Xarelto)
      ii. Apixaban (Eliquis)
      iii. Edoxaban (Lixiana, Savaysa)

VTE PROPHYLAXIS

Unfractionated Heparin (UFH)

- 5.000 units SQ every 8 hours

Enoxaparin (Lovenox)

- 40 mg SQ once daily or 30 mg SQ once daily if CrCl < 30 mL/min

Fondaparinux (Arixtra)

- 2.5 mg SQ daily if CrCl > 30 mL/min and actual body weight > 50kg

Rivaroxaban (Xarelto) - Surgical VTE Prophylaxis

- Knee replacement: 10 mg once daily for 12 days
- Hip replacement: 10 mg once daily for 35 days
- Initial dose should be taken at least 6-10 hours after surgery once hemostasis has been established
- Avoid use if CrCl < 30 mL/min

Apixaban (Eliquis) - Surgical VTE Prophylaxis

- Knee replacement: 2.5mg BID for 12 days
- Hip replacement: 2.5mg BID for 35 days
- Initial dose should be given 12 to 24 hours after surgery once hemostasis has been established
- No dose adjustment with moderate renal impairment for above Apixaban VTE indications
- Not studied in patients with CrCl < 25 mL/min

VTE TREATMENT

Unfractionated Heparin (UFH)

- Bolus 80 units/kg followed by infusion of 18 units/kg/hr

Enoxaparin (Lovenox)

- 1 mg/kg SC every 12 hours or
- 1.5 mg/kg SC daily: "suggested over twice-daily regimen"

Fondaparinux (Arixtra)

- Weight <50 kg: 5 mg SQ daily
- Weight 50-100 kg: 7.5 mg SQ daily
- Weight >100 kg: 10 mg SQ daily

ARIXTRA is contraindicated:

- Creatinine clearance <30 mL/min
- DVT prophylaxis if weight < 50 kg

Rivaroxaban (Xarelto)

- 15 mg BID x 21 days
- On day #22 transition to 20 mg once daily

Reduce Risk of Recurrent DVT or PE

- Following 6 months of treatment, 20 mg once daily

Apixaban (Eliquis)

- 10 mg BID x 7 days, then 5 mg BID

Reduce Risk of Recurrent DVT or PE

- Following 6 months of treatment, 2.5 mg BID

Edoxaban (Lixiana, Savaysa)

- >60 kg: 60 mg daily
- <60 kg: 30 mg daily
- Treat with parenteral anticoagulation for 5-10 days (dual therapy)
- CrCl 15 to 50 mL/min: decrease dose to 30 mg daily

Dabigatran (Pradaxa)

- 150 mg BID
- Treat with parenteral anticoagulation for 5-10 days (dual therapy)
- Avoid use CrCl < 30 mL/min

ANTICOAGULATION REVERSAL STRATEGIES FOR SEVERE/ LIFE THREATENING BLEEDING

SEVERE / LIFE THREATENING BLEEDING

1. Acute bleeding associated with a fall in hemoglobin ≥2g/dL
2. Symptomatic or fatal bleeding in a critical area or organ: intraocular, intraspinal, or intramuscular with compartment syndrome, retroperitoneal, intra-articular or pericarddidal bleeding
3. Clinically significant acute intracranial or intraspinal hemorrhage
   a. Glasgow Coma Score (GCS) < 7
   b. Intracerebral hematoma volume > 30mls
   c. Subdural hematomas with a maximum thickness ≥ 10 mm or midlineshift ≥ 5mm
   d. Subarachnoid hemorrhage (SAH) with any evidence of hydrocephalus, infratentorial ICH location, epidural hematomas, or any intraventricular extension of hemorrhage.
4. Bleeding requiring immediate surgical intervention
5. Life threatening bleed defined by the physician

TREATMENT STRATEGIES FOR SEVERE / LIFE THREATENING BLEEDING FROM TSOACS

Direct Factor Xa Inibitors (Rivaroxaban, Apixaban, Endoxaban)	Direct Thrombin Inhibitors Dabigartran (Paradaxa)
Consider **charcoal** - YES (If previous does ingested withing 2-4 hours) Charcoal 50 g PO x 1 dose Consider **Anti-Fibrinolytics** - YES	Consider **Charcoal** - YES (If previous does ingested with 2-4 hours) Charcoal 50 g PO x 1 dose Consider **Anti-Fibrinolytics** - YES
Consider **Hemodialysis** - NO	Consider **Hemodylasis** - YES
PCC4 (Kcentra) 25 units/kg (max 2000 units) x1 • May repeat 25 units/kg (Maximum 2000 units) x 1 • Maximum total dose (including repeat dose) = 4000 units If PCC4 contraindicated give **aPCC (FEIBA)** If antidote available - consider **Andexanet alfa** (Current available literature does not support widespread use of Andexanet alpha in the hospital setting as standard of care)	**Idarucizumab (Praxbind®)** 5 g IV x 1 (administered as two separate 2.5 g doses, no more than 15 minutes apart) • If Idarucizumab is not available, **aPCC (FEIBA)** 50 units/kg/kg x 1 • If bleeding persists after 30-60 minutes from initial aPCC dose, consider a repeat dose of aPCC at 25-30 units/kg x 1

Praxbind (Idarucizumab)

Idarucizumab is a humanized, monoclonal, antibody fragment that specifically binds with high affinity to dabigatran. Dabigatran has an affinity for idarucizumab that is 350 times greater than its affinity for thrombin.

Andexanet Alfa

Antidote for oral direct and injectable indirect Factor Xa InhibitorsAndexanet alfa is a modified recombinant factor Xa molecule administered intravenously. Antidote to reverse the anticoagulant activity of oral direct (apixaban, edoxaban, and rivaroxaban) and injectable indirect (enoxaparin and fondaparinux) factor Xa inhibitors. Andexanet alfa acts as a decoy to target and sequester with high specificity both oral and injectable factor Xa inhibitors.

TREATMENT STRATEGIES FOR SEVERE / LIFE THREATENING BLEEDING - WARFARIN

- INR ≥ 1.4
- Vitamin K IVPB 10 mg + PCC4 25 units/kg (max 1500 units)
- If partial or unsuccessful reversal, may provide additional dose of PCC4 500 units x 1
- Recheck INR 10-30 minutes after PCC4 administration

TREATMENT OPTIONS IF MAJOR BLEEDING STARTS AFTER UNFRACTIONATED HEPARIN (UFH) THERAPY

- Most common cause of drug related death in hospitalized patients = heparin
- Antidote: Protamine; 1 mg of protamine neutralizes 100 units of heparin; administer over 15 minutes
- If dose is unknown, a fixed empiric does of 10 to 50 mg IV may be given
- **PEARL:** Management of Major Bleeding with LMWHs is similar to anticoagulation reversal strategy with UFH

ANTICOAGULATION CASCADE

Contact Activation (intrinsic) Pathway

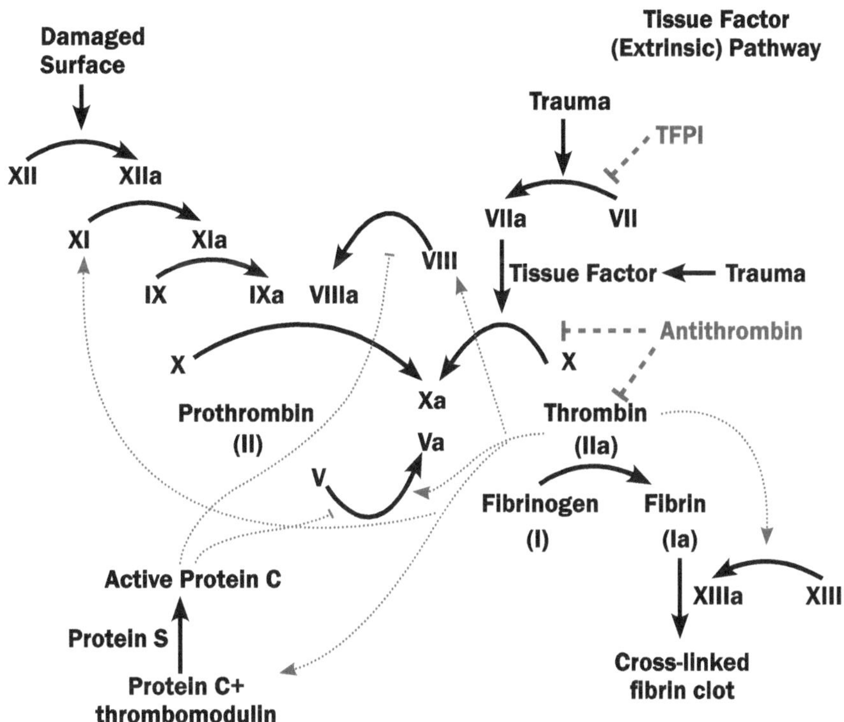

MECHANISM OF ANTICOAGULATION

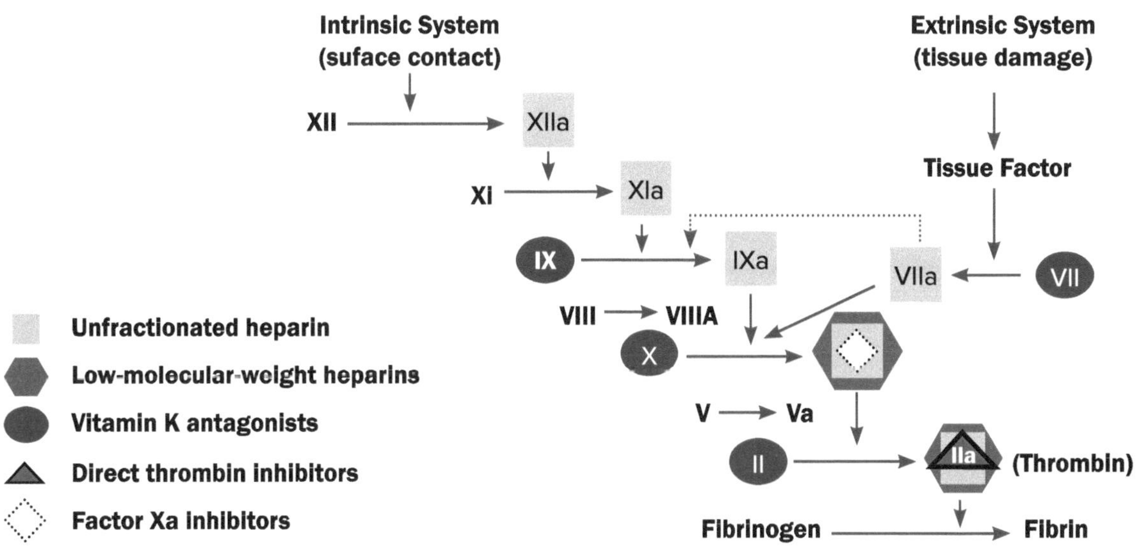

WELL'S CRITERIA FOR ASSESSMENT OF PRETEST PROBABILITY FOR PE

Clinical Signs and Symptoms of DVT	3 points
An alternative diagnosis in less likely than PE	3 points
Heart Rate > 100	1.5 points
Immobilization at least 3 days, or Surgery in the Previous 4 weeks	1.5 points
Previous, objectively diagnosed PE or DVT	1.5 points
Hemoptysis	1 point
Malignancy w/ Treatment within 6 months, or palliative	1 point

Low-risk patients, score < 2 had a mean probability of 3.6% for PE
Intermediate-risk patients, score 2-6 had a mean probability of 20.5% for PE
High-risk patients, score > 6 had a mean probability of 66.7% for PE

Modified Wells Criteria PE
If < 4 Proceed to PERC
If > 4 CT angio or V/Q

PULMONARY EMBOLISM RULE-OUT CRITERIA (PERC)

- Age ≥ 50y
- Tachycardia, HR > 100
- O2 sat < 95%
- Prior DVT or PE
- Recent trauma or surgery
- Hemoptysis
- Exogenous estrogen (hormone use)
- Unilateral leg swelling

If NO criteria are met, PE can be ruled out
If any criteria are met, unable to rule out PE

PERC RULE

MNEMONIC - (HAD CLOTS)

The patient must meet the following:

H	no **H**ormones
A	no **A**ge > 50
D	no **D**VT/PE history

C	no **C**oughing blood
L	no **L**ower extremity swelling unilaterally
O	no **O**2 saturation <95
T	no **T**achycardia >100
S	no **S**urgery/trauma within past 28 days

PULMONARY EMBOLISM - PEARLS

- Most Common **Symptom** = dyspnea, 75% > CP 45%
- Most Common **Sign** = tachypnea, 54% > LE swelling/erythema/tenderness (47%) > tachycardia (24%)
- Triad of Dyspnea, CP and Hemoptysis < 20%
- Most common cause of death from pulmonary thromboembolism = hemodynamic collapse
- Most common cause of upper extremity DVT = catheters
- Most common **ECG** finding = sinus tachycardia and non-specific ST changes

ECG FINDINGS IN PULMONARY EMBOLISM

Mnemonic – (NA STRIPE)

N	**N**on-specific ST changes
A	**A**trial fibrillation, new onset (see mnemonic AFIB)

S	**S**1Q3T3 - Classic finding, however uncommon
T	**T**achycardia - Sinus tachycardia=most common ECG finding
R	**R**AD, RBBB
I	**I**nverted T-wave in V1-V4
P	**P**ulmonale (peaked P waves in lead II)
E	**E**levation - ST segment elevation

The CXR is most often abnormal in PE

- Conflicting literature:
  Most common CXR finding from PIOPED trail = atelectasis
  Most common CXR finding from UPET (Urokinase PE Trail) = elevated hemidiaphragm
- Most common CXR in admitted patients = cardiomegaly
- Most common CXR in outpatient patients = basilar atelectasis
- Other CXR findings: Hampton's hump, (wedge-shaped consolidation in lung periphery), Westermark's sign, (dilation of proximal arteries with collapse of distal vasculature)

PULMONARY EMBOLISM - PEARLS

- **ABG**: acute respiratory alkalosis, hypoxemia, an abnormal AaO2 gradient or normal
- **A-a gradient:** should be widened; Sn 90%, Sp 15%
- A-a gradient = 150 – PaO2 – (PaCO2 x 1.25)
  Normal = 5-20 (calculate on room air)
- Lack of hypoxemia does NOT rule out diagnosis of PE
- **Ventilation-perfusion (V/Q)** nuclear medicine scan (sensitivity 95–99%) is *more sensitive* then spiral computed tomography (CT) chest angiogram Sn = 90% for PE
- New generation **spiral CT chest angiogram** has replaced V/Q scanning as preferred diagnostic study
  - CT Chest Angiogram = High sensitivity
  - Ability to identify alternative diagnoses (pneumonia, aortic dissection, pleural effusions, cancers)
  - CT might miss subsegmental emboli (doubtful clinical significance)
  - V/Q scanning takes time and is not readily available from the ED
- **ECHO**: right heart strain in 40%
- **PEARL: McConnell's sign** = RV hypokinesis in the presence of normal RV apical contractility on ECHO

PULMONARY EMBOLISM – PEARLS PREGNANCY

- Threshold for human teratogenesis = 10 rad; fetus most vulnerable 8 to 15 weeks gestation
- V/Q --- Total fetal exposure to xenon-133 and technetium-99m = 0.5 rad; void bladder x 3
- CXR = 0.00005 rad; CT head < 0.1 rad, **CT chest = < 1 rad**; CT abdomen = 3.5 rad
- **Consider diagnostic strategy below for pregnant patients**
  D-dimer → positive → bilateral lower extremity venous doppler → non-diagnostic
  → CT chest over V/Q to diagnose PE

TREATMENT OPTIONS IN PULMONARY EMBOLISM

- Heparin: bolus (80U/kg) then infusion (18U/kg/hr)
- LMWH: Enoxaparin (Lovenox): 1mg/kg SQ or IV every 12 hours or 1.5mg/kg q 24 hours
- tPA: You will find three different protocols for tPA
  - Use in massive PE (hemodynamic instability, severe hypoxia)
  - 100 mg over 2 hours (FDA approved regimen, most textbooks) *or*
  - 15 mg bolus, then 85 mg continuous infusion over 2 hours or
  - Accelerated infusion regimen used in AMI
- **tPA for PE Associated with Cardiac Arrest**
  - 50 mg bolus over 2 minutes
  - If no response to initial bolus or if patient continues to deteriorate 15 minutes after initial bolus → Bolus #2 = 50 mg bolus over 2 minutes

- **Tenecteplase (TNKase) for PE**
  - IV bolus over 5-10 seconds (max 50 mg)
  - < 60 kg: 30 mg
  - ≥ 60 to < 70 kg: 35 mg
  - ≥ 70 to < 80 kg: 40 mg
  - ≥ 80 to < 90 kg: 45 mg
  - ≥ 90 kg: 50 mg

Hold heparin during fibrinolytic infusion. At the conclusion of alteplase infusion begin heparin infusion without a bolus when aPTT has decreased to < 80 seconds.

- Hypotension
  - 0.9% NS cautiously because ↑ RV wall stress can → ↓ the ratio of RV oxygen supply to demand → may result in ischemia, deterioration of RV function, and worsening RV failure and → further ↑interventricular septal shift toward the left ventricle, thereby worsening left ventricular compliance and filling. Consider only 500 to 1,000mL

  - Norepinephrine and dobutamine → permits increased myocardial contractility, while minimizing both vasodilation and the risk of hypotension

- Morphine 4 to 6mg IV PRN

Massive PE = arterial hypotension + cardiogenic shock
- Hypotension: SBP < 90 mm Hg or drop in SBP of at least 40 mm Hg for at least 15 minutes
- Shock = tissue hypoperfusion & hypoxia, altered LOC, oliguria, or cool, clammy extremities

TREATMENT OPTIONS IF MAJOR BLEEDING STARTS AFTER THROMBOLYTIC THERAPY

- Stop the lytic agent
- FFP and cryoprecipitate ASAP
- Aminocaproic acid (Amicar) Inhibits plasminogen activators - 5 gm bolus infused over 1 hr then infusion of 1 gm/hr until bleeding has stopped; rapid administration may result in hypotension, bradycardia and arrythmias

CAUSES OF DYSPNEA

Mnemonic: (SPACE) 2

Dyspnea = a subjective shortness of breath with abnormal and uncomfortable awareness of breathing

S	**S**pontaneous pneumothorax	**S**hock ↑ hemodynamic stimulation
P	**P**neumonia	**P**ulmonary edema (CHF/ARDS)
A	**A**sthma	**A**telectasis
C	**C**OPD (bronchitis/emphysema)	**C**ardiac (CHF, AMI, valvular, AS, MS, AMR)
E	**E**mbolism-pulmonary (PE)	**E**ffusions (pulmonary)

PEARL - Pneumothorax is caused by the presence of free air in intrapleural space

ULTRASOUND FINDINGS IN PNEUMOTHORAX

- Bar code sign (Stratosphere sign)
- US in M-mode
- Normal pattern of "lung sliding" between the visceral and parietal pleura creates significant artifact; dynamic = seashore sign
- When "lung sliding" is ABSENT, there is no artifact; static; the M-line tracing appears as a number of horizontal lines with the appearance of a bar code or planes fumes in stratosphere
- Lung point = most specific finding for pneumothorax: location of transition between the presence and absence of lung sliding

CAUSES OF STRIDOR

Mnemonic: (FACT AIDE) [Mnemonic from Dr. Nicole Colucci]

Problem is at the level of the cords or just below in the trachea

F	**F**oreign Body	**A**	**A**llergy
A	**A**bscess	**I**	**I**rritant/Burn
C	**C**roup	**D**	**D**iptheria
T	**T**racheitis	**E**	**E**piglottitis

FB at level of bronchus / lower respiratory tract = Wheezing
FB in esophagus or lower laryngo-pharynx (BELOW vocal cords) = Drooling
FB in the higher laryngo-pharynx or larynx AT the level of the cords or ABOVE vocal cords = Hoarseness
FB is at the level of the cords or just below in the trachea = Stridor

CAUSES OF PLEURAL EFFUSIONS

Mnemonic: **B (CHAMPS) 3**

B	**B**oerhaave syndrome (left sided)

C	**C**HF Most common cause of effusions in Western countries	**C**irrhosis (with ascites)	**C**hylothorax	
H	**H**emothorax	**H**ypothyroidism	**H**epatic infection (with upward spread)	
A	**A**FB positive = TB Most common cause of effusions developing countries	**A**sbestos	↓ **A**lbumin	**A**ortic dissection (on left side)
M	**M**alignancy	**M**ETS	**M**eig's Syndrome	
P	**P**neumonia "parapneumonic effusion"	**P**E (with infarct)	**P**ancreatitis (on left side)	
S	**S**LE (also RA) 12%	**S**aline overload	**S**ide effect of drugs (NSAIDS, etc.) (see below)	

CAUSES OF PLEURAL EFFUSIONS - SIDE EFFECTS OF DRUGS

Mnemonic: (MAP)

M	(**M**acrodantin, Macrobid) Nitrofurantoin
A	(**A**presoline) Hydralazine
P	**P**rocainamide

DRUG INDUCED LUPUS-LIKE SYNDROME

Mnemonic: (MAPS ID)

M	(**M**acrodantin, Macrobid) Nitrofurantoin
A	(**A**presoline) Hydralazine
P	**P**rocainamide
S	**S**ulfonamides

I	**I**soniazid (INH)
D	**D**ilantin (Phenytoin)

PEARL: Amiodarone (Cordarone) causes pulmonary toxicity by pulmonary fibrosis
PEARL: Amiodarone (Cordarone) can cause chemical epididymitis, hypothyroidism, interstitial lung disease (pulmonary fibrosis), blue-grey skin discoloration, corneal microdeposits; bradycardia, heart blocks, dysrhythmias, prolonged QT, hypotension

PARANEUMONIC EFFUSIONS

Parapneumonic effusion = pleural effusion that forms in the pleural space adjacent to a pneumonia; remember from medical school: lung, visceral pleural, pleural space, outer parietal pleura

a) Simple (uncomplicated): free-flowing sterile effusion; neutrophils, without organisms on Gram stain or culture; treat pneumonia; does not need drainage
b) Complicated: infected with bacteria or other micro-organisms; + neutrophils, elevated LDH; bacteria are cleared rapidly from pleural space = sterile effusion; requires drainage for resolution
c) Empyema: collection of pus within the pleural space; invasion of pleural space from adjacent pneumonia or in the absence of adjacent pneumonia (from direct inoculation after blunt /penetrating trauma, esophageal rupture, surgical complications or after chest tube placement)
d) Complex effusion: effusion with internal loculations
e) Uniloculated effusion: without internal septae (free-flowing or fixed)

PLEURAL EFFUSION PEARLS

Transudative pleural effusions

- Protein content < 3 gm/dl
- Pleural fluid vs. Serum protein RATIO < 3
- Pleural fluid vs. Serum LDH RATIO < 0.6
- LDH content less than 200

Transudative pleural effusions = CHF, cirrhosis, starvation (↓albumin), constrictive pericarditis, nephrotic syndrome and SVC obstruction

Exudative effusions have high amounts of protein and LDH; pH < 7.3
Examples: paraneumonic effusion, malignant effusion, RA effusion, TB effusion or systemic acidosis

- **Ex**udates – **Ex**ceed (**high** amounts of protein and LDH effusion to serum ratios)
- Effusion protein/serum protein > 0.5
- Effusion LDH/serum LDH > 0.6

PEARL: Pleural effusions need 200 cc of fluid to be seen on PA or lateral CXR. <50 cc of fluid if lateral decubitus film

EMPYEMA

- Definitions of an empyema is based on pleural fluid analysis
  - Gram stain: presence of bacteria
  - Gross inspection: fluid is purulent and cloudy
  - Elevated WBC (> 50,000)
  - Decreased glucose
  - pH < 7.2
- Diagnosis: Thoracentesis
- Treatment: chest tube, antibiotics
- Goal: drain and prevent formation of loculations

Thoracentesis Pearl

- Therapeutic thoracentesis: fluid collection stopped once the patient experiences chest discomfort or coughing or has worsening of their vital signs
- Patients tolerate removal of larger volumes of pleural fluid provided they remain asymptomatic
- Diagnostic thoracentesis, a predetermined, minimal amount of fluid may be taken before stopping the procedure

PULMONARY HEMORRHAGE

- Intubate - unaffected lung
  - If left lung problem: intubate right mainstem bronchus
  - if right lung problem: bronchoscopy
- Place patient bleeding side DOWN
- CXR will be abnormal in 3/4 of patients

HEMOPTYSIS

- Life-threatening hemoptysis: approximately 250 mL of blood expectorated in a 24-hour period or bleeding at a rate ≥100 mL/hour
- Most case of hemoptysis are NOT life threatening

CAUSES OF HEMOPTYSIS

Mnemonic: (BIC2) 5

	Common Causes	Less Common Causes			
B	**B**ronchitis (Acute or chronic)	**B**ronchiectasis - including Cystic Fibrosis, Bullous Emphysema	**B**echet's Syndrome and other Alveolar hemorrhage syndromes	**B**roncho-vascular fistula (eg, aortic aneurysm with erosion into airway)	**B**ronchus Met
I	**I**nfection (TB, lung abscess, bronchitis,pneumonia) Parasitic (Paragonimus westermani); Mycetoma and other fungal infections; Yerinia pestis (plague)	**I**nfarct (PE) Only 30% of patients with PE present with hemoptysis, iatrogenic	**I**diopathic Cryptogenic hemoptysis Common = 28%	**I**njury = Blunt chest trauma (bronchial rupture, lung contusion)	**I**diopathic Plumonary Hemosiderosis (IPH)*
C	**C**ancer	**C**ardiac Valves (MS and TV Endocarditis) CHF = 75% of cardiac cases	**C**ocaine "Crack lung"	**C**ongenital Heart Disease	**C**ystic Fibrosis

**Idiopathic Plumonary Hemosiderosis (IPH) = Triad of hemopysis, iron deficiency and other diffuse pulmonary infiltrates*

Other causes

- Alveolar hemorrhage syndromes: Bechet's Syndrome, Goodpasture syndrome and Granulomatosis with polyangiitis (GPA) (formerly called Wegener's) Amyloid and SLE
- Hematologic: platelet dysfunction, anticoagulant therapy and uremia (platelet dysfunction); Thrombocytopenia (ITP, TTP, HUS)
- **Pearl**: Burkholderia cepacia = uncommon respiratory pathogen seen primarily in patients with Cystic Fibrosis
- Catamenial hemoptysis due to ectopic endometrial tissue in the pulmonary system (endometriosis)
- Genetic defect in collagen: Ehlers-Danlos vascular type
- von Willebrand Disease

- Iatrogenic
  - Tracheo-innominate fistula: erosion of tracheal tube into the innominate (brachiocephalic) artery
  - Aorto-bronchial fistula due to aortic graft or stent
  - Bronchoscopy with biopsy or needle aspiration
- TB: cough is the most common presenting symptom, not hemoptysis; hemoptysis is usually minor in acute infection; later → major cause of massive hemoptysis;
- Aspergilloma as a superinfection with TB can also cause massive hemoptysis
- HIV patient with hemoptysis: consider *Strep. pneumo.* or TB
- Children with TB, most common CXR findings = hilar adenopathy, mediastinal lymphadenopathy or consolidated pneumonia

EVALUATION OF HEMOPTYSIS

CXR: bnormal in 70-85%; if neoplasm → abnormal in 80-90%
Massive bleeding: rigid bronchoscopy
Less severe bleeding: fiberoptic bronchoscopy
CT chest

COMMUNITY ACQUIRED PNEUMONIA (CAP)

CAP PATHOGENS

"Typical" pathogens

- *Streptococcus pneumoniae*
- *Moraxella catarrhalis*
- *Haemophilus influenzae, nontypeable*

"Atypical" pathogens are not detectable on GS or cultivatable on standard bacteriologic media

- *Mycoplasma pneumoniae*
- *Chlamydophila pneumoniae*
- *Legionella*

ULTRASOUND FINDING IN PNEUMONIA

- Sonographic appearance of frank consolidation looks remarkably liver-like and is also termed **hepatization**

MILD (AMBULATORY) CAP

The most common pathogens

- *Strep. pneumoniae, M. pneumoniae, C. pneumoniae, and H. influenzae*
- *Mycoplasma* = most common among patients <50 years of age without significant comorbid conditions or abnormal vital signs, whereas *Strep. pneumoniae* was the most common pathogen among older patients and among those with significant underlying disease.
- *Hemophilus* infection was found in 5%—mostly in patients with comorbidities

Treatment

- The use of fluoroquinolones to treat ambulatory patients with CAP without comorbid conditions, risk factors for DRSP, or recent antimicrobial use is discouraged because of concern that widespread use may lead to the development of fluoroquinolone resistance.
- No Comorbidities, no risk factors for Pseudomonas or MRSA: Amoxicillin 1gm po tid x 5-7 days OR Doxycycline 100mg pm bid x 5-day
- Comorbidity present (Chronic heart, lung, liver or renal disease or DM or alcohol disorder, neoplastic disease or asplenia) = Amoxicillin-clavulanate 875 mg/125 mg bid, Cefpodoxime 200 mg bid or Cefuroxime 500 mg bid) for 5 to 7 days + Azithromycin ("Z-Pak") or Clarithromycin 500 mp bid for 5 to 7 days OR Levofloxacin 750 mg po daily x 5 days

TREATMENT FOR NON-ICU – CAP

- Ceftriaxone *or* Cefotaxime *or* Unasyn *or* Ertapenem (Invanz) + Macrolide
- A respiratory fluoroquinolone can be used for penicillin-allergic patients in non-ICU CAP

TREATMENT FOR ICU – CAP

- Therapy with a respiratory fluoroquinolone alone is not established for severe ICU CAP
- Ceftriaxone *or* Cefotaxime *or* Unasyn **plus** either azithromycin or a respiratory fluoroquinolone
- For penicillin-allergic patients → respiratory fluoroquinolone + aztreonam

PNEUMONIA SEVERITY SCORE FOR ELDERLY PATIENTS

CHARACTERISTIC	POINTS
Historical Findings	
Age - Men	Men (years) Women (years - 10)
Nursing home resident	10
Coexisting disease	
Neoplastic disease	30
Liver disease	20
Congestive heart failure	10
Cerebrovascular disease	10
Renal disease	10
Physical Examination Findings	
Altered mental status (acute)	20
Respiratory rate > 30	20
Systolic BP < 90 mmHg	20
Temperature < 35oC or > 40oC	15
Pulse > 125/min	10
Diagnostic Testing Findings	
Arterial pH < 7.35	30
BUN > 30 mg/dL	20
Sodium < 130 mmol/L	20
Glucose > 250 mg/dL	10
Hematocrit < 30%	10
PaO2 < 60 mmHg (or SaO2 < 90%)	10
Pleural effusion	10

Risk Class	Point Score	Mortality (%)	Disposition
2	< 70	0.6	Outpatient
3	71-90	2.8	Brief Inpatient
4	91-130	8.2	Inpatient
5	> 130	29.2	Inpatient

Fine and colleagues developed a *prognostic model*, the Pneumonia Severity Index (PSI), **for thirty day mortality** in patients with CAP. Patients are assigned to one of five risk classes (1=lowest risk and 5=highest risk) based upon a point system. Outpatient management is suggested for Class 1 and 2, brief inpatient for class 3 and traditional hospitalization for Classes 4 & 5. Severe pneumonia may require intensive care unit (ICU) admission. Guidelines should not supersede clinical judgment

SEVERITY OF ILLNESS SCORE

Mnemonic: (CURB 65)

C	Confusion	1 Point
U	Uremia - BUN > 19 mg/dl	1 Point
R	Respiratory rate - RR> 30/min	1 Point
B	Blood pressure, low - BP < 90/60	1 Point
65	Age > 65	1 Point

If score = 1, outpatient ok; If > 1 hospitalize. The higher the score the higher the mortality

EPIDEMIOLOGIC CONDITIONS AND/OR RISK FACTORS RELATED TO SPECIFIC PATHOGENS IN CAP

Most common pathogens of childhood pneumonia with Cystic Fibrosis = Staph aureus and Haemophilus influenzae; by the age of 18 80% of patients with CF are colonized with Pseudomonas

CONDITION	COMMONLY ENCOUNTERED PATHOGEN(S)
Alcoholism	*Streptococcus pneumoniae*, oral anaerobes, Acinetobacter species, *Mycobacterium tuberculosis, Klebsiella pneumoniae*
COPD and/or smoking	*Haemophilus influenzae, Pseudomonas aeruginosa*, Legionella species, *S. pneumoniae, Moraxella cararhalis, Chlamydophila pneumoniae*
Aspiration	Gram-negative enteric pathogens, oral anaerobes
Lung abscess	CA-MRSA, oral anaerobes, endemic fungal pneumonia, *M. tuberculosis, atypical mycobacteria, Klebsiella pneumoniae*
Exposure to bat or bird droppings	*Histoplasma capsulatum* - (Fungal pneumonia; endemic in the Mississippi and Ohio River valley. Transmitted through the droppings of birds and bats)
Exposure to birds	*Chlamydophila psittaci* (if poultry: avian influenza) hyperpyrexia, severe HA

Exposure to rabbits	*Francisella tularensis* - Transmission: contact with infected animals or vectors (ticks) increased LFT's, fever with relative bradycardia
Exposure to farm animals or parturient cats	*Coxiella burnetti* (Q fever) Increased LFT's, fever with relative bradycardia
HIV infection (early)	*S. pneumoniae, H. influenzae, M. tuberculosis*
HIV infection (late)	The pathogens listed for early infection plus Pneumocystis jirovecii, Cryptococcus, Histoplasma, Aspergillus, atypical mycobacteria (especially Mycobacterium kansasii), P. aeruginosa, H. influenzae
Hotel or cruise ship stay in previous 2 weeks	Legionella species - Increased LFT's, fever with relative bradycardia.
Travel to or residence in SW United States	Coccidioides species. Coccidioidomycosis is caused by Coccidioides immitis = fungal infection, ranges from self-limited acute pneumonia (Valley Fever) to disseminated disease, especially in immunosuppressed patients. Hantavirus - rodents, SW US, Viral syndrome or Hanta-Virus pulmonary (HPS) hemorrhagic fever + AKI, circulatory collapse, MR 15%
Travel to or residence in SE and East Asia	*Burkholderia pseudomallei*, avian influenza, SARS
Influenza active in community	Influenza, *S. pneumo, Staph aureus, H. influenzae*
Cough >2 weeks with whoop or posttussive emesis	*Bordetella pertussis* Pneumonia = most common cause of death due to complications of pertusis
Structural lung disease (e.g., bronchiectasis)	*Pseudomonas aeruginosa, Burkholderia cepacia, S. aureus* - Burkholderia uncommon cause of pneumonia - seen in patient with Cystic Fibrosis
Injection drug use	*S. aureus, anaerobes, M. tuberculosis, S. pneumoniae*
Endobronchial obstruction	Anaerobes, *S. pneumoniae, H. influenzae, S. aureus*
In context of bioterrorism	*Bacillus anthracis* (anthrax), *Yersinia pestis* (plague), *Francisella tularensis* (tularemia)

FOUR ORGANISMS THAT CAUSE PNEUMONIA WHICH PRESENT WITH FEVER & RELATIVE BRADYCARDIA ("FAGET SIGN")

1. Legionella pneumophilia (Legionellosis)
2. Coxiella burnetii (Q-fever)
3. Chlamydia psittaci (Psittacosis)
4. Francisella tularensis (Tularemia)

All 4 organisms also cause transaminitis (Elevated LFTs)

FEVER PEARL

- Each 1°F increase = HR increases 10 bpm
- 101°F = 100 bpm
- 102°F = 110 bpm
- 103°F = 120 bpm
- 104°F = 130 bpm
- An increase of < 10bpm = relative bradycardia

SARCOIDOSIS

- Autoimmune disease associated with helper T cells that activate and cause the formation of granulomas
- Most commonly affected organ system = **lungs**
- Pulmonary fibrosis, bilateral hilar lymphadenopathy, cough, hemoptysis, DOE
- **Cardiac**: AV block, CHB, bundle branch blocks, SVT, VT and sudden death; pericarditis, restrictive cardiomyopathy can be early, which can progress to a dilated cardiomyopathy, valve dysfunction, and CHF
- **Neurologic / eyes**: Bell's Palsy (CN VII - unilateral, bilateral; recurrent), peripheral neuropathies, CRVO
- **Endocrine:** Diabetes insipidus
- **Skin**: Lupus pernio (chronic, violaceous, raised plaques and nodules commonly found on the cheeks, nose, and around the eyes) = **pathognomonic for sarcoidosis**
- **Ophthalmologic**: Uveitis, conjunctivitis
- **Lymphadenopathy**
- **Carpal tunnel** syndrome more common vs the general population
- More common in African American
- **Labs**: hypercalcemia; elevated Serum angiotensin converting enzyme (ACE)
- **CXR**: hilar adenopathy
- **Biopsy**: non-caseating granulomas
- **Treatment**: steroids

TUBERCULOSIS

- World's leading cause of infectious death
- Caused by *Mycobacterium tuberculosis*
- Airborne spread

Primary TB (Primary TB infection is usually asymptomatic and identified by PPD)

- Active TB
- Latent TB
- Reactivation TB
- Increase in TB cases in 1980's due to HIV epidemic
- Host defense leads to formation of tubercles (tuberculous nodules, or tuberculomas) and dormant organisms in low oxygen areas
- Latent infection reactivates in immune-compromised states → active infection (reactivation)

Latent tuberculosis infection (LTBI)

- No test that definitively establishes a diagnosis of LTBI
- LTBI is a clinical diagnosis established by demonstrating prior TB infection and excluding **active TB disease** (night sweats, fever, lymphadenopathy, productive cough or hemoptysis; diagnosis = sputum smear for acid fast bacilli (AFB)

Available tests to demonstrate prior TB infection include the tuberculin skin test (TST) and interferon-gamma release assays (IGRAs)

- Two availbale IGRAs include: QuantiFERON®-TB Gold In-Tube test (QFT-GIT) and T-SPOT®.TB test (T-Spot)
- These measure immune sensitization (type IV or delayed-type hypersensitivity) to mycobacterial protein antigens that might occur following exposure to (and infection by) mycobacteria

The goal of testing LTBI: to identify individuals who are at increased risk for the development of active TB disease and therefore would benefit from treatment of LTBI

Treatment of Latent TB: INH for 9 months, rifampin for 4 months, or INH/rifapentine for 3 months
Pyridoxine (B6) with INH to prevent peripheral neuropathy

CXR IN TB

1. Primary TB Ghon Complex: Ghon lesion (tuberculoma) +ipsilateral mediastinal lymphadenopathy
2. Active/reactivation - Upper lobes, cavitary lesions
3. Miliary TB: small fibronodular lesions ("miliary" because they resemble scattered millet seeds
4. Other less "classic" findings
   a. Pleural effusion
   b. Non upper lobe infiltrates

Add specialized views of the chest: apical lordotic projection to evaluate the lung apices or a lateral decubitus to evaluate for presence of pleural effusion

PEARL: skin rash with TB = erythema nodosum
Primary TB infection is usually asymptomatic and identified by PPD
TB skin test is read differently for different at-risk groups
The > risk of disease, the smaller the induration needs to be to be considered a positive test

PPD Criteria

- No risk, positive test = 15mm
- High risk, homeless, health-care workers, IVDA, foreign born positive test = 10mm
- Immunosuppressed, recent TB contact, abnormal CXR, steroid use positive test = 5mm
- **PEARL:** If exposed to TB - Immediate Purified Protein Derivative (PPD) testing, followed by repeat testing in 3 months
- **PEARL:** PPD is often negative in late HIV infection

TB in HIV/AIDS Patients

- TB 200 to 550x greater in AIDS patients
- CXR: nonspecific
- PPD may be nonreactive

Treatment of Active TB or Reactivation TB (RIPE)

- R = Rifampin
- I = Isoniazid (INH)
- P = Pyrazinamide
- E = Ethambutol

Treatment of Latent TB = INH for 9 months

Side Effects of RIPE Therapy (most common side effect of therapy = hepatitis)

R	**R**ifampin	Orange or red-orange discoloration of body fluids (tears, sweat, saliva, urine, or feces). Hepatotoxicity is infrequent, however is more commonly observed in patients with concomitant administrations of hepatotoxins
I	**I**soniazid (INH)	Hepatotoxicity, peripheral neuropathy, lupus-like rash; in overdose: seizures, AG acidosis
P	**P**yrazinamide	Hepatotoxicity
E	**E**thambutol	Ocular toxicity (blindness or color blindness or scotomas)

ASTHMA

- Defined as a reversible airway obstruction secondary to an inflammatory response
- Patient's perception of exacerbation, intensity of wheezing, and pulse oximetry are POOR predictors of severity
- Increased use of beta agonists: predicts the highest risk of sudden DEATH in adult
- Other risk factors: illicit drugs (heroin, cocaine), recent steroid use, hospitalization or intubation within last year and sensitization to mold
- Smoking was not found to have increase risk of death in asthmatics (patients were more likely to have diagnosis of COPD as cause of death rather then asthma)
- Bedside spirometry at presentation can predict response / disposition with > 85% sensitivity and specificity
- ABG is usually NOT helpful in clinical decision-making

CXR indications in asthma

- Focal rhonchi or crackles
- Fever > 39°C (102.2 F)
- Severe disease
- Persistent CP or hypoxemia after treatment of the asthma exacerbation
- Spontaneous pneumomediastinum is uncommon in children, but when it does occur, it is most often in the setting of an asthma exacerbation

US findings with pneumomediastinum

- "Air gap" or echogenic interface anterior to the heart that obscures the views of the cardiac structures

Treatment in moderate and severe exacerbations

- Steroids, beta agonists and anticholinergics (atrovent)
- Steroids (decrease inflammation) in the ED will reduce relapse rates and hospital admissions
- Inhaled steroids control patient's risk of death from asthma
- Magnesium and heliox should be considered in severe exacerbations
- Albuterol β 2 agonist → ↑ cAMP → bronchodilation
- Atrovent is an anticholinergic agent that → ↓cGMP → bronchodilation
- Epinephrine 1:1000 IM in the thigh (vastus lateralis) results in higher and more rapid maximum plasma concentrations

Albuterol, ipratropium, magnesium sulfate and methylprednisolone are all safe options for the management asthma during pregnancy. Avoid epinephrine →may cause uterine vasoconstriction and reduced fetal oxygenation (typically reserved for pregnant patients with anaphylaxis, otherwise avoid epinephrine)

Mechanical Ventilation In Asthmatics

- 3 to 5% of asthmatics will require mechanical ventilation
- Goal of mechanical ventilation in asthmatics = maintain peak pressure < 30 cm H2O to reduce risk of barotrauma and cardiovascular collapse
    - Permissive hypercapnia: RR and TVs are decreased
    - Maximize expiratory time by decreasing I:E ratio = 1:4 (avoid breath stacking/hyperinflation of lungs → this will prevent increasing peak pressure and barotrauma)
    - Inspiratory flow: 80 L/min as an initial upper limit; HIGHER inspiratory flows may be necessary to DECREASE inspiratory time and allow more time for exhalation in selected patients with more severe airflow obstruction
    - Low respiratory rate (RR): 10 to 12 breaths /min (allows for longer expiratory time phase)
    - Low tidal volumes (TV): 6 to 8 mL/kg of predicted or "ideal" body weight
    - Low Minute Ventilation: TV x RR → Goal in asthmatics < 115 mL/kg

- Maintain plateau pressure < 30 cmH20
- Use larger bore ETT → reduce resistance in airway tubing (reducing peak pressures)
- Heavy sedation → avoid patients breathing over the ventilator asynchronously → leading to incomplete exhalation → lung hyperinflation → increased peak pressures

- Adding "extrinsic" positive end-expiratory pressure (PEEP) to offset "intrinsic" PEEP
- Increased "intrinsic" PEEP (auto-PEEP) = breath-stacking and dynamic hyperinflation → barotrauma
- Normally, the end-expiratory pressure = 0 or = to any extrinsic PEEP ("applied" PEEP) delivered by the ventilator
- One consequence of "intrinsic" PEEP is that initiation of the next breath by the patient requires sufficient negative pressure to overcome the intrinsic PEEP and trigger the ventilator
- Intrinsic PEEP can be detected by using ventilator-generated flow vs time graphs to determine whether inspiratory flow begins before expiratory flow reaches 0
- To obtain a numeric value for intrinsic PEEP, extrinsic PEEP is subtracted from airway pressure measured during a breath-hold at end-expiration
  Ideally, intrinsic PEEP should be < 10 cm H2O
- A small amount of applied PEEP (3 to 5 cm H2O) is used in most mechanically ventilated patients to mitigate end-expiratory alveolar collapse
  Increasing the extrinsic PEEP (up to 80% of the intrinsic PEEP) can offset the adverse effects of intrinsic PEEP and reduce the effort necessary to trigger inspiration during patient-initiated breaths
  However, the amount of intrinsic PEEP must be measured accurately to avoid administering excess extrinsic PEEP and exacerbating air-trapping and high inspiratory pressures

Ventilator Pearls

- Minimize risk of ventilator lung injury
- Low tidal volumes: 6 to 8 mL/kg of predicted body weight
- **Predicted body weight** (also known as ideal body weight (IBW)
- Formula for men: PBW (kg) = 50 + 2.3 (height (in) – 60)
- Formula for women: PBW (kg) = 45.5 + 2.3 (height (in) - 60)

ASSESS OF OXYGENATION / VENTILATION PROBLEMS POST INTUBATION: (DOPE)

D	**D**isplacement of ETT
O	**O**bstruction
P	**P**neumothorax
E	**E**quipment failure

ACUTE RESPIRATORY AND METABOLIC ACIDOSIS AND ALKALOSIS

- Normal ABG values
- pH:7.35 – 7.45
- PaCO2: 35 – 45
- HCO3: 22 – 26
- Respiratory Acidosis pH: < 7.35; PaCO2: > 45; HCO3: Normal
- Respiratory Alkalosis pH: > 7.45; PaCO2: < 35; HCO3: Normal
- Metabolic Acidosis pH: < 7.35; PaCO2: Normal; HCO3: < 22
- Metabolic Alkalosis pH: > 7.45; PaCO2: Normal; HCO3: > 26

CHRONIC OBSTRUCTIVE PULMONARY DISEASE (COPD)

- COPD is a spectrum of diseases including chronic asthma, chronic bronchitis, and emphysema
- COPD is an obstructive process; pulmonary function tests: increased residual volume (RV), increased total lung capacity (TLC), and a decreased FEV1/FVC
- Cigarette smoking accounts for 80 to 90% of cases, but only 15% of all smokers develop clinically significant disease
- **Emphysema patient:** ("pink puffers") develops increased lung destruction, expanding chest cavity, weight loss; patients are hunched forward with pursed slips
- **Chronic bronchitis patient:** ("blue bloater") develops polycythemia, plethora, cyanosis, hypertension
- Most common cause of cor pulmonale
- Definition: mucus-producing cough most days of the month, 3 months of a year for 4 years in a row without other underlying disease to explain the cough
- FEV1 is the best predictor of outcome
- CXR abnormal in most cases; CXR findings of COPD: flat diaphragm, ↑ AP diameter, enlarged retrosternal space, blebs
- Treatment: Similar to asthma with exception of liberal use of empiric antibiotics; Limit oxygen administration

Non-invasive ventilation (NIV) = decrease work of breathing

- Non-invasive ventilation (NIV) = very useful to recruit alveoli and reduce dead space.
- Contraindications to noninvasive positive pressure ventilation
- AMS
- Obtunded patient
- Hemodynamic instability
- Inability to tolerate oral secretions
- Recent trauma or injury to the face
- Poor mask fit

TRACHEOINNOMINATE FISTULA BLEEDING

- Tract forms between the trachea and the innominate (brachiocephalic) artery
- Risk factors: prior radiation, excessive neck movement, low tracheostomy placement, and prolonged intubation
- Usually occurs within the first 3 weeks after a tracheostomy has been placed
- May initially present as a self-limited sentinel bleed
- After massive bleeding has begun mortality = high
- **Management**
  - 1) Attempt tamponade with overinflation of the tracheostomy cuff; if unsuccessful —> step #2
  - 2) Tracheostomy should be removed and endotracheal intubation should proceed to secure airway
  - 3) Digital compression via stoma can be attempted
  - 4) Transport to the operating room for surgical exploration

PULMONARY PEARLS

- Adequate sputum specimen must have > 25 PMN's and < 10 squamous epithelial cells
- Sputum cultures are low yield, however recommended
- Most common cause of bacterial pneumonia = ***Strep pneumoniae*** √ rusty/blood sputum. Single shaking rigor; pleuritic CP
- Most common non-bacterial pneumonia in adults < 50 y/o = ***Mycoplasma pneumonia***
- Most common cause of **bullous myringitis** = Viral; Bullous myringitis can also be seen with Mycoplasma

- A common cause of pneumonia in alcoholics = ***Klebsiella pneumonia***, √ "currant jelly" sputum. *Strep pneumoniae* = most common cause of bacterial pneumonia in alcoholics
- ***Klebsiella pneumoniae***
  - **CXR**: Infiltrate often in the upper lobes (most commonly the right); Bulging fissure; Untreated: infiltrate will progress into a necrotizing lesion with air-fluid levels, and can ultimately lead to development of an empyema
  - Treatment: 3rd-generation cephalosporin +aminoglycoside
- **Haemophilus**: COPD, debilitated patient, green sputum, diffuse rales
- **Staphylococcus:** debilitated patient, post influenza, purulent sputum, necrotizing cavitary lesion or empyema on CXR
- **Legionella**: GI symptoms (elevated LFTs), hyponatremia, neuro symptoms (AMS), relative bradycardia, pleuritic CP, unilateral patchy alveolar lower lobe infiltrates, contaminated water
- **Chlamydia**: mucoid green sputum; lose quarters outbreaks, young, follows pharyngitis
- **Neonatal pneumonia**: GBS, *E. coli* and *Klebsiella*
- Most common cause of pneumonia in children < 6 months and 3-5 years old = **RSV and parainfluenza**
  Children > 5 y/o and young adults ***Mycoplasma*** is common
- Most common cause of viral pneumonia in adults = ***Influenza***
  - *Strep pneumoniae* = most common cause of bacterial pneumonia .... However → also consider *Staph* pneumonia during outbreaks of influenza
- The majority of deaths from viral pneumonia occur during winter months
- Most common source of infection in **septic** patient = respiratory system
- Organisms that cause pneumonias which present with **fever and relative bradycardia** = Legionella, Q fever, Psittacosis and Tularemia (note: all 4 also ↑LFTs)
- Most common pathogens to generate **cavitary lesions:** TB, anaerobic bacteria, aerobic gram-negative bacilli, *S. aureus,* and fungal disease
- Most common complication of **cavitary TB:** endobronchial spread (seen on x-ray as 5 to 10 mm poorly defined nodules clustered in dependent portions of the lungs
- Carcinoma suspected on CXR → remember **L.A.** (Los Angeles) is located on the periphery of the US → **L**arge cell and **A**denocarcinoma present as peripheral masses on CXR; Squamous cell and Small cell (most malignant) present as central or hilar tumors.
- Most common cause of cancer deaths in males and females = bronchogenic CA
- **Paraneoplastic syndromes:** ↓Na+/ SIADH, ↑Ca2+/ parathormone, ↓Ca2+/ Calcitonin, ↑ACTH/ Cushing syndrome, gynecomastia/ gonadotropins, ↑Serotonin/ Carcinoid syndrome)
- **CXR findings of COPD:** flat diaphragm, ↑AP diameter, enlarged retrosternal space, blebs
- If you suspect chest pain is due to **pneumothorax**, ask for **inspiratory** and **expiratory** views on chest film
- Albuterol β 2 agonist ↑ **cAMP** → bronchodilation
- Atrovent is an anticholinergic agent that ↓ **cGMP** → bronchodilation
- Epi 1:1000 IM in the thigh (vastus lateralis) results in higher and more rapid maximum plasma concentrations
- Most common occupational lung disease worldwide = **Silicosis** (found in sand, granite, sandstone, flint, slate, and in coal and metallic ores. Cutting, breaking, crushing, drilling, grinding, or abrasive blasting of these materials may produce fine silica dust
  - Fever, SOB, CP, Cor pulmonale and cyanosis
  - Susceptible to TB (silicotuberculosis) suspect silica damages pulmonary macrophages, inhibiting their ability to kill mycobacteria
  - Silicosis is an irreversible condition with no cure
  - Treatment: Lung transplantation

RENAL / UROLOGY

Success in Medical School and Beyond / Mnemonics and Pearls

CAUSES OF HEMATURIA

Mnemonics: (IN STITCHES2) [ANK]

I	**I**nfection (pyelonephritis, hemorrhagic cystitis, prostatitis, TB, Schistosomiasis)
N	**N**ecrosis = Papillary Necrosis (sickle cell disease)

S	**S**tones, Kidney **S**tricture of the urethra
T	**T**oxins (direct kidney injury or rhabdo) (Arsenic and many more) **T**oxemia of pregnancy
I	**I**ntrinsic Kidney Disease (glomerulonephritis, PKD, Medullary Sponge, IgA nephropathy, (Berger's disease) hereditary nephritis, (Alport syndrome), Acute Tubular Necrosis (ATN) **I**atrogenic (post procedure)
T	**T**rauma **T**hrombosis of renal vein or renal artery embolism
C	**C**oagulopathy (Hemophilia, ↑coumadin or heparin toxicity) **C**ancer (renal, bladder, prostate, Wilms' tumor/nephroblastoma)
H	**H**emoglobinopathy (sickle cell disease) **H**uge prostate (BPH)
E	**E**ndocarditis **E**xpanding AAA may erode into urogenital tract; also Aortic Dissection
S	**S**LE (50% nephritis) other immunologic disease = (ITP, HSP (IgA complexes), Goodpasture syndrome, polyarteritis nodosa (PAN); nonimmune causes = TTP, HUS **S**erum sickness, Strep: Post-streptococcal golmerulonephritits+, Granulomatosis with PolyAngitis (GPA)

Don't confuse Berger's Disease with Buergers's disease (thromboangiitis obliterans) = recurring inflammation and thrombosis of small and medium arteries and veins of the hands and feet. Strongly associated with smoking

+Triad of sinusitis, pulmonary infiltrates, and nephritis = Granulomatosis with PolyAngitis (GPA), formerly known as Wegener's Granulomatosis (WG)

ALPORT SYNDROME

- X-linked hereditary disorder
- Sensorineural hearing loss
- Glomerulonephritis
- Progression to chronic kidney disease
- Eye findings = anterior lenticonus (lens becomes cone-shaped); abnormal coloration of the retina (dot-and-fleck retinopathy), possible vision loss

ACUTE KIDNEY INJURY (AKI)

- Defined as a rise in serum Cr of at least 0.3 mg/dL over a 48-hour period and /or ≥ 1.5 times the baseline value within the 7 previous days)
- Pre-renal disease and acute tubular necrosis (ATN) account for 65-75% of cases of AKI

1) Pre-renal disease = results from decreased renal blood; causes =
a) True volume depletion (dehydration, hemorrhage, diuretics, pancreatitis)
b) Renal perfusion reduction (cirrhosis; shock = cardiac, septic, hemorrhagic or hypovolemic)

- FENa < 1%
- Urine osmolality > 500 mOsm
- Bland urine sediment

2) Intrinsic Renal Disease = intrinsic kidney insults = ATN; AIN; glomerular injury from HTN and vascular causes **(microvascular causes** = TTP, HUS, HELLP syndrome, atheroembolic disease, SLE, Granulomatosis with polyangiitis (GPA, formerly called Wegener's), polyarteritis nodosa (PAN), HSP, Goodpasture's; **macrovascular causes** = renal artery occlusion, abdominal aortic disease

- FENa > 2%
- Urine osmolality 250 to 300 mOsm
- active urine sediment

3) Post-renal Disease = obstruction leads to restricted output of urine flow which leads to decreased renal function and azotemia (prostate, bladder or cervical cancers; bilateral hydronephrosis, neurogenic bladder or medications that cause urinary retention and urethral strictures)
Ultrasound (US) = examine for hydronephrosis and bladder size

- **Fractional Excretion of Na (FENa)** = 100x (Plasma Cr x Urinary Na) / (Plasma Na x Urinary Cr)

INTRINSIC RENAL DISEASE - ACUTE TUBULAR NECROSIS (ATN)

Most common cause of AKI (50%) in the hospital setting

Three (3) major causes

a) Renal Ischemia = decrease blood flow to kidney usually secondary to a drop in BP (any of the same process that cause pre-renal failure, however most common in patients with hypotension (surgery, OB complications, sepsis)
b) Nephrotoxic = NSAIDs, ACE inhibitors and ARBs, aminoglycosides,camphotercin B, cisplatin, contrast agents, myoglobinuria due to rhabdomyolysis
c) Sepsis = own category as it causes normal pre-renal factors such as decreased renal perfusion from systemic hypotension, however sepsis-associated high cardiac output may also be observed and direct injury of cytokines (TNF, interleukins etc)

Labs / UA

- BUN to creatinine ratio of < 20
- FENa > 2%
- Inability to concentrate urine (urine osmolality = serum osmolality)

URINE MICROSCOPY = muddy brown granular casts and epithelial casts

PEARL: Red blood cell casts = glomerular damage, glomerulonephritis (GN), vasculitis
PEARL: Granular cast = glomerular damage, glomerulonephritis (GN), vasculitis
PEARL: White blood cell casts = pyelonephritis, AIN, Nephrotic syndrome, post-strep GN
PEARL: Hyaline Cast = most common, Tamm-Horsfall protein; = dehydration or exercise

ACUTE INTERSTITIAL NEPHRITIS (AIN)

- Second most common cause of AKI following ATN
- Results from immune-mediated inflammation of the interstitial space
- Eosinophiluria (eosinophils in urine) and eosinophilia (eosinophils in blood)
- Causes = Allergic reaction to medications (penicillins, antibiotics and
- diuretics that contain sulfa, NSAIDs and PPIs) or infections
- Clinical: rash, fever, and vague constitutional symptoms
- Treatment = Withdrawal of offending medication
- Some cases of AIN are treated with steroids

KIDNEY STONES

3 x more common males > females

Calcium oxalate or Ca phosphate stones

- Most common 75%; radio-opaque
- Causes
  - Hypercalciuria → GI = reabsorption; Bone = resorption (primary hyperPTH); Kidney = Ca2+ leak
  - Idiopathic, sarcoid, hyper-thyroidism,
  - Paget's disease, increased incidence from genetic predisposition, PUD taking antacids, IBD

Magnesium-ammonium-phosphate (Staghorn or struvite stones)

- 15%, associated with alkaline urine (pH > 7.6),
- secondary to recurrent infections: Proteus, Pseudomonas, Klebsiella
- Urea → split to NH3 by Urease → binds H+ → NH4+

Uric acid

- 10%, radiolucent, associated with acidic urine; 25% patients with gout get stones

Cystine stones

- 1%, 2 0 inborn error in metabolism → ↑secretion of cystine → form staghorns

Medications That Can Cause Stones

- Indinavir (Crixivan) - radiolucent stones; HIV med, protease inhibitor
- Radiolucent and require IV contrast for visualization

Kidney Stone Pearls

90% stones < 4 mm pass spontaneously
50% stones 4 to 6mm pass spontaneously
10% stones > 6mm pass spontaneously

- Diagnostic test = non-contrast spiral CT – may find alternate diagnosis .... AAA or appy consider Ultrasound to evaluate for hydronephrosis/ hydroureter in patients with known history of kidney stones
- Most common location of stone at first diagnosis = distal ureter 70%
- Most common site = ureterovesical junction (UVJ)
- Treatment: Fluid, NSAIDs decrease ureteral spasm, narcotics and Tamsulosin (Flomax)

BLADDER STONES

- Almost exclusively in elderly men; complication of other urologic disease
- Most common cause = infection of residual bladder urine with urea-splitting organisms.
- Disorders predisposing to the formation of bladder stones = bladder neck obstruction, neurogenic bladder, vesical diverticula, damage from irradiation, and schistosomiasis
- Clinically, patients most often complain of pain on voiding and hematuria
- A classic complaint is the sudden interruption of the urinary stream
- CT scan is the most sensitive diagnostic study
- Bladder stone = sign of an underlying problem; remove the stone and treat of the underlying abnormality

NEPHRITIC SYNDROME

Mnemonics: (PHARAOH) [ANK, Mnemonic provided by Dr. Justino Dalio]

P	**P**roteinuria
H	**H**ematuria
A	**A**zotemia
R	**R**BC casts
A	Immunoglobulin **A** (IgA) nephropathy (Berger disease) = Most common cause of glomerulonephritis worldwide. 50% present with gross visible hematuria, often accompanying an upper respiratory infection (URI); Post Strep GN = Most common infectious cause of acute glomerulonephritis
O	**O**liguria
H	**H**TN

NEPHROTIC VS NEPHRITIC SYNDROME

- Nephrotic syndrome involves the loss of a lot of protein; common risk for nephrotic syndrome = hypercoagulable state and infection risk; can lead to AKI
- Nephritic syndrome involves the loss of a lot of BLOOD

TESTICULAR CANCER

- painless, unilateral mass; cannot be transilluminated;
- a germ cell tumor which secretes hCG.

TESTICULAR TORSION

- Absent cremasteric reflex
- Pain may be constant, intermittent but is *not* positional
- Manually detorsion of testicle → stand at patient's feet → detorsion in similar fashion to opening a book → patient's right testicle → rotated counterclockwise; left testis → clockwise (external rotation of the testes - medial to lateral)
- Manually detorsion is not curative, attempt while waiting for surgery
- If you cannot exclude torsion by H&P and imaging studies → surgery for scrotal exploration, *regardless* of time since onset of symptoms
- "Blue-dot sign" on testicular exam = Torsion of the testicular appendix
- Salvage rate at 4-6 hours = 96%. Drops to 20% after 12 hours.
- Color flow doppler US of the scrotum is as accurate as radionuclide scanning and much faster to rule out torsion.

PENILE FRACTURE

- Traumatic rupture of the tunica albuginea and corpus cavernosum urologic emergency.
- Sudden blunt trauma of the penis in an erect state causes rupture in one or both corpora.
- Concomitant urethral injury may also occur.
- Clinical diagnosis: Patients usually hear a "popping" or "cracking" sound, followed by significant pain, immediate flaccidity and skin hematoma/ecchymosis.
- Conservative management has fallen out of favor because of high complication rates.
- Surgical repair is necessary to expedite relief of pain and to prevent potential complications → surgical evacuation of hematoma and suture apposition of the disrupted tunica albuginea
- Complications of conservative management include: missed urethral injury, penile abscess, nodule formation at the site of rupture, permanent penile curvature, painful erection, painful coitus, erectile dysfunction, corporal urethral fistula, arterial venous fistula and fibrotic plaque formation.

PRIAPISM

Erection lasting > 2 hours
Engorgement of the corpora cavernosa. Ventral corpora spongiosum and glans penis usually remain flaccid

Two types

- **Low-flow (ischemic) priapism** (most common) 95%
  - Veno-occlusion; painful
  - Most common cause = Sickle cell anemia
  - Ischemic priapism is a compartment syndrome of the penis → emergent aspiration
  - **Diagnosis of ischemic priapism**
    - Cavernosal blood gas that is acidemic (pH < 7.25)
    - Hypoxic (partial pressure oxygen < 30 mm Hg)
    - Hypercapnic (partial pressure carbon dioxide > 60 mm Hg)

- **Arterial (non-ischemic) high-flow** priapism
  - Secondary to a rupture of a cavernous artery; results from a fistula between the Cavernosal Artery and Corpus Cavernosum
  - Rare; usually not painful; Causes = penetrating penile trauma or a blunt perineal injury

Other Causes of Low-flow priapism

- **Idiopathic**
- **Medications**
  - Injectable medications to induce an erection = papaverine, phentolamine (non-selective alpha-1, alpha-2 adrenergic-receptor **antagonist**), and prostaglandin E1
  - Psychotropic medications = chlorpromazine, trazodone, quetiapine, thioridazine and citalopram (SSRI)
  - Rebound hypercoagulable state with anticoagulants = heparin and warfarin
  - Hydralazine, metoclopramide, omeprazole, hydroxyzine (atarax; vistaril), prazosin, tamoxifen, and androstenedione
  - Cocaine, marijuana, ecstasy, and ethanol

- **Neurologic**
  - Spinal cord injury and anesthesia
  - Cauda equina syndrome
  - C5 Fracture

- **Neoplastic**
    - Primary or metastatic; leukemia and multiple myeloma

- **Infection**
    - Mycoplasma pneumoniae (Mechanism is thought to be a hypercoagulable state induced)
    - Malaria

First Line Treatment of Low-Flow priapism
- Cavernosal aspiration at 2 or 10 o'clock position (removes the stale blood, decreasing penile pressure and allowing fresh blood to perfuse the penis)
- Dorsal penile nerves located = At the one (1) and 11-o'clock positions below Buck's fascia

Second Line Treatment of Low-Flow (vaso-occlusive) priapism
- Terbutaline 0.25 to 0.5 mg SQ in deltoid, may be repeated in 20 to 30 min
- Oral pseudoephedrine, 60-120 mg orally due to its alpha-agonist effect (sympathomimetic amine → ↑endogenous norepinephrine from storage vesicles in presynaptic neurons)
- Injection of alpha-1-adrenergic agent (agonist) phenylephrine (Neo-Synephrine)
- In adults, phenylephrine should be diluted with normal saline to provide a final concentration of approximately 100 mcg to 500 mcg per mL [http://www.uptodate.com/contents/priapism]
- Phenylephrine (Neo-Synephrine) 10mg/mL which = 10,000 mcg/mL
- Dilute 10mg/mL Phenylephrine in 100mL of normal saline → 100 mcg/mL of Phenylephrine (Neo-Synephrine) solution → draw up 1 to 5 mL to get recommended treatment dose of 100 mcg to 500 mcg per mL

Treatment High flow
- Observation alone may be sufficient as erectile function is usually unimpaired.
- Compression therapy may be successful in certain cases, especially children

Most common sequela of priapism = impotence

TYPES OF OBSTRUCTION

Mnemonics: (PENIS) [ANK, from Drs.Lusiak / Colucci]

P	**P**rostate/ Phimosis BPH = Most common cause of urinary retention in men.
E	**E**ctopic Ureter
N	**N**eoplasm
I	**I**nfection
S	**S**tone

URETHRAL TRAUMA

- Most common urethral injury = posterior (90%), above the urogenital diaphragm, associated with pelvic fractures (high riding or absent prostate on rectal exam)
- Anterior urethral injury = 10%, direct trauma (kicks or straddle injuries)
- Blood at meatus = urethral trauma, or bladder trauma- perform retrograde urethrogram and cystogram; do not insert foley
- Retrograde urethrogram = Toomey syringe into urethral meatus → inject 60 ml contrast over 30 to 60 seconds → xray during the last 10ml contrast injection

- Retrograde cystogram / retrograde CT cystography = after normal retrograde urethrogram → allow 300 to 400 ml contrast to flow by gravity from a Toomey syringe through a Foley catheter into bladder → clamp foley → AP and lateral films or CT of bladder taken → unclamp Foley → postevacuation film / CT
- 95% of patients with bladder injuries will have gross hematuria; most common mechanism = blunt trauma suprapubic and lower abdominal pain, inability to urinate, pelvic fracture and blood at the meatus.

BLADDER TRAUMA

- Contusion = most common bladder injury → incomplete tear of bladder mucosa; large hematomas can alter bladder shape on cystogram = "pear-shaped" bladder
- Extraperitoneal bladder ruptureheal spontaneously in 14 days with Foley
  - Most common type of bladder rupture 80% (rupture usually at bladder neck)
- Intraperitoneal bladder rupture (injury is in the dome posteriorly, the only portion of dome covered by the peritoneum) → surgical repair
- Bladder dome is the weakest portion of the bladder

RENAL TRAUMA

- Microscopic hematuria is defined as a >10 RBCs per high-power field (HPF) without evidence of gross blood
- Most experts believe that there is limited utility for exact quantification of RBC content by microscopic analysis unless associated with systolic hypotension
- In general, however, the presence of microscopic hematuria is not considered indicative of severe underlying renal trauma and such patients can be safely discharged with urology follow-up
- CT scan with contrast is recommended in the setting of:
  - Gross hematuria
  - Signs of shock
  - Suspicion of an intra-abdominal injury
  - Hemodynamic instability
  - Mechanism that includes rapid deceleration
- Most common urologic injury = renal; 80% have concurrent injuries
- Most common renal injury = contusion 90% (Grade I)
- Renal injuries are Graded I to V
- Surgery: Uncontrolled hemorrhage, penetrating injuries, avulsed major renal vessel, extensive urine extravasation, Grade V injury (shattered kidney with avulsed hilum)

RENAL TRAUMA GRADE 1-5

Grade 1	Contusion/bruise Subcapsular haematoma with an intact capsule
Grade 2	Minor laceration-superficial parenchymal laceration <1cm
Grade 3	Major laceration >1cm without collecting system disruption/extravasation
Grade 4	Laceration through the cortex, medulla and collecting system Contained renal artery or vein injury
Grade 5	Completely shattered kidney Or Complete vascular avulsion

BENIGN PROSTATIC HYPERTROPHY

Treatment:

- **Anticholinergic agents**
  - Oxybutynin (Oxytrol)
  - Fesoterodine (Toviaz)
  - Darifenacin (Enablex)
  - Tolterodine (Detrol, Detrol LA)

- **Phosphodiesterase type 5 (PDE-5) inhibitors**
  - Tadalafil (Cialis)
  - Sildenafil (Viagra)

- **Alpha-1 blockers**
  - Silodosin (Rapaflo)
  - Terazosin (Hytrin)
  - Alfuzosin (Uroxatral)
  - Doxazosin (Cardura)
  - Tamsulosin (Flomax)
  - Alpha-blockers work by reducing smooth muscle tone

- **5-reductase inhibitors**
  - Finasteride (Proscar) (Propecia)
  - Dutasteride (Avodart)
  - 5-reductase inhibitors reduce prostate volume

- **Surgery (TURP)**

MANAGEMENT OF ACUTE URINARY RETENTION

- Prompt bladder decompression
- Urethral catheterization is contraindicated in patients who have had recent urologic surgery (eg, radical prostatectomy or urethral reconstruction)
- A suprapubic catheter may be necessary when obstruction precludes a urethral catheter and is also preferred in patients who are expected to require longer-term catheterization
- Transient hypotension after initial bladder decompression normalizes without intervention and does not progress to clinically significant hypotension

Hematuria after initial bladder decompression = 2 to 16% of patients and is rarely clinically significant

ACUTE BACTERIAL PROSTATITIS

- The most common cause = Escherichia coli. Other less common causes = Klebsiella, Pseudomonas, Enterobacter and Proteus
- Fever, LBP, perineal pain, malaise, myalgias and arthralgias, urinary frequency, urgency, dysuria, urinary retention
- Prostate exam: tender, swollen and boggy prostate (Prostatic massage should be limited - palpation may lead to bacteremia and sepsis)
- Urine culture usually reveals the causative pathogen
- Nontoxic patients = discharged 4-6 week of oral ciprofloxacin or trimethoprim-sulfamethoxazole
- Systemic toxicity = admitted, IV ciprofloxacin or ceftriaxone with or without gentamicin. Urology consult

UROLOGY PEARLS

- Most common cause of hematuria in females = infection
- Most common cause of hematuria in men = BPH → urinary retention
- Most common cause of hematuria worldwide = Schistosomiasis → *Schistosoma haematobium* (blood fluke) *S. mansoni & S. japonicum* = espophageal varices; Dx = eosinophilia and identification of eggs in first-morning urine or stool or biopsy; Treatment = Praziquantel
- Degree of hematuria after blunt trauma does not correspond to degree of renal injury
- Pseudo-hematuria = blood tinged but *no* RBC's on UA consider myoglobinuria (from trauma, seizures, burns, sepsis – any cause of rhabdo), pyridium, rifampin, porphyria
- Spontaneous complete drainage of distended bladder ok, no need to clamp. Transient gross hematuria or hypotension is usually insignificant
- If urinary retention is chronic (not acute) → there is a risk for post-obstructive diuresis → recommendation is to observe patient in ED for 4 to 6 hours.
- Fournier's gangrene = surgical debridement, fluid and antibiotic cover aerobic/anaerobic Polymicrobial infection; Causative organisms mostly bacteria from the distal colon; the most common are B. fragilis and E. coli.
- Acute hydrocele is most likely associated with = testicular cancer (7-25% of patients)
- Hydrocele = collection of fluid between the parietal and visceral layers of the tunica vaginalis
- Acute Right-sided varicocele is most likely associated with = IVC thrombosis or compression of IVC by tumors
- Acute Left-sided varicocele is most likely associated with = Renal cell CA or obstruction of left renal vein. Most common 80-90%

Paraphimosis inability to reduce the retracted foreskin over the glans, manual decompression; dorsal slit

- Options to reduce swelling before manual reduction
- Compress swollen glans with an elastic bandage for 10 minutes prior to reduction
- Mannitol-soaked gauze or sugar application for 30 minutes (reducing swelling via osmosis)
- Injecting hyaluronidase into the foreskin (facilitating diffusion of edema)
- Aspirating corporal blood, and puncturing the foreskin with a hypodermic needle (facilitates expression of edema) The latter two methods are not routinely recommended and should be reserved for refractory cases
- Avoid ice it can help reduce swelling but can also result in decreased blood flow
- If manual reduction does not work → dorsal slit

Phimosis inability to retract the foreskin to visualize the glans; topical steroids 4-6 weeks; circumcision = definitive treatment

Balanitis inflammation of the glans penis; Candida 40%, *Group B Strep.*, Gardnerella and anaerobes; occurs in 1/4 male sex partners of women infected with candida

Treatment = Fluconazole 150 mg po x 1

Posthitis inflammation of the foreskin; consider adding 1st generation cephalosporin for bacterial infection

Balanoposthitis is inflammation of both the glans penis and surrounding foreskin

Recurrent Balanoposthitis can be the sole presenting symptom of = diabetes mellitus

UROLOGY PEARLS – STDS

Epididymitis

- < 35 y/o GC (ceftriaxone 250 mg IM) and Chlamydia (doxy 100 mg po bid x 10 day ***not*** zithro x1)
- > 35 y/o *E. coli* (quinolone x 10 to 14 days)
- Prehn's sign = scrotal elevation → ↓pain in epididymitis and not in torsion; know sign for test then forget it, since insensitive to distinguish from epididymitis from testicular torsion
- **Pearl:** Amiodarone can cause chemical epididymitis Also causes hyper/hypothyroidism, interstitial lung disease, blue-grey skin discoloration, corneal microdeposits, Bradycardia, heart blocks, dysrhythmias, prolonged QT, hypotension

Chancroid

- *Haemophilus ducreyi*, gram-negative bacillus = painful chancres ***(Do Cry with H. ducreyi)***
- High rates of HIV infection among patient who have chancroid
- 10% of persons who have chancroid acquired in the US are co-infected with *T. pallidum* or HSV
- Treatment
  - Azithromycin 1 gm orally or
  - Ceftriaxone 250 mg IM in a single dose or
  - Ciprofloxacin 500 mg twice daily x 3 days

Granuloma Inguinale (Donovanosis)

- Klebsiella granulomatis; Rare in US, seen in developing countries
- Beefy-red, velvety, painless ulcer with rolled border
- Diagnosis = organism within macrophages (Donovan bodies) in biopsy specimens taken from the advancing edge of the ulceration. Macrophages engulf clusters of organisms that look like microscopic safety pins = Donovan bodies
- Treatment = Doxy 100 mg po bid x 3 weeks minimum, Cipro, Azithromycin or Bactrim

Lymphogranuloma Venereum (LGV)

- Chlamydia trachomatis serotypes L1-3
- Painless papules, vesicles, or ulcers
- Typically unilateral, painful inguinal lymphadenopathy ("groove" sign)
- HIV and Syphilis testing should be performed on all patients with LGV
- Evaluate sexual partners with contact within 60 days before onset of symptoms and treat Sumter presumptively for Chlamydia trachomatis with Azithromycin 1 g PO single-dose or Doxycycline 100 mg po bid x 7 days
- Treatment = Doxy 100 mg po bid or Erythromycin base 500 mg four times daily x 3 weeks, Azithromycin 1gm po once weekly x3 weeks

SYPHILIS DIVIDED INTO CLINICAL STAGES

Caused by spirochete Treponema Pallidum

Primary	Painless chancre - Absence of systemic signs or symptoms
Secondary *(5-8 weeks after resolution of primary syphilis)*	Maculopapular, copper-colored rash. Involves palms and soles. Starts on trunk and spreads outward (centripetal). Associated fever, malaise, and myalgias, Lymphadenopathy Condyloma lata
Latent	Asymptomatic - Early latent syphilis = <1 year from inoculation; Late latent (>1 year from inoculation)
Tertiary	Manifestations 10-20 yrs following primary infection CNS, CV, skin, and/or bone (gummas) may be involved

- Diagnosis - corkscrew-like spirochetes under dark field microscopy; serologic tests (VDRL, RPR) FTA-ABS (Fluorescent treponemal antibody absorption)
- Treatment - Primary, Secondary, Early Latent = Benzathine Penicillin G, 2.4 million units IM. Single does IM Doxycycline, tetracycline and erythromycin can be used in penicillin allergic patients.
- Treatment of Teriary or late latent syphilis = weekly Benthazine penicillin G IM x 3 weeks.
- Jarisch-Herxheimer reaction = acute onset of fever, rigors, HA, myalgias and possibly hypotension may occur within 24 hours of initiating treatment
- Condyloma lata = raised, flat, grayish papular lesions which are found in moist areas of the body including the anus, vulva, and scrotum; seen in secondary syphilis

Pearl

- Condyloma acuminatum = broad-based, pedunculated, cauliflower-like warts caused by human papillomavirus (HPV)
- Condyloma lata = broad-based, raised, flat grayish, moist papules due to Treponema pallidum

Trichomoniasis

- Parasite *Trichomonas vaginalis*
- Treatment = Metronidazole 2 gm orally in a single dose
- Diagnosis = saline microscopy of vaginal secretions on wet slide prep (motile, flagellated trichomonads)
- Sensitivity = 60-70%
- Immunochromatographic capillary flow dipstick technology, and a nucleic acid probe test performed on vaginal secretions; more sensitive than vaginal wet preparation, however ↑false positives
- Culture if need definitive diagnosis

Bacterial Vaginosis (BV)

- Polymicrobial infection
- Clue cells on saline microscopy (bacteria adhered to vaginal epithelial cells)
- Metronidazole 500 mg twice daily for 7 days
- All symptomatic pregnant women with BV should be treated, regardless of trimester
- Woman's response to therapy and the likelihood of relapse or recurrence **not** affected by treatment of sex partner

Urine Dipstick analysis

- Leukocyte esterase (LE) = enzyme found in neutrophils which are not normally present in urine unless an infection is present
- Sensitivity = 75-96% in detecting pyuria associated with a UTI
- Most sensitive for a UTI on urine dipstick testing
- Nitrite = produced by nitrate reductase of gram-negative bacteria acting on urinary nitrate
- In order to generate a positive test, the bacteria must act on the urine for 6 hours

Pregnancy UTI

- Treat
- Cephalosporins, nitrofurantoin
- Complications: ↑ Risk of preterm birth, low birth weight, perinatal mortality

Pregnancy - Treatment of Asymptomatic Bacteriuria - IDSA Guidelines:

- Recommended approach is to obtain a urine culture and wait for results before treating. Culture results will guide narrow/targeted antibiotics to treat the cultured bacteria. This avoids exposure to broad-spectrum agents and potential side effects. Since these patients are asymptomatic/ hemodynamically stable and culture results should return in 24-48 hours, waiting for results is an acceptable approach (https://www.idsociety.org/practice-guideline/asymptomatic-bacteriuria/)

Cystitis

- Most commonly cause = Escherichia coli; #2 Staphylococcus saprophyticus
- Colony-forming units (CFU's) necessary for a positive urine culture:
- Non-catherized specimen = Colony count > 100,000 cfu/mL
- Urine collected by catheterization

DIALYSIS CRITERIA

Mnemonic: (AEIOU)

Note: Mnemonic AEIOU also used in "Causes of Coma"

A	**A**cidosis
E	**E**lectrolyte abnormalities: hyperkalemia, hypercalcemia (calcium >18 or neurologic symtoms); patients who can't get fluids (congestive heart failure or renal failure patients)
I	**I*ngestion of toxins (**I**sopropanol, **B**arbiturates, **A**mphetamines, **I**NH, **L**ithium, **T**heophylline, **E**thylene glycol, **A**SA, **M**ethanol)
O	**O**verload-fluid
U	**U**remic Pericarditis

*INDICATIONS FOR DIALYSIS OF TOXINS

Mnemonic: (I BAIL TEAM)

Dialysis can BAIL your medical TEAM out of a life threatening situation

I	**I**sopropanol (isopropyl alcohol, rubbing alcohol; note: normal AG ↑ osmolar gap)

B	**B**arbiturates → long acting (charcoal hemoperfusion); Beta blockers (water soluble = atenolol)
A	**A**mphetamines
I	**I**NH
L	**L**ithium (level > 4 mEq/L or 2-4 if poor clinical condition) Level: 2.5 mEq/L in chronic ingestion. End organ damage: AKI, seizures, coma: inability to handle aggressive hydration (CHF, CKD)

T	**T**heophylline (charcoal hemoperfusion)
E	**E**thylene glycol serum concentration > 50 mg/dL Serum glycolic acid > 8 mmol/L AG > 20 regardless of drug level pH < 7.3 regardless of drug level End-organ damage = AKI, CNS

A	**A**SA Level > 100 or > 90 mg/dL if impaired renal function in acute ingestion Level > 40 mg/dL in chronic ingestion End-organ damage: AKI, liver failure, AMS (sign of cerebral edema), seizure Severe acidemia: systemic pH ≤ 7.20 Worsening acid-base status despite aggressive treatment Rapidly rising ASA level Clinical deterioration despite aggressive management
M	**M**ethanol Serum methanol levels > 50 mg/dL End-organ damage: Visual, CNS, AKI Electrolyte disturbances unresponsive to supportive care pH < 7.25; High anion gap regardless of drug level **M**ushrooms: Amanita (charcoal hemoperfusion)

Note: dialysis has NOT been shown to be effective in Benzodiazepine, Clonidine, Digoxin, Dilantin, MAOI OD, Heroin (↑ Vd), Organophosphate poisonings. TCA OD-highly bound and high volume of distribution; Iron

Drugs Which Can Be Dialyzed Have

- Small molecular weight
- Small volume of distribution
- Water Solubility
- Lack protein binding

OVERDOSES WHERE BICARB MAY BE A TREATMENT OPTION

Mnemonic: (LCD BITS)

Sodium bicarbonate 1 to 2 mEq/kg bolus

L	**L**amictal (Lamotrigine)
C	**C**ocaine overdose: treat if wide-complex tachycardia
D	**D**iphenhydramine **D**arvon: Propoxyphene (similar to type IA antidysrhythmic agents)

B	**B**arbiturates - Long acting only, eg phenobarbital and barbital; 25% of phenobarbital is excreted in urine; alkaline urine pH → ↑ excretion
I	**I**NH (Isoniazid); treatment: pyridoxine (B6)
T	**T**CAs: treat if wide-complex tachycardia, hypotension and ventricular arrhythmias
S	**S**alicylates: favors the formation of ionized salicylate → ↓ ASA reabsorption → ↑ exertion

PEARL: Propranolol has sodium channel blocking properties and may widen QRS complex and lead to ventricular dysrhythmias; Consider bicarb early in toxicity with widen QRS

Normal duration (interval) of QRS complex

- 0.08 to 0.1 seconds
- 80 to 100 milliseconds (ms)

Normal QT interval

- 0.4 to 0.44 seconds
- 400 to 440 ms

CHARCOAL INEFFECTIVE

Mnemonic: **(NO CHARCOAL)**

NO	**NO** Airway (Airway is not intact); **N**SAIDs. (no evidence to support the use of activated charcoal in NSAID oversdose)

C	**C**austics / **C**orrosives
H	**H**eavy metals (Iron, lead, mercury, zinc and arsenic
A	**A**lcohol and glycols (ethanol, methanol, isopropyl alcohol, ethylene glycol and acetone)
R	**R**apidly absorbable substances (liquids)
C	**C**yanide
O	**O**rganophosphates
A	**A**liphatic hydrocarbons: Most common complications of hydrocarbon ingestion = aspiration pneumonitis; CXR could be normal for up to 6 hours
L	**L**ithium

WHOLE BOWEL IRRIGATION

Mnemonic: **(SLIMS)**

S	**S**ustained release
L	**L**ithium
I	**I**ron - Kids eat (pica) lead chips
M	**M**etals (heavy)
S	**S**tuffers

RADIOPAQUE SUBSTANCES

Mnemonic: **(BET A CHIP)**

B	**B**arium
E	**E**nteric coated ASA
T	**T**CA's

A	**A**ntihistamines

C	**C**hloral hydrate
H	**H**eavy metals (Iron, lead, etc. Note: MVI with Iron-not seen on x-ray) Treatment: whole bowel irrigation
I	**I**odine
P	**P**henothiazine: Chlorpromazine (Thorazine), Prochlorperazine (Compazine), Mesoridazine (Serentil), Thioridazine (Mellaril) and Promethazine (Phenergan)

CAUSES OF NON-ANION GAP ACIDOSIS

Mnemonic: (A HARD CUP)

A	**A**ddison's Disease
H	**H**yperalimentation
A	**A**cetazolamide (Diamox)
R	**R**TA (proximal)
D	**D**iarrhea
C	**C**holestyramine
U	**U**terosigmoidostomy
P	**P**ancreatic fistulas

Causes of ↓ AG = Acetazolamide, Ammonium Cl, Bromide, Iodide, Lithium, Polymyxin B, Spironolactone, Sulindac

CAUSES OF ANION GAP ACIDOSIS

Mnemonic: (CAT MUDPILES)

Anion Gap = Na - (Cl + HCO3)

C	CO, **C**N (inhibit cytochrome oxidase a-a3 → ↑ lactate)
A	**A**lcoholic ketoacidosis
T	**T**oluene (secondary) to acidic metabolites
M	**M**ethanol, **M**etformin
U	**U**remia
D	**D**KA
P	**P**araldehyde
I	**I**NH (Isoniazid, inhibits lactate ↔ pyruvate, therefore → ↑ lactate; **I**ron (hypovolemia and anemia → tissue hypoperfusion → ↑ lactate)
L	**L**actic acidosis
E	**E**thylene glycol
S	**S**alicylates

Salicylates

- Inhibit Kreb's cycle dehydrogenases → ↑ lactate. Also, uncouple oxidative phosphorylation → ↑ heat (fever) and ↑glycolysis → hypoglycemia → ↑lipid metabolism → ↑ketones → ↑ acidosis

ETOH

- Normal AG and ↑ osmolal gap; however if ETOH ketoacidosis, AG is↑

Causes of Lactic Acidosis

- CO, CN, ASA, INH, Fe toxicity, ETOH abuse, hypoxemia, metformin, ritodrine, seizure and shock

METHANOL AND ETHYLENE GLYCOL

- Both inhibit mitochondrial respiration → ↓ intracellular NAD/NADH ratio → ↑ anaerobic glycolysis → ↑ lactate

METHANOL (WINDSHIELD WASHER FLUID)

- ADH formaldehyde → Formic acid → accounts for most of the AG metabolic acidosis and ocular toxicity; symptoms may be delayed for up to 12 to 18 hrs

Methanol Treatment

- ETOH or Fomepizole (4-methylpyrazole)
- **Folate** (Folic Acid) (B9) 50 mg IV q 6 hours for several days
- Bicarb for severe acidosis
- Fomepizole →
    - 15 mg/kg over 30 minutes
    - 10 mg/kg q 12 hours x 4 doses
    - More frequent dosing required during dialysis (Fomepizole is removed with dialysis)
    - FO, FO, FO ... Not Ho, Ho, Ho
        - **FO**rmic Acid - accounts for ocular toxicity
        - **FO**mepizole
        - **FO**late

Methanol Indications for dialysis

- pH < 7.25
- Electrolyte disturbances unresponsive to supportive care
- Serum methanol levels > 50 mg/dL
- Evidence of end organ damage (visual or CNS dysfunction; AKI)
- High anion gap metabolic acidosis, regardless of drug level

ETHYLENE GLYCOL

- Used as de-icer, antifreeze and solvents, automobile coolant
- ADH Glycoaldehyde → Glycolic acid → Formic acid and Oxalic acid
- **GO** = Toxic metabolites
    - **G** - Glycolic Acid → main player for ↑ Anion gap metabolic acidosis
    - **O** - Oxalic Acid → Binds calcium (Ca 2+) → urine crystals (classic boards question)

Ethylene Glycol 3 Phases of Toxicity

Patients are sick so a CCN (Critical Care Nurse) will follow 3 Phases of EG Toxicity

C	**C**NS	1 to 12 hrs; ataxia, slurred speech, hallucinations, seizures, nystagmus, coma, death
C	**C**ardiopulmonary	2 to 24 hrs; ↑HR, ↑BP, ↑RR = most common; CHF, ARDS, CV collapse
N	**N**ephrotoxic	24 to 72 hrs; flank pain, ATN, **Ca 2+ Oxalate crystals** → ↓Ca 2+ Flank pain, hematuria, oliguria

Ethylene Glycol - Lab Findings

- Anion gap metabolic acidosis
- Osmol gap
- Hypocalcemia
- Acute renal failure
- **Maltese crosses** in urine; florescent urine under Wood's lamp

Ethylene Glycol Treatment

- ETOH or Fomepizole
- Thiamine (B1) 100 mg and Pyridoxine (B6) 100 mg IM or IV (cofactors needed in the metabolic pathway of ethylene glycol for the conversion to → nontoxic compounds)
- Replace Ca 2+ if necessary; 1 amp Ca Gluconate
- Bicarb for severe acidosis

PEARL: Babesiosis disease = **Maltese Crosses** on peripheral smear
Babesia parasites reproduce in RBCs, where they can be seen as cross-shaped inclusions (four merozoites asexually budding, but attached together forming a structure looking like a "Maltese cross")

Ethylene Glycol Indications for Dialysis

- Ethylene glycol serum concentration > 50mg/dl
- Serum glycolic acid > 8 mmol/L
- Evidence of end-organ damage (signs of nephrotoxicity or CNS dysfunction)
- Metabolic acidosis
  - Anion gap (AG) > 20 regardless of drug level
  - Initial pH <7.3 regardless of drug level

SUBSTANCES CAUSING AN OSMOLAL GAP

Mnemonic: (I MADE GAS)

Note: You would too, if you ate GYROS everyday!

I	**I**sopropyl alcohol
M	**M**ethanol / **M**annitol
A	**A**lcohol (ETOH) Ethanol intoxication = mosts common cause of elevated osmolal gap
D	**D**KA (due to acetone)
E	**E**thylene Glycol
G	**G**lycerol
A	**A**cetone
S	**S**orbitol

Ketoacidosis, lactic acidosis, and chronic kidney disease can also cause an elevated osmolal gap

RESPIRATORY COMPENSATION FOR METABOLIC ACIDOSIS

$PCO2 = 1.5 [HCO3] + 8 \pm 2$

Winter Formula

If measured PCO2 is > Winter Formula PCO2 = concomitant respiratory ACIDOSIS
If measured PCO2 is < Winter Formula PCO2 = concomitant respiratory ALKALOSIS

Anion Gap = Na – (CL + HCO3)	*Normal: <11
Osmolarity = 2 [Na] + glucose/18 + BUN/2.8	Normal: 280-290
Osmolal Gap = Lab determined osmolarity – calculated osmolarity	Normal: 5-10

Note: every 4.2mg/dl of alcohol = 1 milliosmol; therefore if Osmolal Gap is elevated, order serum ethanol level and make correction; if Osmolal Gap still elevated think of the mnemonic, "I MADE GAS"

**Each lab should determine its own reference range for AG*

Acute Respiratory and Metabolic Acidosis and Alkalosis

Normal ABG values

- pH: 7.35 – 7.45
- PaCO2: 40 +/- 5
- HCO3: 24 +/- 2

Respiratory Acidosis pH: < 7.35; PaCO2: > 45; HCO3: Normal
Respiratory Alkalosis pH: > 7.45; PaCO2: < 35; HCO3: Normal
Metabolic Acidosis pH: < 7.35; PaCO2: Normal; HCO3: < 22
Major unmeasured anion in serum = albumin
Baseline AG must be adjusted downward in patients with hypoalbuminemia. The expected AG will fall by 2.5 mEq/L for every 1 g/dL (10 g/L) reduction in the serum albumin concentration

DRUGS THAT INCREASE DIGOXIN LEVELS

Mnemonic: (VAN – PQ)

V	**V**erapamil (Isoptin, Calan: Sustained release = Isoptin SR, Calan SR, Verelan, Covera)
A	**A**miodarone (Cordarone)
N	**N**ifedipine (Procardia, Adalat)

P	**P**rozac
Q	**Q**uinidine

POISONING ASSOCIATED WITH FEVER

Mnemonic: (SAL$_2$T$_3$ ASAP)

S	**S**alicylates		
A	**A**mphetamines		
L	**L**SD (rare)	**L**ithium	
T	**T**CA's	**T**heophylline	**T**hyroxine

A	**A**nticholinergics (antihistamines, phenothiazine, TCA's)
S	**S**ympathomimetics (cocaine, amphetamines)
A	**A**ntihistamines
P	**P**CP (may be hypo-or hyperthermic)
MAO Inhibitor overdose	

POISONING ASSOCIATED WITH HYPO-THERMIA

Mnemonic: (COOLS)

C	**C**arbon monoxide
O	**O**piates
O	**O**ral hypoglycemics, insulin
L	**L**iquor
S	**S**edative hypnotics (barbiturates, benzodiazepines, chloral hydrate, etc.)

DIAPHORETIC SKIN

Mnemonic: (SOAP)

S	**S**ympathomimetics
O	**O**rganophosphates
A	**A**SA (salicylates)
P	**P**CP

SIGNS AND SYMPTOMS OF CHOLINERGIC EXCESS

Mnemonic: (SLUDGE BAM)

S	**S**alivation
L	**L**acrimation
U	**U**rination
D	**D**iaphoresis
G	**G**I – motility (diarrhea)
E	**E**mesis

B	1) **B**radycardia	2) **B**ronchoconstriction → **B**ronchospasm	3) **B**ronchorrhea
A	**A**bdominal cramps		
M	1) **M**iosis	2) **M**uscle cramps, weakness and fasciculations	

ACETYLCHOLINESTERASE (ACE) INHIBITORS

- **Examples of acetylcholinesterase inhibitors include:** organophosphate and carbamate insecticides, nerve gases (sarin, soman, tabun and VX) and therapeutic agents (edrophonium/tensilon, pyridostigmine, physostigmine, and neostigmine)
- **Organophosphate Poisoning:** the insecticides' phosphate radicals covalently bind to active serine sites on ACHE → enzymatically inert proteins; **irreversible** inhibition. Examples include: isoflurophate, echothiophate, pesticides such as malathion and parathion and toxins such as sarin and other nerve gases
- **Carbamates** → carbamylation of ACHE → **reversible** inhibition, because the bond spontaneously breaks within 4 to 8 hours with regeneration on ACHE to the active form. Examples include: pyridostigmine, physostigmine, neostigmine and pesticides like carbaryl
- Net result of ACHE inhibition = cholinergic excess

TREATMENT CHOLINERGIC TOXIDROME

1) **ABC's**
2) Decontamination
3) **Atropine** 3 mg IV, (peds 0.05 mg/kg IV), large amounts (10-20 mg) may be needed over 24 hours. Atropine blocks the action of acetylcholine at *muscarinic* (**SLUDGE BA** presentation), not nicotine receptors responsible for **M**uscle cramps, weakness and fasciculation and tachycardia

4) **Pralidoxime (2-PAM)** adults 1-2 gm IV, (peds 23-30 mg/kg over 3-5 minutes) 2-PAM reverses the cholinergic *nicotinic* effects that are unaffected by atropine alone.
   Use in carbamate poisoning is controversial
   Mechanism:
   - Reactivation of cholinesterase by cleaving the phosphorylated active sites
   - Direct detoxification of unbound organophosphate and
   - Endogenous ANTI-cholinergic effect

PEARL: Seizures, anxiety, or fasciculation: diazepam 10-20 mg IV; recurrent seizures: consider longer-acting agents (such as phenobarbital)
RSI PEARL: avoid succinylcholine - it is degraded by acetylcholinesterase and may result in a long duration of paralysis

SIGNS AND SYMPTOMS OF ANTI-CHOLINERGIC TOXICITY

- Dry as a bone (dry skin first symptom)
- Hot as Hades (hyperthermia)
- Blind as a bat (mydriasis)
- Mad as a hatter (delirium, hallucinations)
- Red as a beet (flushing with hyperthermia)
- Tachycardia, urinary retention, hypoactive or absent bowel sounds

ANTI-CHOLINERGIC TOXICITY EXAMPLES

- Anti-parkinsonian drugs, anti-histamines (H1-receptor blockers), phenothiazine, some mushrooms, TCAs, atropine, scopolamine, Atrovent and chemically related drugs to TCA's such as carbamazepine (Tegretol), cyclobenzaprine (Flexeril), Jimson weed (Datura stramonium) and deadly nightshade (Atropa belladonna)
- **PEARL:** sympathomimetics present with similar symptoms as anti-cholinergic excess .... however, **sympathomimetics → sweating and + bowel sounds**
- Treatment: Physostigmine 1-2 mg IVP slowly over 5"
- If Physostigmine is given too fast → SLUDGE BAM or seizures
- Also, most common side effect of physostigmine = seizures; other side effects: ↓HR,↓BP and SLUDGE BAM
- t ½ = 30-60 minutes, may repeat in 20 minutes if no effect

SUBSTANCE CAUSING NYSTAGMUS

Mnemonic: (PCP To PETS MEALS)

If you want to see your pets go crazy and demonstrate nystagmus, add PCP to your pets' meals

PCP	**PCP** (Phencyclidine)
To	**T**hiamine depletion
P	**P**henytoin
E	**E**TOH
T	1) **T**egretol 2) **T**hiamine depletion
S	**S**olvents
M	**M**ethanol
E	**E**thylene glycol
A	**A**lcohols (isopropyl alcohol)
L	**L**ithium
S	**S**edative hypnotics

MIOSIS

Mnemonic: (COPS) 2

C	**C**lonidine	**C**holinergics
O	**O**piates	**O**rganophosphates
P	**P**henothiazine	**P**ilocarpine
S	**S**edative hypnotics	**S**troke (pontine bleed)

PEARL: PCP Intoxication (cholinergic) = **miosis** (2.1%) or (anticholinergic findings) = **mydriasis** (6.2%)
PEARL: Horner syndrome = miosis

MYDRIASIS

Mnemonic: (4 - AAAA)

A	**A**ntihistamines
A	**A**ntidepressants (TCAs)
A	**A**NTI-cholinergics
A	**A**mphetamines & other Sympathomimetics (cocaine)

CAUSES OF SEIZURES

Mnemonic: (U HIT)2 (OTIS CAMPBELL) 3 Hemlock

MEDICAL			
U	**U**remia	**U**sed up oxygen (hypoxia)	
H	**H**ypo's (Na, Ca, Mg)	**H**ypo-glycemia	
I	**I**nfection	**I**diopathic	
T	**T**rauma (SAH, etc.)	**T**umor (brain)	
TOXICOLOGY *- Otis Campbell = The "town drunk" on "The Andy Griffith Show"*			
O	**O**rganophosphates	**O**piates	**O**lanzapine (Zyprexa)
T	**T**CA's	**T**heophylline	**T**ramadol (Ultram)
I	**I**NH	**I**ron	**I**nhalants
S	**S**ympathomimetics	**S**alicylates	**S**SRIs
C	**C**ocaine	**C**O	**C**N and **C**amphor
A	**A**mphetamines	**A**nticholinergics	**A**nesthetics - local
M	**M**DMA (Ecstacy / Molly)	**M**eperidine (Demerol)	**M**ushrooms (Gyromitra esculenta)

P	**P**CP	**P**hysostigmine	**P**ropoxyphene (Darvon)
B	**B**-blockers	**B**enadryl	**B**upropion (Wellbutrin, Zyban)
E	**E**TOH withdrawal	**E**tomidate	**E**phedra
L	**L**ithium	**L**SD	**L**exapro (Escitalopram)
L	**L**ead	**L**idocaine	**L**indane Avoid patients <50 Kg Children < 2 years
Hemlock	**Hemlock** (water hemlock, Accidental ingestion - can be mistaken for parsnips; treament hemodialysis)		

SEIZURE HISTORY

Mnemonic (B COLD)

B	**B**ladder or Bowel incontinence

C	**C**haracter (type of seizure)
O	**O**nset (when did it start, what was the patient doing)
L	**L**ocation (where did the activity start)
D	**D**uration (how long did it last)

Also, previous episodes of seizure activity, previous medical history, meds and trauma history.

MORE CAUSES OF SEIZURES

Gamma-Aminobutyric acid (GABA), the principal inhibitory neurotransmitter in the cerebral cortex, maintains the inhibitory tone that counterbalances neuronal excitation.
When this balance is perturbed, seizures may ensue

Treat INH (isoniazid) seizures with IV pyridoxine (Vitamin B6), 1 mg for each mg INH, if unknown amount ingested, give 5 mg IV; HCO3, for alkaline diuresis; consider dialysis

Decrease B6 → decrease GABA → refractory seizues with AG metabolic acidosis

Water Hemlock *(Cicuta douglasii)* → intractable seizures occur 1hr after ingestion; ↑ mortality; Treatment: hemodialysis

Anti-Epileptics That May Cause Seizures:
Lamictal (lamotrigine), Phenytoin, Fosphenytoin, carbamazepine (Tegretol)

CAUSES OF SEIZURES – WITHDRAWAL

Mnemonic - (BEGS)

B	**B**aclofen
E	**E**TOH
G	**G**amma-hydroxybutyrate (GHB)
S	**S**edative Hypnotics

INHALANTS

- Most commonly abused = adolescents
- Most inhalants are volatile hydrocarbons
- **Sniffing**: inhale a volatile substance directly (modeling glue or rubber cement
- **Huffing**: a volatile liquid is poured onto a fabric which is then placed over the mouth or nose while breathing deeply
- **Bagging**: solvent is instilled into a plastic or paper bag so that rebreathing can be performed; Spray paint is most commonly abused by bagging
- **Dusting**: inhalation of compressed air cleaners marketed for cleaning keyboards and electronic components
- Majority of deaths from inhalants = cardiotoxicity; cardiac dysrhythmias → "sudden sniffing death"
- ECG: Afib, VF, PVCs, QT interval prolongation, and U waves.
- Effects of volatile hydrocarbons: euphoria, visual and auditory hallucinations, HAs and dizziness
- With increased toxicity: slurred speech, confusion, tremors, and weakness, transient CN palsies
- All neurologic effects of acute use generally resolve spontaneously
- Chronic abuse can lead to leukomalacia, dementia, ataxia, eye movement disorders, and anosmia
- Neurobehavioral deficits will include inattention apathy, impaired memory and visuospatial skills
- Hepatotoxicity and AKI
- Dermatologic and upper airway lesions may develop due to chemical irritation and when compressed air is used
- Cold injuries from decompressive hypothermia can lead to frostbite
- Lead to life-threatening edema of the posterior oropharynx and epiglottis

NON-CARDIOGENIC PULMONARY EDEMA

Mnemonic - (MOP CD)2 ASAP

M	**M**ethamphetamine smoking meth	**M**ountain sickness (**HAPE**=**h**igh **a**ltitude **p**ulmonary **e**dema) Also patchy alveolar infiltrates, most commonly involving the right middle lobe. Treatment: descent
O	**O**piates (heroin, methadone)	**O**verwhelming Sepsis (ARDS)
P	**P**henobarbital	**P**ancreatitis

C	**C**arbon Monoxide / Chlorine	**C**VA (neurogenic pulmonary edema) Treatment: Decrease ICP

D	Drugs	Drowning

A	ASA (Salicylates - more common in chronic poisoning and adults more > common than peds)
S	Sympathomimetics (smoking cocaine or methamphetamines)
A	APAP
P	Phosgene

PEARL: ANTI-cholinergic toxicity = *cardiogenic* pulmonary edema secondary to depressed myocardial contraction

Choking Agents
Phosgene and Chlorine = non-cardiogenic-pulmonary edema
Delayed symptoms with phosgene; *immediate* symptoms are noted with chlorine

ACUTE RESPIRATORY DISTRESS SYNDROME (ARDS)

- Diffuse bilateral inflammatory lung injury
- Accumulation of excess fluid in the interstitium and alveoli, leads to decreased lung compliance, impaired gas exchange, and rapidly worsening respiratory status

Diagnosis of ARDS requires
1) Diffuse bilateral pulmonary infiltrates on CXR
2) Exclusion of a cardiac etiology (normal ECHO, BNP, or right heart catheterization)
3) PaO2 / FiO2 < 200
    - Example: PaO2 = 100 and FiO2 = 80
    - PaO2 / FiO2 = PaO2 100 / FiO2 0.8 = 125
    - Diagnosis = ARDS

Supportive measures to decrease mortality
- Low tidal volume ventilation
- High positive end-expiratory pressure (PEEP)
- Prone positioning (improves gas exchange)
- (Low TV ventilation and high PEEP prevent alveolar overdistension and collapse

LITHIUM TOXICITY

Three Types of Lithium Toxicity: Acute, Chronic and Acute on Chronic
- **Acute Toxicity**
    - Hand tremor 65%
    - GI : N / V/ D, anorexia, abdominal cramping → common early
    - Fever in severe acute toxicity
    - Acute overdose GI toxicity >> CNS toxicity
    - ECG: flat T waves, ↓ST, ↓HR, U waves, ↑QTc (inhibits Na/K pump → ↓K+ in cell), ventricular arrhythmias, sinus arrest, asystole
- **Chronic Toxicity**
    - CNS: lethargy, confusion, spasticity, cogwheel rigidity, nystagmus, ↑DTRs, coma and seizures
    - Polyuria → nephrogenic diabetes insipidus (DI) → inhibits arginine vasopressin (Antidiuretic hormone, ADH); more common in chronic toxicity

- **Acute on Chronic Toxicity**
  - Elevated Lithium levels in acute toxicity in patients already taking Lithium.
  - Morbidity can be significant.
  - Clinical presentation: GI + CNS effects

- **PEARL:** Normal range 0.6 to 1.2 mEq/L (Lithium is slowly eliminated from cells, half-life = 24 +/- 12 hours, therefore patients may be toxic with levels in therapeutic range)
- **PEARL:** Serum levels do NOT predict CNS levels (brain may → 2 to 3x higher concentrations)
- **PEARL:** Lithium is cleared by the kidneys

LITHIUM TOXICITY TREATMENT

Mild/moderate toxicity

- Aggressive hydration with **0.9% NS** (if dehydrated kidney reabsorbs lithium preferentially)
- **Kayexalate** 15gm po (risk for hypokalemia)
- **Charcoal** is *ineffective* → consider charcoal in polydrug toxicity. Avoid diuretics
- **Whole-bowel irrigation** → helpful, especially if sustained-release lithium products

Severe toxicity → Hemodialysis

- Coma, seizures, renal failure, inability to handle aggressive hydration (CHF, CKD)
- Level > 3.5 or 4.0 mEq/L in acute overdose. Level > 2.5 mEq/L in chronic ingestion
- Patients with minimal change in their levels after 6 hours of hydration
- Seizures: BZP, Phenobarbital; Dilantin ↓ renal excretion of lithium and is ineffective
- If patient is asymptomatic after 6 hours of treatment of acute, non-sustained release, ingestions → psych consult

Lithium PEARLS:

- Careful with fluid resuscitation in cirrhosis, heart failure and renal failure patients (consider dialysis)
- Monitor electrolytes, particularly sodium, in patients with concomitant diabetes insipidus
- Forced diuresis with loop diuretics is con*traindicated (enhances the retention of lithium)*
- Therapeutic lithium levels can result in hyperparathyroidism (parathyroid hyperplasia → mild ↑Ca 2+)
- Therapeutic lithium levels can result antithyroid effect → blocks thyroid hormone release → myxedema coma

***PEARL:** Interesting trivia provided by Dr. Bryan Bluhm → when the soft drink 7-UP was introduced in 1929 it originally contained Lithium; fyi the molecular weight of Lithium = 7*

IRON TOXICITY - 5 STAGES

Stage 1 (Gastrointestinal) Within 6 hours of ingestion

- N /V/ D abdominal pain; GI bleeding common
- Ask about # of emesis episodes - patients without vomiting 6 hours will not have major toxicity; check X-ray: most pills are radiopaque
- Significant volume could lead to hypovolemic shock

Stage 2 (Latent) usually occurs 6-12 hours after ingestion and may lasts 24 hours

- Resolution of GI symptoms
- This deceptive phase as the patient appears to improve and recover
- Metabolic abnormalities during this phase may include ↓BP, metabolic acidosis, and coagulopathy
- Uncoupling of oxidative phosphorylation → anaerobic metabolism → AG metabolic acidosis

Stage 3 (metabolic/cardiovascular – systemic toxicity) starts as early as 6-8 hours, lasts up to 2 days

- Most patients die during this phase
- Multi-system organ failure - SHOCK
- Acute Renal Failure
- Recurrent GI bleeding
- Cardiomyopathy with CV collapse
- Coagulopathy worsens bleeding; leukocytosis
- CNS symptoms: lethargy, encephalopathy and coma
- Anion-Gap metabolic acidosis (intracellular iron disrupts cellular metabolism)
- Combination of fluid and blood loss, with additional third-spacing → hypovolemia or shock
- Acute lung injury (ALI)

Stage 4 (hepatic) Fulminant hepatic failure, 1 to 4 days after exposure

- ↑ LFTs, BILI and ↑coagulopathy (hepatic injury → ↓factor production / hepatic failure)
- Hepatic injury → ↓ Glucose (hypoglycemia)
- ↑ Ammonia → encephalopathy, coma

Stage 5 (delayed) Usually → 4 to 6 weeks after a severe poisoning

- Gastric outlet obstruction or proximal bowel scarring / pyloric scarring

IRON PEARLS

- Serum Fe levels drawn 4 to 6 hours after ingestion
- Symptomatic patients and patients with a large exposure
- Serum iron concentrations of < 500 µg/dL 4 to 8 hours after ingestion suggest a low risk of significant toxicity
- Concentrations of > 500 µg/dL at 6 hours = Significant toxicity
- Elemental Iron of > 60 mg/kg at 6 hours = Significant toxicity
- Ferrous **F**umarate = 33% elemental iron
- Ferrous **S**ulfate = 20% elemental iron
- Ferrous **G**luconate = 12% elemental iron
- **F - S - G** - rhymes with MSG = order of Iron preparations with most to least amount of elemental iron 33 > 20 > 12%
- Iron does not cross the placenta but it causes severe maternal metabolic derangements and shock, which are associated with adverse fetal outcomes
- Deferoxamine does not cross the placenta

IRON TOXICITY TREATMENT

- Fluid, vitamin K, FFP, blood, antiemetics
- Whole-bowel irrigation - whole-bowel irrigation with a polyethylene glycol electrolyte lavage solution (PEG-ELS) is routinely recommended
- EGD to remove pills
- Deferoxamine 90 mg/kg IM (up to 1 gm in PEDS), q 4 to 6 hours as clinically indicated; binds directly to free iron; change in urine color (vin rosé urine) → should not be the sole factor in deciding toxicity
- Gastric lavage is not recommended in iron toxicity because it does NOT effectively remove large numbers of pills → consider EGD
- Charcoal does NOT bind iron
- **Deferoxamine indications**
    - Iron level > 500 mcg/dL or > 60 mg/kg (peds) regardless of symptoms
    - Other indications: signs of systemic toxicity: intractable vomiting or diarrhea, shock, severe AMS, and elevated anion gap metabolic acidosis

TRICYCLIC ANTIDEPRESSANT (TCA) PATHOPHYSIOLOGY

1) **Inhibition of amine uptake** → ↑ serotonin → serotonin syndrome and ↑ norepinephrine, dopamine → early sympathomimetic effects (↑ HR, early mild HTN, followed by hypotension, arrhythmias)
2) **Anticholinergic effects** → only muscarinic, NOT nicotinic → central anticholinergic symptoms delirium, hallucinations, seizures, sedation and coma peripheral symptoms please see anticholinergic toxicity
3) **Inhibition of adrenergic post-synaptic receptors (α1 and α2)** → ↓ BP and reflex ↑ HR. Inhibition of ocular α adrenergic receptors → **miosis** which frequently offsets anticholinergic-induced **mydriasis**
4) **Na+ channel blockade** → Bradycardia, QRS prolongation, RAD, hypotension & seizures
   - Na+ channel blockade → negative chronotropic → ↓ **HR** (the ↑ HR from anticholinergic activity partially offsets the ↓ HR; if patients has ↓ HR and **wide QRS** = ↑ toxicity/Na channel blockade)
   - Na+ channel blockade → ↓ Na+ influx and delayed depolarization → ↑ ***QRS & PR*** on ECG
   - ↓ rapid Na+ influx → ↓ release of intracellular Ca++ → ↓ myocardial contractility → ↓ **BP**
   - Na+ channel blockade → (other: VT/VF, heart blocks, **seizures**)
5) **K+ channel antagonist** → ↓ K+ efflux during repolarization → ↑ ***QT*** → torsades
6) **GABA antagonism → seizures**

CARBON MONOXIDE (CO) POISONING – PATHOPHYSIOLOGY

- The affinity of CO for hemoglobin is 250x > than the affinity of O2 for hemoglobin →↓ of the O2 carrying capacity in the blood → tissue hypoxia
- Shifting of the oxygen-hemoglobin dissociation curve → **LEFT** →↓ O2 available at cellular level →↓tissue hypoxia
- Binds to cytochromes A, and P450 → inhibit cellular (mitochondrial) respiration→lactic acid
- Binds to myoglobin →↓the O2 available to myocardium → ischemia / arrhythmias
- Brain lipid peroxidation → neuronal damage
- See mnemonics, atrial fibrillation, seizures and non-cardiogenic pulmonary edema
- Classic *cherry red* skin is rarely seen
- Visual disturbances are frequent and *correlate with the duration of exposure*. Flame-shaped retinal hemorrhages, bright red retinal veins, papilledema, blindness is uncommon.
- Rhabdomyolysis → renal failure
- Check ECG, cardiac enzymes, ABG, lactate and COHB level
- N/V/D, hepatic necrosis, hematochezia, melena, non-pancreatic ↑amylase, DI, ↑glucose, ↓Ca, ↑BUN/Cr, DIC, ↑WBC. CO Poisoning is known to cause delayed neurologic sequelae
- CO is removed almost exclusively via the pulmonary circulation through competitive binding of hemoglobin by O2
- Serum elimination half-life of carboxyhemoglobin (COHb)
  Remember: ↓ 1/3 → 1/3 → 1/3
  Breathing room air = 180 minutes → 100% O2 = 60 min → 20 min with HBO [Rozen's 12, 6th ed., pg. 1240]
  Breathing room air = 5 hours → 100% O2 = 90 min → 30 min with HBO [Up to Date 2020]

HYPERBARIC OXYGEN (HBO)

- HBO therapy has been shown to decrease neurocognitive sequelae due to CO poisoning at 6 weeks and 12 months. No data suggesting benefit if HBOT is started over 12 hours post exposure
- **Definite Indications**
  - ↓BP
  - Coma
  - Seizure
  - Myocardial ischemia- dysrhythmia
  - ↑ Prolonged exposure
  - LOC or near syncope
  - Any symptomatic pregnant patient. Pregnancy with COHB > 15%; fetal distress
  - MS changes and /or abnormal neuro exam
  - COHb > 25%
  - Persistent symptoms affer hours of treatment

HYDROFLUORIC ACID (HF)

Fluoride ions bind calcium and magnesium → cause profound hypocalcemia and hypomagnesemia

- Hypocalcemia can cause QTc prolongation and precipitate ventricular dysrhythmias, which is the most common cause of death from hydrofluoric acid exposure
- Hydrofluoric acid also penetrates deeply into tissue and can cause severe pain out of proportion to physical exam findings.
- Onset of symptoms from dermal exposure to low concentrations of HF may be delayed up to 24 hours
- Deaths due to cardiac arrest have been reported with HF exposures involving less than 5% body surface area
- **Treatment** of choice: Calcium
- Calcium gluconate can be administered: topically, intradermally or systemically
- If persistent pain after 1 hour of topical application or direct injection, calcium can be given via an artery or vein

ACETAMINOPHEN (N-ACETYL-PARA-AMINOPHENOL, OR APAP) OVERDOSE PEARLS

- Replaced viral hepatitis as the most common cause of acute hepatic failure in the US
- 90% of APAP is metabolized in the liver to ***sulfate*** and ***glucuronide*** conjugates
  Conjugated metabolites lack biologic activity and are not hepatotoxic → excreted in urine
- 5% remaining APAP is → excreted unchanged in the urine and
- 5% remaining is metabolized via the hepatic **cytochrome P450 pathway** to a hepatotoxic metabolite → N-acetyl-p-benzoquinone-imine (NAPQI)
- The amount of NAPQI formed during the metabolism of APAP at therapeutic doses can be detoxified by conjugation with hepatic glutathione → nontoxic NAPQI conjugates → excreted in urine
- At *toxic doses,* acute ingestion = **150 mg/kg peds, 7.5 grams adults** → *sulfate* and *glucuronide* conjugation become saturated → ↑APAP is shunted into the cytochrome P450 pathway for further metabolism → ↑ NAPQI → ***glutathione*** stores are depleted → hepatic necrosis

Conditions that decrease glutothione stores - enhance APAP toxicity

- Old age
- Hepatic disease
- Renal disease
- Compromised Nutritional status
- Prolonged Fasting
- Malnutrition
- Cystic Fibrosis
- Gastroenteritis
- HIV disease
- Chronic ETOH abuse

Conditions that decrease glucuronidation - enhance APAP toxicity

- Hepatic glucuronidation depends on carbohydrate reserves
- Prolonged fasting and malnutrition → deplete carbohydrate reserves → Glucuronidation is reduced → more APAP is metabolized down P450 pathway → increased production of NAPQI

Drugs that stimulate/induce the P450 pathway may enhance APAP toxicity:

- Chronic use of: antihistamines, Phenytoin, Phenobarbital, barbiturates, Carbamazepine, INH, Rifampin, Nafcillin, Trimethoprim-sulfamethoxazole (TMP-SMZ), Zidovudine, smoking, and chronic ETOH abuse)

Drugs that inhibit the P450 pathway protect against APAP toxicity: cimetidine (Tagamet)

PEARL: *Acute* ingestion of ETOH protects against APAP toxicity by competitive inhibition via the cytochrome P450 pathway → ↓ amount of NAPQI produced

PEARL: children are less susceptible to hepatoxicity than adults (increased rate of sulfation and increased relative size of liver affords hepato-protective effects to pediatric patients)

P450 CYCLOSPORINE PEARLS

- Cyclosporine Pearl #1: Drugs that inhibit cytochrome P450 enzymes increase cyclosporine half-life and drug toxicity (nephrotoxicity)
- Cyclosporine Pearl #2: Drugs that induce cytochrome P450 enzymes decrease the half-life of cyclosporine which leads to a reduced immunosuppressant effect, precipitating acute rejection
-

APAP (Metabolized in the liver)

90%

Excreted unchanged in urine

Sulfate and **glucuronide** conjugates

Cytochrome P450 pathway
NAPQI + ***glutathione*** →
Non-toxic NAPQI

Excreted in Urine

At **toxic doses** sulfate and glucuronide pathways become saturated → ↑APAP metabolized by cytochrome P450 enzymes. Once glutathione stores are depleted → ↑ NAPQI → hepatic injury

FOUR STAGES OF ACETAMINOPHEN POISONING

Stage	Time Following Ingestion	Characteristics
I	First day	Anorexia, N/V/malaise, lethargy, pallor, diaphoresis
II	1 to 3 days	Abdominal pain, liver tenderness, elevated LFT's, lipase, oliguria (ATN)
III	3 to 4 days	Peak LFT's and ↑ PT/INR, jaundice, confusion (hepatic encephalopathy), ↑ammonia, lactic acidosis Hypoglycemia
IV	4 days to 2 weeks	Resolution of hepatoxicity or progressive failure

- The serum APAP concentration should be measured at 4 and 24 hours after a single large overdose of an immediate-release preparation. The level should be evaluated according to the **Rumack-Matthew nomogram** to determine the risk of hepatotoxicity and need for therapy.
- There are no early symptoms that can predict APAP toxicity
- Other labs: serum tox, urine tox, pregnancy, UA, LFTs, lipase, coags, CBC, electrolytes, glucose, BUN/

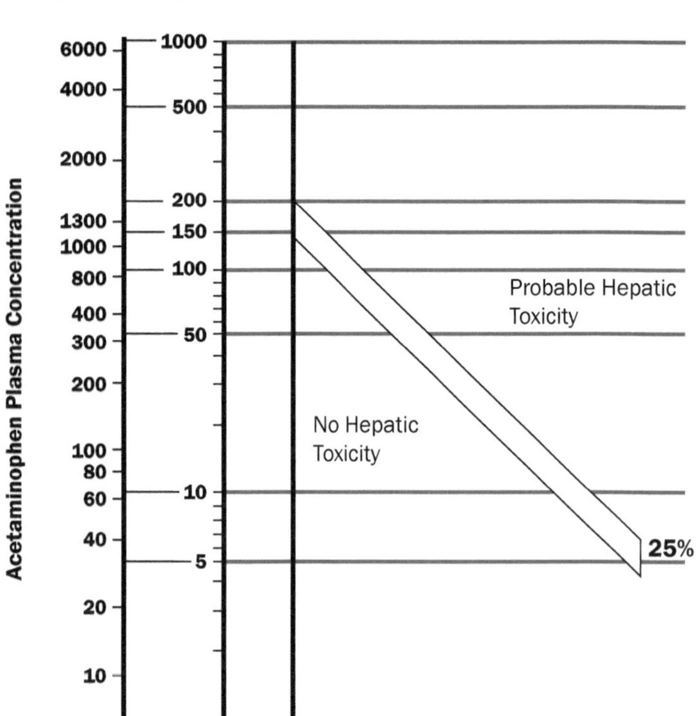

Rumack-Matthew nomogram for the single acute acetaminophen poisoning. Semilogarithmic plot of plasma acetaminophen levels versus time. Caution s for use of this chart: (1) The time coordinates refer to time of ingestion. (2) Serum levels drawn before 4 hours may not represent peak levels. (3) The graph should be used only in relation to a single acute ingestion. (4) The lower solid line 25% below the standard nomogram is included to allow for possible errors in acetaminophen plasma assays and estimated time from ingestion of an overdose. (Adapted from Rumack BH, Matthew H: Pediatrics 55:871-876, 1975.)

Cr; (evaluate for hepatorenal syndrome); severe overdoses – ammonia level

- Alcoholic hepatitis and chronic APAP poisoning AST (GOT)/ALT (GPT) ratio > 2
- ***Acute*** APAP poisoning hepatitis AST/ALT ratio < 2
- Lipase: See mnemonic, "Drugs that cause pancreatitis"
- Glucose: impaired hepatic gluconeogenesis → hypoglycemia
- Elevated PT / INR indicate impaired synthetic liver function
- ABG: evaluate for acidosis
- UA: proteinuria and hematuria may indicate acute tubular necrosis (ATN)
- CXR: Non-cardiogenic pulmonary edema may develop in severe APAP poisoning
- ECG: coingested cardiotoxic substances
- APAP crosses the placenta, which places the fetus at potential risk of hepatotoxicity
- NAPQI does not cross the placenta
- The fetus metabolizes APAP → hepatotoxicity

PROGNOSTIC INDICATORS – NEED FOR LIVER TRANSPLANTATION

King's College Criteria

- Arterial pH < 7.3 after fluid resuscitation
- PT > 100 seconds or > 1.8x control or INR > 6.5
- Serum creatinine > 3.4 mg/dL (300 µmol/L)
- Grade III or IV hepatic encephalopathy

While not part of the King's College Criteria, hyperphosphatemia and hyperlactatemia are strong predictors of poor prognosis for survival without transplantation

- Lactate – level > 3.5 after fluid resuscitation – predictive of poor prognosis for survival without transplantation
- Phosphate – also used as early predictor of outcome

Acetaminophen Antidote: N-acetylcysteine (NAC)
Trade names: Mucomyst (oral) and Acetadote (IV)

- If given within 8 hours NAC almost 100% effective in preventing hepatotoxicity
- Although some controversy persists regarding mechanism of action, most toxicologists believe N-acetylcysteine prevents APAP-induced hepatic injury by restoring glutathione stores (acts as a glutathione precursor or substitute)
- **PEARL:** Can also use NAC in mushroom toxicity - Amanita

N-Acetylcysteine (NAC) 72 hour oral protocol

1. **140 mg/kg po** loading dose
2. Next, give 70 mg/kg every 4 hours x 17 doses

N-Acetylcysteine (NAC) 21 Hour intravenous (IV) protocol

1. 150 mg/kg IV over 60 minutes followed by
2. 50 mg/kg IV over 4 hours followed by
3. 100 mg/kg IV in 1,000cc D5W over 16 hours

A major limitation of IV N-acetylcysteine is anaphylactoid reactions

- The majority of these reactions consist of mild skin flushing and rash and usually occur
- within the first hour of treatment.
- Mild reactions are treated with antihistamines
- More serious reactions are managed by slowing or temporarily stopping the infusion and administering antihistamines, IV fluids and steroids.
- These reactions do NOT preclude subsequent doses

Endpoints of Antidote Treatment

- Check serum ALT and APAP 18 hours after starting treatment
- Serum APAP level < 10 mcg/mL AND
  a) No evidence of liver injury
    - ALT is decreasing or in normal range
    - Decrease by > 50% from peak measurement OR
    - 3 consecutive decreasing values (all below 1000 IU/L)

  b) Encephalopathy and coagulopathy have resolved
  c) Liver transplant is performed
  d) Death
- If ALT is elevated OR if the APAP concentration is detectable
  - Continue treatment with N-acetylcysteine at 6.25 mg/kg/hr (for IV protocol)
  - 70 mg/kg every four hours (for oral protocol)
  - Obtain serum APAP and ALT measurements every 12 hours thereafter
- If ALT is elevated after 18 hours re-check INR
- INR should be < 2.0

Activated charcoal - Actively binds APAP

- Binds NAC, however the reduction in NAC absorption is insignificant
- Dose of charcoal = 1 gm/kg (max dose 50 mg)
- Give charcoal if presentation within 4 hours; significant treatment benefit if administered within 1 hour post ingestion; asymptomatic patients who present > 4 hours are unlikely to benefit from AC unless co-ingestants

Hemodialysis

- Because of its low volume of distribution and minimal protein binding, acetaminophen can be removed via hemodialysis
- However, considering N-acetylcysteine is so effective in the management of acetaminophen toxicity, the role for dialysis is ***minimal***

Gastric lavage

- No proven efficacy in isolated acetaminophen overdose

ACETAMINOPHEN OVERDOSE PEARLS

(N-acetyl-para-aminophenol, or APAP)

The 150 Rule

- Toxic dose is 150 mg/kg
- Give NAC if level is >150 mcg/mL four hours post-ingestion
- Initial loading dose of NAC is 150 mg/kg IV (140mg/kg PO)

August 2013 FDA issued safety announcement on acetaminophen-associated skin reactions

1. Stevens-Johnson syndrome (SJS)
2. Toxic epidermal necrolysis (TEN)
3. Acute generalized exanthematous pustulosis

SALICYLATE METABOLISM

At therapeutic levels, 90% of salicylate is protein bound and therefore limited to the vascular space
In ASA toxicity → the degree of protein binding falls → more drug reaches the tissues

ASA is metabolized in the liver and excreted in the urine
In ASA toxicity → normal hepatic detoxification is saturated and the ability of the liver to metabolize the drug diminishes

A small amount of ASA is excreted unchanged in the urine
In ASA toxicity → more ASA is dependent on (slow) renal excretion
In the face of dehydration and decreased GFR, drug clearance is further *impaired*

Salicylate toxicity is associated with significant fetal morbidity and mortality

ASPIRIN PEARLS

CHOP ASPIRIN

C	Cardiac depression (from acidosis) -→ hypotension -→ VT/VF
H	Hypoglycemia
O	Oxidative phosphorylation – uncoupled
P	Platelet dysfunction and prolonged PT/INR

A	Acidosis - metabolic acidosis
S	Sweating / diaphoresis
P	Pulmonary edema (non-cardiogenic)
I	Increase VS = temperature (fever), RR (respiratory alkalosis)
R	Ringing in the ears (tinnnitus); deafness
I	Irritable / AMS (cerebral edema) / vertigo; irritable myocardium
N	Nausea / Vomiting

SALICYLATE OVERDOSE PATHOPHYSIOLOGY

1) Krebs cycle inhibition → ↑ lactate → ↑ ***metabolic acidosis***
2) Uncouples oxidative phosphorylation in the mitochondria
   → ↓ ATP production → release of energy in form of ↑ heat (*fever*)
   → ↓ ATP production → ***cerebral edema***
   → ↓ ATP production → acidosis → ***cardiac*** depression / hypotension / VT/VF
   → ↑ anaerobic glycolysis → ***hypoglycemia*** → ↑ lipid metabolism → ↑ ketones →
   ↑ ***metabolic acidosis (Lactic acidosis)***
3) Stimulates respiratory centers in brain stem (medulla) → Kussmaul breathing → ***respiratory alkalosis*** (predominates early) (tachypnea – rapid shallow breathing and hyperpnea – exaggerated deep breaths)
4) Stimulates medulla →nausea and vomiting, diaphoresis, tinnitus, vertigo, deafness, agitation, delirum, and hallucinations

5) ↑ pulmonary capillary permeability→ noncardiogenic pulmonary edema /**ARDS**
   a. More common in adults > peds
   b. More common in chronic > acute ASA poisoning
6) ↓clotting factor VII synthesis, → prolonged ↑ PT /INR
7) Inhibition of cyclooxygenase → decrease in prostoglandins, prostacyclin and thromboxane → platelet dysfunction and gastric mucosal injury
8) Kidney = increased renal HCO3 (bicarbonate) excretion → Metabolic acidosis

SALICYLATE OVERDOSE

- Order serum tox (ASA, APAP, TCA, ETOH) and urine tox
- Acute ingestion of **150 to 300 mg/kg** produce mild/moderate toxicity: N/V/diaphoresis/↑RR/tinnitus / vertigo (often first symptom reported)
- **300 – 500 mg/kg** = severe toxicity; hyperthermia, AMS / coma, non-cardiogenic pulmonary edema
- **> 500 mg/kg** = potentially lethal
- Repeat ASA level every 2 hours until it is declining
- Peak ASA levels could be delayed due to :
  - Pylorospasm
  - Bezoar formation
  - Use of extended-release enteric-coated formulations
- ABG: presence of primary respiratory alkalosis and metabolic acidosis should suggest ASA toxicity
- Repeat ABG every 2 hours until acid-base status stable / improving (keep arterial pH > 7.4)
- Check electrolytes, BUN/Cr, lactate, CBC (thrombocytopenia), LFTs (hepatitis has been described in adults)
- Repeat electrolytes and urine pH every 2 hours
- CXR: evaluate for non-cardiogenic pulmonary edema
- ECG: most common finding = sinus tachycardia; ventricular arrhythmias have described as a preterminal event
- Chronic overdose more commonly lethal (MR 25%) vs acute OD which has a MR of 2%
- Done nomogram has limitations, deceptive utility and not recommended

SALICYLATE OVERDOSE TREATMENT

- Charcoal multiple doses; first dose 1gm/kg orally up to a max of 50gm
  - 25 gm orally every two hours for three doses OR
  - 50 gm orally every four hours for two doses
- Volume resuscitate unless cerebral or pulmonary edema
- Oxygen; avoid intubation
- Fluid resuscitation unless pulmonary edema
- Dextrose drip if AMS, regardless of serum glucose
- Sodium Bicarbonate
  - 1 to 2 mEq/kg (maximum 100 mEq) IVP over 3 to 5 minutes
  - Maintenance therapy: 2 to 3 Amps of Bicarb in 1 L of D5W, run at 250 mL/hour in adults or 2x maintenance in children
  - Alkalemia (arterial pH up to 7.55) is not a contraindication to bicarb therapy
- Bicarb and K+ are needed to produce alkaline urine
- Why K+? → When Na+ is reabsorbed, the kidney preferentially secretes H+ ions into the tubular lumen rather than K+, you need K+ ions to compete with H+ ions → produce more alkaline urine
- Monitor ABG (keep arterial pH > 7.4), electrolytes and urine pH every 2 hours
- Bicarb 1 mEg/kg IV boluses until arterial pH > 7.4
- Continuous IV infusion of 1 L 5% dextrose in water, which is added 50 to 100 mmolNaHCO3 and 40 mmol KCL, started at 2x maintenance rate

- ASA is eliminated by renal excretion
- Ionized ASA cannot be reabsorbed and → **excreted**
- *Alkaline urine* favors the formation of *ionized* salicylate → ↑ excretion
- **Hemodialysis**
  - Profoundly AMS (sign of cerebral edema) seizure activity
  - Pulmonary or cerebral edema
  - Acute kidney injury
  - Liver failure
  - A plasma ASA concentration of > 100 mg/dL in ingestion or > 40mg/dL in chronic ingestion, >90 mg/dL if impaired renal function
  - Clinical deterioration despite aggressive management
- Severe acidemia: systemic pH ≤ 7.20
- Worsening acid-base status despite aggressive treatment
- Rapidly rising ASA level

METHEMOGLOBINEMIA

- A form of hemoglobin wherein the ferrous (Fe^{2+}) has been oxidized → ferric (Fe^{3+}) Leftward shit of oxyhemoglobin dissociation curve.
- The oxidized hemoglobin is incapable of carrying oxygen
- Causes: benzocaine, lidocaine, prilocaine, dapsone, sulfonamides, nitrofurantoin, phenazopyridine (Pyridium), antimalarials (primaquine, chloroquine), nitrites and nitrates, acetaminophen, acetanilid, phenacetin, celecoxib, Gyromita mushroom poisoning
- Gas can accumulate within silos filled with decomposing grain. Gas often appears reddish-brown and contains nitrogen oxides Nitrogen oxides ——> can induce methemoglobinemia "Silo filler's disease"
- Most common cause of methemoglobinemia = overaggressive use of benzocaine spray during local procedures (intubation, nasogastric tube insertion, EGD)
- Cyanosis is usually the first presenting symptom
- Blood sample = chocolate in color → turns red on exposure to air
- Presentation: Hypoxic, cyanotic, unresponsive to supplemental oxygen, SOB
- Symptoms of severe toxicity = hypotension, pulmonary edema, and hemoptysis
- Treatment: Methylene Blue 1-2mg/kg, one 10 ml 10% solution (100mg) is initial adult dose treat if symptomatic or levels above > 25%

Methemoglobin (MetHb) and carboxyhemoglobin (COHb) → ABG = normal PaO_2 and calculated oxygen saturation, because the dissolved oxygen is unaffected, hence normal PaO_2. Pulse oximetry will be low

The calculated oxygen saturation is based on the PaO_2, therefore, will also be normal

You must order MEASURED oxygen saturation (measures the % hemoglobin bound to oxygen) – abnormally low ↓

MUSHROOM POISONING

- Mushrooms symptom onset
  - If onset < 6 hours after ingestion clinical course benign
  - If onset > 6 hours possible hepatotoxic, nephrotoxic, and erythromelalgic (hemolytic anemia) syndromes
- ***Amanita* species** (Cyclopeptides) = nearly **all** mushroom fatalities; 3 phases of illness:
  1) GI → 2) quiescent → 3) hepatic failure → hepatorenal syndrome
  Onset of symptoms delayed 6 to 24 hours; does not cross placental barrier
  No specific antidote, however **treatment options** include:
  - Activated charcoal (Multidose)

- IV Vitamin C
- N-acetylcysteine (NAC)
- If IV Silymarin is not available consider high-dose IV Penicillin G (PCN G) and oral silymarin or similar milk thistle product
- IV Silymarin (silibinin) /hepatoprotective – occupies receptor sites
- Cimetidine
- Liver transplant

- ***Gyromitra esculenta*** → CNS and hepatotoxic; Methemoglobinemia; onset < 6 to 24 hours; heat labile; more toxic/fatal then Amanita however fewer fatalities because poisoning much less common.
  - Treatment: High dose Pyridoxine (70 mg/kg intravenously up to 5 g); benzodiazepines Methylene blue (1 to 2 mg/kg slowly infused over five minutes) if the methemoglobin level is 20% or causing symptoms.
- ***Psilocybe Cubensis*** → structurally similar to LSD → psychedelic effects; onset < 30 min
  - Treatment: Benzodiazepines; supportive care
- ***Cortinarius orellanus*** → norleucine toxin = nephrotoxic → delayed onset renal failure
- ***Inocybe and Clitocybe*** → muscarine → onset < 30 min SLUDGE BAM; treatment: atropine
- ***Amanita pantherina*** (panther mushroom) → anticholinergic symptoms treatment of severe cases = physostigmine
- ***Coprinus*** → inky cap" or "shaggy mane": disulfiram (Antabuse) reaction with ETOH onset 2 to 72 hours and < 30 min after ETOH (HA, flushing, SOB, ↑RR, ↑HR)
  Treatment: beta-blockers for SVT, Norepinephrine for refractory ↓ BP
- **GI toxins with onset of symptoms** < 2 hours = most commonly ingested mushroom
  N/V/D (occasionally bloody) / abdominal pain
  - *Chlorophyllum molybdates* (green gill) – most common
  - *Omphalotus illudens* (jack-o'-lantern)
  - *Boletus piperatus* (pepper bolete)
  - *Agaricus arvensis* (horse mushroom)

PEARL: Hypoglycemia is one of the most common causes of death in mushroom toxicity

PEARLS - COCAINE, OPIATE, BARBITURATE, PCP, GHB, NMS, SYMPATHOMIMETICS

- **Tox Psychosis**
  - Alcohol-induced psychosis = typically *auditory* hallucinations
  - Cannabis-induced psychosis = severe anxiety, persecutory delusions and emotional lability
  - Cocaine psychosis = often paranoia and can persist for *weeks*
  - Most medication induced psychosis resolve shortly after discontinuing of the offending agent
  - Amphetamine or cocaine-induced psychosis = *formication* (tactile hallucinations - feeling of bugs crawling on or under the skin)
- **Cocaine** acts as a type IA sodium channel blocker → prolongs the QT
- **Urine cocaine screening assay** tests for the primary metabolite of cocaine, benzoylecgonine, not the parent compound; detectable within 4 hours, remains detectable up to 8 days; detectable in hair.
- **Treatment of hypertension caused by cocaine toxicity:** benzodiazepines and phentolamine
- **Cocaine** overdose: beta-blockers are contraindicated → unopposed a-adrenergic receptor stimulation → will worsen cocaine-induced coronary and peripheral vasoconstriction
- **Cocaine** use is a common cause of strokes in young adults (3rd and 4th decades of life), and is the most common cause of drug-associated stroke

- **Opiate**-induced pulmonary edema: treatment with diuretics is not effective. Use of naloxone and supportive treatment is all that usually is needed, and typically clears rapidly in 24-36 hours
- **Opioid toxidrome:** respiratory depression, sedation, and miosis; signs of more severe toxicity can include bradycardia, hypotension, and hypothermia
- **Methadone ingestion:** classic opioid toxidrome; Methadone ECG finding = prolonged QTc interval (risk of torsades de pointes)
- Miosis is a well-known side effect of opiate use however **meperidine** causes mydriasis instead
- **Naloxone (Narcan):** 0.4 mg IV initial test dose should be given (avoid violent withdrawal symptoms). every three minutes up to 10 mg total IV
- Clinical effects of **opiate** reversal with naloxone: 30-60 minutes

Symptoms of Opioid Withdrawal

- Dysphoria, restlessness, rhinorrhea, lacrimation, myalgias, arthralgias, N /V / D, abdominal cramping, tachycardia, HTN, yawning, lacrimation, piloerection, mydriasis, and increased bowel sounds.
- **Treatment:**
    - Clonidine (alpha-2 adrenergic agonist)
    - Subaxone

- Cutaneous bullae occur in 4-6% of patients with **barbiturate** coma and in 50% of patients who die from barbiturate overdose.
- **Phencyclidine (PCP):** dissociative agent; Patients exhibit bizarre behavior, agitation, and extreme violence; blank or catatonic stare; vertical, horizontal, and rotary nystagmus
- Haloperidol (Haldol) use in **PCP** overdose may trigger a syndrome similar to neuroleptic malignant syndrome; consider benzodiazepines for sedation to avoid this potential complication
- Bruxism, or jaw clenching, is seen in nearly 100% of **MDMA** (Ecstasy) users. They often resort to use of pacifiers or lollipops to relieve jaw tension.
- Hallmark of **GHB** overdose: rapid and profound CNS depression; deep levels of anesthesia last only 1-4 hours and spontaneously resolve with only supportive treatment
- **Sympathomimetics** present with similar symptoms as **anti-cholinergic** excess.... however, sympathomimetics → sweating and + bowel sounds.

NEUROLEPTIC MALIGNANT SYNDROME

- **NMS caused by**
    A) Drugs that antagonzie dopamine receptors Antipsychotics (Haldol) and Prolixin (Fluphenazine) = most common
    B) NMS can occur predictably from abrupt cessation (withdrawal) of dopamine agonists such as those to treat Parkinson disease (Levodopa and carbidopa combo)
    C) Antiemetics can cause NMS Metoclopramide (prochlorperazine) and promethazine (phenergan)
- NMS - central dopamine depletion, lead pipe rigidity, (elevated CPK), fever, AMS, autonomic instability
- Both **Neuroleptic Malignant Syndrome** (NMS) and **Serotonin Syndrome**: autonomic instability, fever, altered MS and muscle rigidity
- Rigidity in NMS more severe ("lead pipe" rigidity) >>> vs Serotonin Syndrome
- NMS Treatment
    - NMS medical treatment options – controversial, include:
    - Dantrolene, a direct-acting skeletal muscle relaxant; 1 to 2.5mg/kg IV in adults, can be repeated to a maximum dose of 10 mg/kg/day. Dantrolene antagonizes the excessive release of Calcium from the sarcoplasmic reticulum
    - Bromocriptine, a dopamine agonist, restores lost dopaminergic tone. 2.5 mg (through nasogastric tube) every six to eight hours are titrated up to a maximum dose of 40 mg/day

NEUROLEPTIC MALIGNANT SYNDROME TREATMENT

Mnemonic DAB PARTY

D	**D**antrolene
A	**A**mantadine
B	**B**romocriptine
Party	**P**aralyze

- If severe consider a nondepolarizing paralytic agent (Vecuronium, Rocuronium or Pancuronium)
- Hyperreflexia and clonus can coexist in Serotonin Syndrome, which is *not* typical in NMS

SEROTONIN SYNDROME

- Presentation
    - Altered mental status (AMS), tachycardia, hyperthermia, diaphoresis, mydriasis, myoclonus, inducible CLONUS, hyperreflexia, and seizures
    - Results from elevated serotonin
- Causes of Serotonin Syndrome
    - Drugs that inhibit serotonin breakdown: monoamine oxidase inhibitors (MAOIs)
    - Block serotonin reuptake: selective serotonin reuptake inhibitors (SSRIs), cocaine, meperidine, dextromethorphan
    - Enhance serotonin release: MDMA (ecstasy)
    - Serve as serotonin precursors or agonists: tryptophan, lithium

EXCITED DELIRIUM SYNDROME

- Previously referred to as Agitated Delirium
- AMS, paranoia, fever, high pain tolerance, tachypnea, tachycardia, sweating, agitation/combative
- Sudden death in police custody
- Mirror or glass attraction
- Usually males, history of mental illness, acute/chronic drug abuse (cocaine), alcohol withdrawal

MALIGNANT HYPERTHERIMA

- Pathology is beyond the neuromuscular junction (NMJ)
- Inappropriate release of Calcium from the sarcoplasmic reticulum in the skeletal muscle in response to medications (ie succinylcholine and certain inhaled anesthetics (halothane)
- Treatment: Dantrolene (antagonizes the excessive release of Ca from the sarcoplasmic reticulum)
- Since the pathology is beyond the NMJ, paralytic agents will not reverse the rigidity

DEXTROMETHORPHAN

- Ingredient in cold preparations
- Opiod with similar structure to phencyclidine (PCP)
- Euphoric and dissociative properties: drug of abuse
  - a) NMDA receptor antagonist
  - b) Inhibits serotonin reuptake
- Overdose clinical findings:
  - Diaphoresis, fever,
  - HTN, tachycardia,
  - mydriasis, rotary NYSTAGMUS slurred speech, lethargy, agitation/mania, dysarthria, ataxia, psychoses, less respiratory depression to other opiods
- Intoxication resembles LSD: euphoria and visual hallucinations
- Dextromethorphan when ingested with a SSRI or a MAOI → serotonin syndrome
- Treatment: Supportive, IV hydration, benzodiazepines, and cooling measures
- Naloxone to reverse respiratory coma
- Dystonic reactions reported in children after therapeutic administration

ETHANOL

- 20 md/dL of Ethanol (ETOH) is eliminated from the blood per hour in persons who are NOT alcohol tolerant
- ETOH metabolism rates are higher in alcoholics
- Hepatic alcohol dehydrogenase is the major enzyme responsible for initial ethanol metabolism

ARSENIC TOXICITY

- Ingestion, absorption, or inhalation (arsine gas)
- Triad of sublethal arsine exposure: abdominal pain, hematuria and jaundice
- Arsenic forms arsine gas during the production processes used in semiconductor facilities
- Arsine gas is a clear, odorless and highly toxic gas (garlic smell)
- Toxicity: vertigo, HA, N / V, severe hemolysis, renal failure, jaundice, anemia, hypotension, seizures, hypoxia, pulmonary edema, and death
- Treatment: exchange transfusion, urinary alkalinization, and hemodialysis if renal failure
- Ingestion treatment: chelation with Dimercaprol (British anti-Lewisite (BAL)
- **PEARL**: BAL is not effective in arsine gas toxicity

PEARLS - TODDLER TOX KILLERS

- Even a small amount of following can result in death: B-blockers, especially Inderal (propranolol), CCBs, camphor, ethylene glycol (tx dialysis), lomotil (tx naloxone), Amanita phalloides, Methyl salicylate, sulfonylureas (D5W & octreotide), TCAs and theophylline and antimalarials
- Liquid nicotine commonly used in e-cigarettes now recognized as "one pill killer"

SULFONYLUREA OD, WITHDRAWAL SYNDROMES, CLONIDINE, LEAD, HEMLOCKS, DIG

- Treatment option of refractory hypoglycemia after sulfonylurea OD = **Octreotide** → somatostatin analog → inhibits insulin secretion from the pancreas that are a result of both the sulfonylurea and dextrose
- **NSAID overdose** typically does not cause serious toxicity; Charcoal ineffective; symptomatic overdoses can occur in ingestions >100 mg/kg and should develop within 4 hours

- **Acute Alcohol withdrawal**: anxiety, tremulousness, agitation, autonomic hyperactivity (↑HR, HTN, arrhythmias), hallucinations, and/or seizure
- **Heroin withdrawal**: yawning, N/V/D, abdominal pain, piloerection, restlessness, mydriasis and rhinorrhea
- **Cocaine withdrawal:** simulates depression
- Bluish lines on the gingival: **lead lines** from lead toxicity
  Lead concentrates in metaphyses of growing bones: distal femur, both ends of tibia or distal radius
- **Aldrich - Mees Lines** are horizontal lines of discoloration on the nails of the fingers and toes
  Poisonings: arsenic, thallium; or renal failure
- **Water Hemlock** *(Cicuta douglasii)* → intractable seizures occur 1 hour after ingestion; ↑ mortality.
  - Accidental ingestion can be mistaken for parsnips.
  - Neurotoxin → GABA receptor antagonist → intractable seizures → death; treatment hemodialysis
  - Root contains the greatest concentration of toxin
- **Poison Hemlock** *(Conium maculatum)* was reportedly used to execute Socrates (I had to add a Greek pearl).
  - Accidental ingestion can be mistaken for wild carrots.
  - Nicotinic receptor over-stimulation → respiratory failure
  - Root contains the greatest concentration of toxin
- **Digoxin toxicity** presentation: weakness, fatigue, nausea/vomiting/diarrhea, confusion, and a visual disturbance hallmarked by yellow/green halos around objects: dysrhythmias, hypotension, cardogenic shock
  - Lily of the valley (Convallaria majalis)
  - Foxglove (Digitalis purpurea)
  - Nerium Oleander
  - **Criteria for Digibind**
    - Digoxin level > 10 mg/mL
    - Cardiovascular instability
    - Blocks (Mobitz II, CHB)
    - Ventricular dysrhythmia)
    - K > 5 mEq/L
    - AMS attributed to digoxin
    - Ingestion
    - > 10 mg in adults or
    - > 0.3 mg/kg in children
    - **Treatment in cardiac arrest:** 20 vials of digoxin-specific antibody

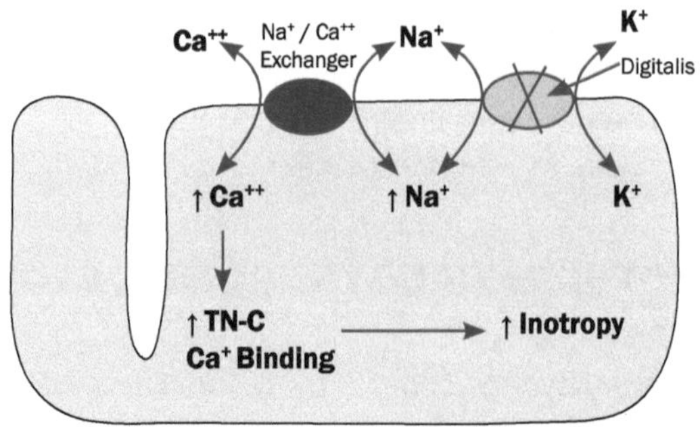

CLONIDINE TOXICITY

- ↓BP, ↓HR, ↓ RR, MS change, and miosis and lethargy → closely mimics opioid toxicity
- Clonidine = centrally acting alpha-2 agonist → inhibits sympathetic outflow by binding to pre-synaptic catecholamine receptors → decreases HR & BP
- Overdose levels = paradoxical transient HTN from peripheral post-synaptic alpha-receptor agonist; As central effects begin to predominate → hypotension, bradycardia, hypoventilation, lethargy and AMS
- Findings may be similar to opioid overdose, however you do not get QTc interval prolongation and torsades de pointes which may be seen with opioid overdose

CHRONIC LEAD POISONING SYMPTOMS

- Subtle, insidious; much more common then acute toxicity
- HA, joint pain, constipation, decrease growth HTN
- Anemia (microcytic hypochromic), basophilic stippling
- Lead lines: increased metaphyseal activity seen X-ray
- Lead lines: blue-purplish lines on gingiva
- Gout
- Cognitive impairment (decreased IQ, learning disability, decreased attention span, hyperactivity)
- Sensorineural hearing loss
- Peripheral neuropathy (wrist or foot drop) in adults

ACUTE LEAD POISONING - SYMPTOMS

- N / V / crampy abdominal pain, constipation, ataxia, AKI
- HA, seizures, acute encephalopathy, coma

LEAD ENCEPHALOPATHY

- AMS, seizure, elevated blood lead level (BLL) > 70 mcg/dL
- Cerebral edema (avoid LP if possible)

LEAD TOXICITY - TREATMENT

- Blood lead levels (BLL) > 70 µg/dL, regardless of symptoms = parenteral chelation
- British anti-lewisite (BAL) (Dimercaprol)
  - First Disodium ethylenediaminetetraacetic acid (CaNa2EDTA)
  - Second CaNa2-EDTA can initially increase the distribution of lead into the CNS, which will worsen encephalopathy
- British anti-lewisite (BAL) prevents this phenomenon and should be administered four (4) hours BEFORE CaNa2-EDTA
- BAL: IM dose every 4 hours x 3 to 5 days
- **PEARL:** British anti-lewisite (BAL) (Dimercaprol) is diluted in peanut oil and should not be given to patients with a peanut allergy
- BLL 45-69 µg/dL treated outpatient with oral Chemet (Succimer), chemical name: meso 2, 3-dimercaptosuccinic acid (DMSA)
- If there is a large burden of lead chips in the gut (usually from pica) - whole-bowel irrigation with polyethylene glycol can decrease absorption

VALPROIC ACID (DEPAKOTE) OVERDOSE

- Vomiting; CNS: ataxia, cerebral edema, respiratory depression, coma, death (rare)
- Elevated serum ammonia level, hypocalcemia, metabolic acidosis, elevated Na
- Treatment: Supportive, activated charcoal
- Naloxone and dialysis - limited data - only few case reports
- L-carnitine mainstay of treatment

PEARLS - BETA-BLOCKER, CCBS, SEIZURES, ANESTHETICS, STRYCHNINE, ODORS

- **Treatment options for Beta-blocker and CCBs Overdose**
    - Glucagon 3 mg IV (max 10mg), then begin infusion 3 to 5 mg/hour
    - Glucagon → enhances Ca entry and usage in cell → ↑ cardiac inotropy
    - High dose insulin 1.0 unit/kg bolus with Dextrose bolus (0.5g/kg IV); Insulin drip 0.5 unit/kg/hr with D25W
    - With CCB OD give Ca Gluconate or Ca Chloride (central line)
    - Vasopressors
    - Milrinone (Primacor) or Inamrinone (Inocor)
    - Intravenous lipid emulsion
    - Charcoal
    - Whole bowel irrigation for sustained release preparations
- **Beta-blocker toxicity:** bradycardia, hypotension that typically develops within 6 hours of ingestion; Heart block and hypoglycemia
- Beta-blocker cause seizures (see seizure mnemonic) while CCBs *rarely* cause seizures
- Children can have significant life-threatening toxicity from minor accidental ingestions of B-blockers/ CCBs
- **Treatment options for local anesthetic toxicity:** Intravenous lipid emulsion. Also referred to intravenous fat emulsion. Intravenous lipid emulsion can be considered in Beta Blocker CCB, TCA toxicities if standard therapies are not working.
- Most common cause of **drug-induce seizures** = Bupropion (Wellbutrin, Zyban)
- **Isopropyl alcohol** → "pseudo renal failure" = early clue for diagnosis. ↑ Cr, normal BUN and ↑ acetone level
- **Intoxications that improve with Narcan**: heroin, clonidine, tramadol, captopril, ethanol and valproic acid, Dextromethorphan
- **Strychnine** poisoning resembles = tetanus infection; Strychnine blocks glycine receptor (glycine is an inhibitory neurotransmitter) → absorbed rapidly → acute generalized seizure like skeletal muscles contractions.
    - No "off switch" → muscle spasms, hyperthermia, rhabdomyolosis, acidosis and respiratory failure
    - **Treatment:** supportive care BZPs, cooling and hydration
- The most commonly abused substance among adolescents presenting to the ED = **alcohol**
- In non-diabetic children ages 2 to 10, the most common drug induced cause of hypoglycemia = alcohol (Other causes, Reyes, sepsis, aspirin, adrenal insufficiency, hypothyroidism)
- **Toxic odors:**
    - Fruity – isopropanol, DKA
    - Pear like – chloral hydrate
    - Garlic – arsenic, organophosphates, DMSO, selenium, Mustard agent
    - Mustard – Mustard (blister) agent
    - Rotten Eggs – hydrogen sulfide, sulfur dioxide
    - Fresh hay – phosgene
    - Wintergreen mint – methylsalicylate
    - Moth balls – camphor, naphthalene

CONTRAINDICATIONS TO GASTRIC LAVAGE

- Unprotected airway
- Hydrocarbon ingestion (unless intubated)
- Corrosive ingestion
- FB ingestion
- Bleeding diatheses
- Known esophageal strictures
- History of Gastric Bypass Surgery
- Small Children

CONTRAINDICATIONS TO ROMAZICON (FLUMAZENIL)

- Chronic BZP use
- Presence of proconvulsant coingestant
- History of Seizures
- TCA overdose

BODY PACKERS ("PACKING" TO GO ON A TRIP); "MULES" OR "SWALLOWERS"

- Most often swallowed, but they may be insert into rectum or vagina
- Sealed drug-filled packets (heroin, cocaine or amphetamine) in an attempt to smuggle drug across secure borders
- After ingestion, antimotility drugs (loperamide or diphenoxylate-atropine) = slow intestinal motility
- Once they arrive at their destination, use promotility drugs (magnesium hydroxide or magnesium citrate) to promote packet expulsion and retrieval
- Present to ED with law enforcement refer for evaluation, intestinal obstruction or drug toxicity if packet ruptures
- **Treatment**
  - Cardiac monitor, continuous pulse oximetry, large-bore IVs
  - Whole bowel irrigation with polyethylene glycol (PEG, 2 L/h plus promotility agent = speed gastrointestinal passage of the packets
  - Activated charcoal 1g/kg
  - Endpoint of therapy: contrast-enhanced abdominal CT (or barium-enhanced radiography) to document clearance of all packets from the GI tract
  - If packets rupture → drug toxicity → fatal
  - If rupture: emergent OR → remove packets

BODY STUFFERS

"Stuff" everything down mouth when caught by police

MERCURY TOXICITY

Mercury exists in three different forms

1) **Elemental** (thermometers, paint, smelting, fluorescent light bulbs); liquid at room temperature
   - Elemental mercury is minimally absorbed through the GI tract; toxic when inhaled; acute inhalation: fever, SOB, interstitial pneumonitis, N / V, and vision changes

2) **Inorganic** (leather processing; mercury salts; outside US inorganic mercury salts have been used in cosmetic skin creams)
   - Inorganic mercury: corrosive; absorbed via ingestion to a much lesser extent than organic mercury; gastrointestinal hemorrhage/perforation, shock, and renal failure (RF)

3) **Organic** (pesticides, seafood, thimerosal preservative) - no effective treatment; if ingestion try charcoal; AVOID Dimercaprol (British anti-Lewisite [BAL])
    - Organic mercury is readily absorbed via the gastrointestinal tract causing acute GI, followed by neurologic symptom (crosses blood-brain barrier) causing permanent neurologic disability

- **Clinical Presentations**
    - Acute and chronic exposures can both present with paresthesias, tremor, ataxia, memory problems, weakness, vision changes, and hearing loss
    - Chronic mercury toxicity: delirium, emotional lability, gingivitis, stomatitis, neuropathy, ataxia, renal failure, and acrodynia (painful swelling and pink hue affecting the hands and feet)
- **Diagnosis**
    - 24-hour urine mercury levels: diagnose elemental and inorganic mercury toxicity (toxic if > 100mcg/L)
    - Blood mercury levels = used only for organic mercury
- **Treatment** depends on the form of mercury and is subdivided into decontamination and enhanced elimination
    - Chelating agents: Dimercaprol (British anti-Lewisite [BAL]), D-penicillamine (rarely used GI side effects) and succimer (dimercaptosuccinic acid [DMSA])
    - The preferred agent: succimer (DMSA) in the United States
    - Dimercaprol (British anti-Lewisite [BAL]) is absolutely contraindicated in organic mercury poisoning as it can increase mercury levels and worsen neurologic symptoms
    - Hemodialysis can also be used in conjunction with chelation when patient exhibits signs of renal failure
    - Physically exposed to mercury: all clothing removed and skin washed with soap and water (decon)
- **PEARL:** Latex and nitrile gloves do NOT protect the wearer from organic mercury

BUPRENORPHINE

- Partial agonist at the mu opioid receptor
- Antagonist at the kappa opioid receptor
- Suboxone = Buprenorphine + naloxone (2, 4, 8mg strips, sublingual)
- Naloxone included to avoid abuse
- Patients stayed in treatment 30 days later 78%
- Medication Assisted Therapy (MAT)
- X-waiver
- https://www.acep.org/education/ed-x-waiver-training-corps/

KRATOM

- Grows on trees in Thailand
- Stimulant and opiate like effects
- Eating capsule, drinking in tea
- Used for self-treatment of opioid withdrawal, little published evidence of efficacy and increasing numbers of reports of lethal overdose and other adverse effects
- Adverse Effects: Hepatitis, seizures (observe for 6 hours in ED after seizure), respiratory depression, psychosis, withdrawal (similar to that seen with opioids)
- Treatment of seizures and agitation: benzodiazepines
- Treatment of kratom overdose: consider naloxone; however, the clinical effectiveness of naloxone in reversing the effects of kratom overdose has not been proven

NEUROLOGY

TRUE EMERGENT CAUSES OF SYNCOPE

Mnemonic - **(CRASH - PAT)**

C	**C**ardiac arrhythmia - Check ECG for findings of dysrhythmogenesis (e.g., bifascicular block, intraventricular conduction delay, QT interval abnormalities, Brugada pattern
R	**R**uptured AAA or **R**uptured Ectopic- Young woman + abdominal pain + syncope = ruptured extopic pregnancy. Older male + abdominal / flank pain + syncope = ruptured AAA
A	**A**ortic stenosis: Elderly patient, SAD = Syncope + Angina + Dyspnea
S	**S**AH - Sudden onset severe HA + syncope
H	**H**CM (Hypertrophic cardiomyopathy): adolescent athlete + syncope
P	**P**E: any of Virchow's Triad + sudden onset SOB + syncope
A	**A**ortic Dissection 9% (most common cause = cardiac tamponade; other = cerebral ischemia)
T	**T**amponade (cardiac tamponade): 3D's (distant heart sounds, decreased BP, distended neck veins)

CAUSES OF SYNCOPE

Mnemonic - **(OH MY HEAD AND VESSELS ARE HIN PAIN)**

O	**O**rthostatic hypotension
H	**H**ypovolemia

MY	**M**I

H	**H**ypoxia (CO/Anemia)
E	s**E**izure
A	**A**ortic stenosis
D	**D**rugs

AND	**A**nemia

V	**V**asovagal: prodrome of nausea, sweating, warmth + syncope
E	**E**ctopic
S	**S**AH
S	**S**ensitivity (Hyper)-Carotid Sinus
E	**E**lectrolyte abnormally → dysrhythmia
L	**L**ow SVR (sepsis)
S	**S**ubclavian steal

ARE	**A**nxiety → vasovagal

HIN	**HCM** Hypertrophic cardiomyopathy

PAIN	**P**sychiatric; **P**ericardial tamponade

EVALUATION OF SYNCOPE

- The most sensitive test in evaluation of patient with syncope = H&P
- Cause of syncope determined by thorough H&P in 50 to 85% of patients

SAN FRANCISCO SYNCOPE RULE (SFSR)

Mnemonic - **(CHESS)**

C	**C**HF History
H	**H**ematocrit < 30%
E	**E**CG Abnormal
S	**S**hortness of Breath
S	**S**BP in triage < 90mmHg

A patient with any of the above measures is considered at high risk for a serious outcome (death, MI, arrhythmia, PE, CVA, SAH, significant hemorrhage)

PEARL: Syncope related to paroxysmal atrioventricular block (AVB) or sinoatrial block (SAB) = **Stokes-Adams Syndrome**

ELEMENTS SUGGESTING CARDIAC CAUSE OF SYNCOPE (SLEEP)

Mnemonic - **(SLEEP)**

S	**S**OB
L	**L**ack of prolonged prodrome or postdrome symptoms
E	**E**xertion then syncope
E	**E**CG findings of dysrhythmogenesis (e.g., bifascicular block, intraventricular conduction delay, QT interval abnormalities, Brugada pattern)
P	**P**alpitations at the time of syncope

CAUSES OF HEADACHE

Mnemonic - **(MGM STUDIOS VAPE Post MGM Tension Clusters)** [ANK]

M	**M**igraine
G	**G**laucoma
M	**M**eningitis

S	**S**inusitis
T	**T**emporal arteritis
U	**U**ncontrolbed HTN
D	**D**issection (carotid or vertebral)

I	**I**ritis
O	**O**ptic neuritis
S	**S**AH / SDH / EDH / intercranial hemorrhage
V	**V**enous sinus thrombosis
A	**A**bscess - Cerebral
P	**P**seudotumor cerbri
E	**E**ncephalitis
Post	**Post** LP
M	**M**astoiditis
G	**G**as (Carbon monoxide (CO) poisoning)
M	**M**ass (CNS tumor)
Tension	**T**ension headache
Clusters	**C**luster headache

HEADACHE PEARLS

- Primary Headache syndromes = Cluster, migraine, and Tension.
- Most common recurrent head pain syndrome = **Tension HA**
  Women > men; 75% population affected
- Cluster HA: look for autonomic instability

POST DURAL PUNCTURE HA (PDPH)

- Most common complication of LP 40%
- Aggravated in the upright position and diminished in the supine position
- The amount of time supine does not affect incidence of HA
- Persistent dural leak and subsequent CSF hypotenstion occurs within 24-48 hours after LP

Factors to ↓PDPH

- Orient spinal needle bevel parallel to longitudinal dural fibers (increases chances that fibers will be separated rather than cut by the tip of the needle)
- Smaller diameter needles → will cause less leakage 25 gauge (although a 22 gauge or larger needle is required to determine opening pressure)
- Using atraumatic needles or pencil-point needles (Whitacre or Sprotte needles) which do not cut the dural fibers
- Hydrating the patient with 1 liter normal saline may also help prevent a post lumbar puncture headache
- Stylet should be replaced before the needle is removed.
- Treatment if bed rest and analgesics fail: **epidural blood patch** (autologous blood clot), caffeine, analgesics, IVF

MIGRAINE HEADACHE

- Women > men
- Gradual onset
- Unilateral > bilateral
- Throbbing/pulsating
- **Without Aura** = most common, N/V/ Photo and Phono-phobia
- **With Aura** = visual most common (scotoma, flashing lights) sounds; motor (hemiparesis, aphasia, ophthalmoplegia); sensory (hemiparesthesia); brainstem (vertigo, ataxia)
- Aura then within 30 minutes headache follows

The pharmacologic treatment of migraine headaches is divided into abortive and prophylactic therapies

- **Prophylactic therapies**
  - Beta-adrenergic blocking agents (propranolol) reduce the frequency and severity of migraine headaches and are most widely used for prophylaxis
  - Other medications include: CCBs (verapamil), TCAs (amitriptyline), anticonvulsants (valproic acid, topiramate (topamax) and Botulinum toxin A

- **Abortive therapies**
  - Dihydroergotamine (DHE) and sumatriptan are used for moderate to severe attacks
  - DHE & Triptans contraindicated in HTN or CV disease
  - Ketorolac and other NSAIDS, acetaminophen and antiemetics are used as abortive therapies used for mild to moderate attacks
  - Metoclopramide can treat both the pain and nausea (dopamine receptor antagonist, which is hypothesized to be the mechanism by which it treats migraines)
  - Treatment when systemic medications have failed = **Sphenopalatine ganglion block**

TEMPORAL ARTERITIS (TA) / GIANT CELL ARTERITIS (GCA)

- Most common systemic vasculitis in US
- Monocular vision loss; vision loss transient (amaurosis fugax), HA, jaw claudication, may lead to permanent vision loss
- More common in females > males
- Chronic, segmental, granulomatous vasculitis affecting large and medium sized arteries
- Most commonly affects one or more branches of the carotid artery (temporal artery, ophthalmic artery, and posterior ciliary artery)
- Aorta can also be involved
- Aortic involvement can lead to valvular insufficiency, aortic arch syndrome, and dissection
- Carotid and vertebrobasilar arteries can also be affected = neurologic complications
- Associated with polymyalgia rheumatica

3 of the following 5 items must be present

1. Age > 50 years (Almost never before the age of 50)
2. New-onset headache or localized head pain
3. Temporal artery tenderness to palpation or reduced pulsation
4. Erythrocyte sedimentation rate (ESR) greater than 50 mm/h
5. Abnormal arterial biopsy

- Complications of GCA/TA: visual disturbances, diplopia and blindness
- Diplopia is due to opthalmoplegia usually of CN III or VI
- Blindness is sometimes ***preceded*** by a visual field cut, amaurosis fugax, blurred vision or diplopia
- Blindness in GCA/TA is due to posterior ciliary artery occlusion → ↓ blood flow to optic nerve → ischemia → blindness (less common blindness is due to central retinal artery occlusion or ischemic retrobulbar optic neuritis)
- **Diagnosis** is made by temporal artery biopsy. Biopsy should be done within 1 week of the initiation of steroid therapy
- **Treatment:** Start prednisone 60 mg/day po in the ED for one month followed by slow taper over 6 months, if no vision loss; if vision loss methylprednisone IV
- Improvement of systemic symptoms typically occurs within 72 hours of initiation of therapy

STROKE SIGNS

Mnemonic - BE FAST

American Stroke Association BE FAST signs for spotting stroke

B	**B**alance; loss of balance, headache or dizziness
E	**E**yes; blurred vision; visual disturbances

F	**F**ace dropping
A	**A**rm Weakness
S	**S**peech difficulty
T	**T**ime to call emergency

STROKE SYNDROMES

Anterior Cerebral Artery

- Paralysis of opposite leg > worse than arm
- Sensory deficit paralleling paralysis
- AMS; confusion
- Bowel or bladder incontinence
- Loss of Temporal Lobe Function: lack of judgment or insight into condition and primitive reflexes can reappear (suck and grasp)
- Weakness and sensory findings: contralateral to the affected vessel
- LOWER EXTREMITY > Upper
- Large anterior circulation occlusion treated with tPA, recommend subsequent thrombectomy

Middle Cerebral Artery (Most common)

- Paralysis of opposite body, arm, face > worse than leg
- Sensory deficit paralleling paralysis
- Hemianopsia = Blindness in lateral half of visual field
- Agnosia = inability to recognize objects
- Aphasia (receptive, expressive or both) is present if dominant hemisphere involved
- Weakness and sensory findings = contralateral to the affected vessel
- UPPER EXTREMITY / FACE > Lower
- Gaze deviation toward lesion

Right-handed and 80% left-handed patients are left hemisphere dominant
Non-dominant hemisphere involved = inattention, neglect, dysarthic (difficulty articulating words) but not aphasic

Posterior Cerebral Artery
- Hemianopsia
- AMS
- Cortical blindness
- CN III paralysis

STROKE SYNDROMES

Mnemonic - Brainstem Stroke (5 D's)

Vertebrobasilar arterial system perfuses the medulla, cerebellum, pons, midbrain, thalamus, and occipital cortex

D	**D**iplopia
D	**D**ysphagia
D	**D**ysarthria
D	**D**izziness – vertigo, nystagmus
D	**D**rop attacks (syncope)

Contralateral loss of pain and temperature
Bilateral spasticity
Facial numbness / paresthesias
Ipsilateral CN Deficits
Contralateral weakness

- **Wallenberg Syndrome (Lateral Medullary Syndrome)** = *Ipsilateral* absence of facial pain and temperature, with *contralateral* loss of these senses over the body; ataxia; Horner syndrome; **d**ysphagia and **d**ysarthria (ipsilateral CN V, IX, X, XI involvement)

BASILAR ARTERY OCCLUSION

- Coma
- Severe quadriplegia
- *Locked in syndrome* (pontine lesion → complete muscle paralysis except for upward gaze)

CEREBELLAR INFARCTION

- N/V/HA/Neck pain
- Central Vertigo
- CN abnormalities often present
- Drop attacks
- 6 to 8 hours delay in cerebral edema → ↑ brainstem pressure → decrease LOC

LARGE VESSEL OCCLUSION (LVO) STROKES

Should be clinically suspected if any Cortical Signs are noted on exam:
- Homonymous hemianopia
- Aphasia (expressive vs receptive vs global aphasia)
- Gaze deviation
- Neglect

Mechanical thrombectomy can be completed up to 24 hours after onset of LVO

STROKE PEARLS

- Intracerebral lesions - gaze = TOWARDS the affected side
- Brainstem abnormalities - gaze = AWAY from the affected side
- Pinpoint pupils = Pontine hemorrhage
- Dysconjugate gaze (failure of the eyes to turn together in the same direction)
    - Vertical plane = Pontine or Cerebellar lesions
    - Horizontal plane = drowsiness, sedated states (ETOH intoxication)
- Most ischemic strokes will not be seen on CT for at least 6 hours
- 80% of **strokes** are ischemic. Patients with Afib are 10 to 20x more likely to develop stroke, and the majority of these are embolic events
- 30 day mortality after stoke = 20 – 25%; in-hospital mortality = 15%
- Most common cause of new onset seizures in elderly = strokes
- Acute painless *vision loss* → anterior circulation stroke
  Common Carotid a. → Internal Carotid a. → first branch = ophthalmic artery → CN II (optic) and retina
- Internal Carotid artery terminates by branching → Anterior and Middle Cerebral arteries at the Circle of Willis
- Door to doctor ≤ 10 minutes
- Door to CT ≤ 25 minutes
- Door to CT read ≤ 45 minutes
- Door to to Treatment ≤ 60 minutes
- Access to a neurological expert = 15 minutes
- Access to a neurosurgical expert = 2 hours

CUSHING REFLEX TRIAD

1. HTN (↑BP)
2. Bradycardia (↓ HR)
3. Irregular Respiratory Rate (RR)

STROKE MIMICS

Mnemonic - (MI HEMI) [http://www.jems.com/articles/print/volume-36/issue-3/patient-care/identifying-diseases-mimic-str.html with modification]

MI	**Mi**graine (hemiplegic migraine)
H	**H**ypo or **H**yperglycemia
E	**E**pilepsy (focal seizures)
M	**M**ultiple sclerosis
I	**I**nfections – CNS (encephalitis, meningitis or abscess)

STROKE CAUSES IN YOUNG PATIENTS

Mnemonic - (8 C's) [Step Up to USMLE Step 2, Van Kleunen JP. Lippincott, 2nd Edition 2008 from Dr Postel, with modifications]

C	Cocaine
C	Cancer (brain tumor)
C	Cardiogenic Emboli
C	Coagulation (sickle cell) **PEARL:** Treatment = plasma exchange
C	CNS infection (septic emboli)
C	Congenital vascular lesion
C	Consanguinity (genetic disease like Von Hippel-Lindau (VHL) syndrome , neurofibromatosis)
C	Cervical artery dissection

LACUNAR INFARCTS

- Small vessel strokes (DM, HTN); 80-90% patients have HTN
- More common in African-American patients
- Most common sites: subcortical structures of cerebrum (BG, thalamus, internal capsule),
- & brainstem (pons)
- Most common lacunae syndromes = pure motor or pure sensory strokes or ataxic hemiparesis
- Subcortical, so **rarely** → cognitive deficits, aphasia, LOC, simultaneous motor-sensory findings or memory impairment

ALTEPASE (TPA) IN ACUTE ISCHEMIC STROKE (AIS)

tPA / HEPARIN

- tPA dose = 0.9 mg/kg, max 90mg
- First 10% bolus over 1 min, remaining infused over next **60 min**
- Do *not* administer **heparin** or ASA during the first 24 hrs of fibrinolytic therapy

tPA INCLUSION CRITERIA

- Last known well < 4.5 hours
- Age = or > 18
- Ischemic stroke causing measurable deficit
- No contraindications to tPA

tPA EXCLUSION CRITERIA

- Significant head trauma < 3 months
- Prior stroke < 3 months
- Symptoms suggest SAH
- Arterial puncture in non-compressible site < 7days
- ANY history of previous ICH
- Intracranial neoplasm, AVM or aneursym
- Recent intracranial or spine surgery
- SBP >185 or DBP > 115 mmHg
- Active internal bleeding
- Acute bleeding diathesis

- Platelet count < 100,000 mm3
- Heparin received with 48 hours with elevated PTT
- INR > 1.7 (PT > 15 seconds)
- Use of Direct IIa or Xa inhibitors
- Glucose < 50 or Glucose > 400
- Suspected / confirmed endocarditis
- CT = multilobar infarct (hypodensity > 1/3 cerebral hemisphere)

tPA RELATIVE EXCLUSION CRITERIA

- Minor stroke symptoms
- Rapidly improving stroke symptoms
- Pregnancy
- Seizure at onset with postictal residual neuro symptoms
- Major surgery within previous 14 days
- Serious trauma within 14 days
- Recent GI tract hemorrhage within previous 21 days
- Recent GU tract hemorrhage within previous 21 days
- AMI within previous 3 months

tPA PEARLS

- Intracranial hemorrhage (ICH) after tPA = 6 to 8%
- Patients with the lowest risk of hemorrhage after tPA
    - Low National Institutes of Health Stroke Scale (NIHSS)
    - No history of HTN
    - No history of DM
    - Young age
- Caution is advised with tPA if NIHSS > 22; although there may be some benefit to therapy, there is a significant increase in the risk of intracranial hemorrhage
- Patients > 80 years have poorer outcomes than younger patients, but the incidence of ICH is not higher

TENECTEPLASE (TNKASE) IN ACUTE ISCHEMIC STROKE (AIS)

0.25 mg/kg IV bolus (max 25 mg) over 5-10 seconds

CEREBRAL PERFUSION PRESSURE

- CPP = MAP – ICP
- Ideal CPP = > **70** mmHg
- Normal intracranial pressure **(ICP) < 20 mmHg**
- **Do not agressively treat BP in ischemic stroke if not giving tPA only treat BP if > 220/120**

TIA

- Focal symptoms, usually weakness or numbness, resolve within < 24 hours
- Majority of TIAs last less than 30 minutes
- (New proposed definition = A brief episode of neuro dysfunction caused by focal brain or retinal ischemia with clinical symptoms lasting < 1 hour without evidence of infarction - on neuroimaging)
- Patients who experience TIA are at risk for stroke
- Greatest risk for stroke following TIA = in the first 2 days

ABCD2

A simple score to identify individuals at high early risk of stroke after transient ischemic attack

A	Age	1 point for age > 60 years
B	Blood pressure > 140/90 mmHg	1 point for hypertension at the acute evaluation
C	Clinical features	2 points for unilateral weakness 1 for speech disturbance without weakness
D	Symptom Duration	1 point for 10 to 59 minutes 2 points for > 60 minutes
D	Diabetes	1 point

Total scores ranged from 0 (lowest risk) to 7 (highest risk)
Stroke risk at 2 days, 7 days, and 90 days:

- Scores 0-3: low risk. Consider discharging home
- Scores 4-5: moderate risk
- Scores 6-7: high risk

ABCD2 score of 4-5 points = Moderate Risk
2-Day Stroke Risk: 4.1%.
7-Day Stroke Risk: 5.9%.
90-Day Stroke Risk: 9.8%.

GLASGOW COMA SCORE

Eye Opening (4)
4 = Spontaneous
3 = To voice
2 = To pain
1 = None

Verbal Response (5)
5 = Alert and oriented
4 = Disoriented conversation
3 = Speaking, but not coherent
2 = Moans or unintelligible words
1 = None

Motor Response (6)
6 = Follows commands
5 = Localizes pain
4 = Movement or withdrawal to pain
3 = Decorticate flexion
2 = Decerebrate extension
1 = None

HORNER SYNDROME

Mnemonic - (PAM)

Triad: Ptosis, miosis, and facial anhidros is due to insult to or deficiency or sympathetic innervation

Sympathetic nerve impulses are disrupted and the pupil constricts due to more parasympathetic than sympathetic stimulation

P	**P**tosis
A	**A**nhidrosis face
M	**M**iosis

Causes: internal carotid artery dissection, aortic dissection, CNS tumors, CVA, Pancoast tumor, herpes Zoster, trauma, Wallenberg Syndrome, thorastic neuroblastoma, adrenal neuroblastoma with mets to lung, thyroid adenomas; complication of alveloar nerve block.

ACUTE TRANSVERSE MYELITIS (ATM)

Neuro-inflammatory spinal cord disorder; presents with acute, raid onset of neurologic signs and symptoms

1. Motor - Weakness of legs and arms; rapid paralysis
2. Sensory - Transverse sensory impairment, thoracic clinical sensory level most common; pain dysesthesia and paresthesias
4. Autonomic dysfunction - Bowel and bladder dysfunction (incontinence or constipation/ retention), sexual dysfunction

- 1-8 new cases per million people per year
- All ages with bimodal peaks between the ages of 10-19 and 30-39 years of age
- 1/3 = no sequelae; 1/3 = moderate degree and 1/3 = severe degree of permanent disabilities
- Rapid progression = poor recovery
- Inflammation or demyelination of the spinal cord
- Several segments involved
- Bilateral findings
- Thoracic cord region 60-70%
- **Causes of ATM**
  - Idiopathic
  - Infectious: 30% follow viral infections: West Nile virus (WNV), Herpes, HIV, HTLV-1, Zika; Non-viral causes: Mycoplasma, syphilis, Scleroderma, Sjorgren syndrome and SLE
  - Autoimmune: Ankylosing spondylitis, Behcet disease, Scleroderma, Sjorgren syndrome and SLE
  - Multiple sclerosis (MS) neuromyelitis optica (NMO), acute disseminated encephalomyelitis
  - Other causes: Neurosarcoidosis, paraneoplastic syndromes
- **Evaluation**
  - MRI: spinal cord swelling
    Help exclude compression cord lesion
  - LP: Elevated WBC, increased protein and elevated IgG
- **Treatment for idiopathic ATM**
  - Steroids: methylprednisolone (30 mg/kg up to 1000 mg daily)
  - Add Plasmapharesis if ATM + motor impairment
- **Recurrence**
  - 25 -33% with idiopathic TM
  - 70% with secondary TM

TRAUMATIC SPINAL CORD INJURIES (TSCI)

INCOMPLETE SPINAL CORD INJURIES

CENTRAL CORD SYNDROME

Usually in the elderly when the neck is subjected to hyperextension The ligamentum flavum buckles into the cord → contusion to the central portion of the cord → neurological deficits in ***upper*** extremity >>> lower extremities. Bladder dysfunction and burning dysesthesias may also be present. Most common incomplete spinal cord syndrome

Mnemonic - **(MUDER)**

M	**M**otor > Sensory (paresthesias)
U	**U**pper extremity > Lower extremity (bilateral weakness and sensory changes UE > LE)
D	**D**istal > Proximal
E	**E**xtension injury
R	Retention (urinary retention)

ANTERIOR CORD SYNDROME

Flexion injuries → anterior cord compression → complete paralysis and pain and temperature loss distal to the lesion. **Preservation** of the Posterior Columns (fine touch, conscious proprioception and vibratory sense) PEARL: In addition to injury, may have vascular etiology = secondary to spine ischemia after AAA repair surgery)

BROWN-SEQUARD SYNDROME

Hemisection of the spinal cord usually from penetrating GSW or knife wound, may be seen in lateral mass fractures of cervical spine →

- ***IPSILATERAL*** motor paralysis and loss of position-vibratory sensation. Ipsilateral Motor paralysis (lateral corticospinal tract) Proprioception, vibration and light touch sensation loss (Posterior columns)
- ***CONTRALATERAL*** sensory - pain and temperature - loss (lateral spinothalmic tract)
- **MS PEARL:** multiple sclerosis (MS) can cause symptoms consistent with a Brown-Séquard syndome

COMPLETE CORD INJURY

- Total loss of sensory, autonomic and voluntary motor distal to spinal cord level of injury
- In the acute stage, DTR's are absent
- Males may have priapism
- Bulbocavernosus reflex is usually absent
- Urinary retention

NEUROGENIC SHOCK (SPINAL - SHOCK)

Triad → ↓ BP, ↓HR, and peripheral vasodilation resulting from autonomic dysfunction and the interruption of Sympathetic Nervous System control; warm skin
Treatment: Trendelenburg position and fluid

BULBOCAVERNOUS REFLEX

(reflex contraction of anal sphincter in response to squeezing the glans penis or tugging on an indwelling Foley catheter)

- Associated head injury occurs in about 25% of patients with spinal cord injury
- Judicious fluids – Excess fluids cause further cord swelling and increased damage
- Bradycardia may require external pacing or administration of atropine
- Glucocorticoid therapy is not endorsed by the American College of Surgeons and is not included in Advanced Trauma Life Support (ATLS) guidelines

CORD INJURY SENSORY LEVELS

Clavicle	C5
Thumb	C6
Index & middle finger	C7
Ring & small finger	C8
Nipples	T4
Umbilicus	T10
Medial thigh	L2-3
Knee	L4
Lateral calf	L5
Perineum	S2,3,4

DEEP TENDON REFLEXES

Biceps: C5 /6
Brachioradialis: C6
Triceps: C7
Patella: L4
Achilles: S1
0: Absent
1+: Hypoactive
2+: Normal
3+: Hyperactive
4+: Hyperactive with clonus

PEARL: Testing for Cervical radiculopathy: **Spurling test**
Extend and rotate neck towards the affected side then apply a downward pressure
A positive test = reproducing radicular pain down the affected side due to traction on the nerve roots

SPINAL CORD TRACTS

Mnemonic - (SCALP)

	TRACT	FUNCTION	SITE OF CROSSOVER
S	**S**pinocerebellar tract	Muscle tone Unconscious proprioception	Ipsilateral
C	**C**orticospinal tract	Voluntary motor. 2 divisions of the corticospinal tract. **Lateral corticospinal tract**: controls limbs and digits **Anterior corticospinal tract**: controls trunk muscles	Lateral corticospinal tract: 90% medulla Anterior corticospinal tract: 10% spinal cord
A	**A**nterior Spinothalamic	Crude touch	Spinal Cord
L	**L**ateral Spinothalamic	Pain Temperature	Spinal Cord
P	**P**osterior columns (Dorsal)	Fine touch Conscious proprioception Vibratory sense	Medulla

- The maximum neurologic deficit after blunt spinal cord trauma is seen over many hours and is not seen immediately
- Factors that worsen spinal cord injury
  Hypoxia, hypoglycemia, ↓ BP, hyperthermia, mishandling by medical personnel

CAUDA EQUINA SYNDROME

Causes

- Central disk herniation (most common L4-L5), trauma, malignancy, epidural hematoma, or abscess

Presentation

- Acute onset of back pain and radiculopathies of multiple levels involving both legs
- Flaccidity of lower extremities (lower motor neuron symptoms)
- Loss of DTRs
- Urinary retention = most consistent finding (90%)
- As neurogenic bladder develops, patients will develop overflow incontinence
- Saddle anesthesia (75%)
- Loss of rectal tone (60-80%)
- **Diagnosis**: Emergent MRI
- **Treatment:** Emergent surgery to decompress the nerves
- **PEARL:** The spinal cord ends at L1-L2 vertebrae → The most distal of the spinal cord = **conus medullaris**, distal to this → collection of horsetail-like nerve roots = **cauda equina** (Latin for horse's tail) → Nerve root injury rather than a true spinal cord injury

CONUS MEDULLARIS SYNDROME

- Findings: sudden and bilateral presentation; preserved knee reflexes, altered ankle reflexes; marked lower back pain; numbness localized to the perianal area; symmetric findings in the LE (strength and sensation); impotence
- EARLY-onset urinary retention and fecal incontinence
- **Diagnosis**: Emergent MRI
- **Treatment:** emergency surgery to decompress the nerves

CRANIAL NERVES

Mnemonic - (Oh, Oh, Oh, To Touch A Funky Vest Gives Very Amazing Happiness)

O	I.	**O**lfactory nerve
O	II.	**O**ptic nerve
O	III.	**O**culomotor nerve – EOMs, pupillary constriction via PNS, upper lid elevation (levator palpebrae) CNIII Palsy = On exam eye is "down & out"
T	IV.	**T**rochlear nerve (LR_6SO_4) → superior oblique muscle moves eye downward and laterally. CN IV Palsy - Exam: Patient has their **head tilted**; Causes of CN IV Palsy: compression, MS, HTN, DM
T	V.	**T**rigeminal nerve – chew, face/mouth touch and pain

A	VI.	**A**bducens nerve – lateral rectus muscle moves eye laterally. CN VI Palsy - Exam: When the patient looks straight at your the affected eye is adducted (looking at nose), When patient looks left or right (depending on which eye is affected) the affected eye will fail to Abduct
F	VII.	**F**acial nerve – face muscles, tears, saliva, taste
V	VIII.	**V**estibulocochlear nerve/Auditory nerve – hearing, equilibrium
G	IX.	**G**lossopharyngeal nerve – taste, senses carotid BP
V	X.	**V**agus nerve – senses aortic BP, slows HR, stimulates digestive organs, taste, Unilateral palatal elevation
A	XI.	**A**ccessory nerve/Spinal accessory nerve – trapezius, SCM, swallowing
H	XII.	**H**ypoglossal nerve – tongue motor

CRANIAL NERVE PEARLS

CN III (Oculomotor) palsy causes: Infarction, hemorrhage, neoplasm, aneurysm, abscess, meningitis, vascular disease (DM, microvascular ischemia/atherosclerosis), cavernous sinus mass, thyroid eye disease, uncal herniation

- Exam: Patient is looking down and out

CN IV (trochlear nerve) innervates superior oblique

- Exam: patient has their head tilted

CN VI (abducens nerve) innervates the ipsilateral lateral rectus; binocular diplopia

- Most common ocular motor palsy
- Causes: aneurysm, vascular disease (DM, HTN, atherosclerosis), trauma, neoplasm, MS, MG, meningitis, cavernous sinus thrombosis (CST), thyroid eye disease, ↑ ICP → downward displacement of the brainstem (30% of patients with pseudotumor cerebri have an isolated abducens nerve palsy)

CN VII Bell's Palsy

Mnemonic - (COWS)

Examination of CN VII

C	**C**lose Your Eyes
O	**O**pen your eyes (try to open the patient's eyes)
W	**W**rinkly your forehead
S	**S**mile

- **PEARL:** Bell's Palsy = CN VII Palsy; lose ipsilateral forehead strength; lower motor neuron (LMN) lesion; Treatment: steroids, antivirals
- **PEARL:** Most common CN involved in cephalic tetanus = CN VII (facial nerve)
- **PEARL:** Most common CN involved in Lyme Disease: CN VII (facial nerve)

NERVE INJURIES
Mnemonics - (DR CUMA)

D	**D**rop wrist
R	**R**adial nerve

C	**C**law hand
U	**U**lnar nerve
M	**M**edian nerve
A	**A**pe hand

MEDIAN NERVE

Median nerve innervates all of the muscles anterior compartment of the forearm except the medial/ulnar half of the FDP and the Flexi Carpi ulnaris (innervated by ulnar nerve)

1. Flexor Carpi Radialis (FCR) and Flexor Digitorum Superficialis (FDS) → wrist flexion
2. Flexor Digitorum Superficialis (FDS) → finger flexion
3. Median nerve branches → to the anterior interosseous nerve (AIN) which is a purely motor branch of the median nerve; It innervates: pronator quadratus (PQ), flexor pollicis longus (FPL), and flexor digitorum profundus (FDP)
4. Palmar cutaneous nerve (sensory branch) provides sensation to most of palm
5. Recurrent branch of the median nerve → innervates thenar motor muscles of the thumb → supplies—> "OAF" in "LOAF"
6. Common palmar digital branches → innervate 1st and 2cd (lateral) Lumbricals at the index and middle fingers → Supplies "L" in "LOAF"

Evaluation of Median Nerve

- Test ***anterior interosseus nerve*** → make a circle or, "OK" sign, with thumb/index finger
- Test ***recurrent branch of median nerve*** → Thumb opposition to fiifth finger (recurrent motor branch)
- Test **sensation of palm** – from the thumb to radial half of ring finger. Sensation to dorsum of hand – DIP index and middle fingers, and ulnar 1/2 of distal DIP ring finger
- All the **intrinsic muscles** of the hand are innervated by the Ulnar Nerve, except 4 muscles which are innervated by the Median Nerve → mnemonic:"LOAF"

INTRINSIC MUSCLES OF THE HAND INNERVATED BY THE MEDIAN NERVE
Mnemonic - (LOAF)

L	**L** umbricals; lateral two, 1st and 2cd (Ulnar N. innervates 3rd and 4th, Flex fingers at the MCP
O	**O**pponens pollicis (thumb opposition)
A	**A**bductor pollicis brevis (thumb ABDuction)
F	**F**lexor pollicis brevis (thumb flexion)

ULNAR NERVE

- Provides **sensation** to the little finger and ulnar half of ring finger
- Eponym for ulnar nerve palsy "**Tardy Ulnar Palsy**" – palsy can manifest years after injury. Severe wasting of ulnar aspect of the forearm and intrinsic muscles of the hand
- All the **intrinsic muscles** of the hand are innervated by the Ulnar Nerve, except 4 muscles which are innervated by the Median Nerve (mnemonic:"LOAF")
- Lateral / radial half of the FDP, the flexor carpi ulnaris (FCU) (wrist flexion) and 3rd and 4th lumbricals are Innervated by the ulnar nerve

RADIAL NERVE

- Wrist extension then branches → posterior interosseus nerve → finger extension
- Dorsal hand sensation. Test sensation over the dorsum of the thumb-index finger web space
- Eponym for radial nerve palsy = **"Saturday Night Palsy"** and **"Bridegroom Palsy"**
- **PEARL:** Most common nerve injury after humerus fracture = Radial Nerve

LIFE THREATENING CAUSES OF ALTERED MENTAL STATUS

Mnemonics - (WHHHIMP)

W	**W**ernicke's encephalopathy (give thiamine)
H	**H**ypoglycemia
H	**H**TN encephalopathy
H	**H**ypoxia
I	**I**ntracerebral hemorrhage
M	**M**eningitis
P	**P**oisonings

CAUSES OF COMA OR ALTERED MENTAL STATUS

Mnemonic - (AEIOU SET TIPS)

Note: AEIOU is the mnemonic used for "Dialysis Criteria"

A	**A**lcohol and other drugs – (opiates), **A**cidosis
E	**E**ndocrine (↓↑ glucose, myxedema coma -↓ T3)
I	**I**ncreased BP or NH3 (Hypertensive or Hepatic Encephalopathy)
O	**O**verdose, **O**piates
U	**U**remia

S	**S**AH/Stroke, **S**hunt
E	**E**lectrolytes (Na+, Ca++)
T	**T**rauma, **T**umor

T	**T**emperature (heat stroke)
I	**I**nfection
P	**P**sychiatric, **P**oisoning
S	**S**pace occupying lesions Shock Seizure → Post Ictal

ALTERED LEVEL OF CONSCIOUSNESS TREATMENT OPTIONS

Mnemonic - (DONT)

D	**D**extrose - one AMP of D 50%
O	**O**xygen
N	**N**arcan (Naloxone) 2 mg IV (Start with 0.2mg if history of opiate abuse)
T	**T**hiamine 100 mg IV, give BEFORE glucose

CAUSES OF PERIPHERAL NEUROPATHY

Mnemonic - (HIT DANG SPARTEN)

H	**H**ereditary
I	**I**nfectious (Diphtheria, Mono, syphilis, hepatitis, HIV) INH
T	**T**oxic (heavy metals: lead, arsenic, mercury, thallium)

D	**D**iabetes
A	**A**lcohol
N	**N**utritional Deficiencies: Thiamine (B1), Niacin (B3), Cobalamin (B12), Vit E, Pyridoxine (B6)
G	**G**uillain-Barre syndrome

S	**S**ystemic (SLE, PA, sarcoid, hypothyroid)
P	**P**orphyria
A	**A**myloid
R	**R**enal failure
T	**T**rauma
E	**E**maciation (see nutritional above)
N	**N**o known cause

HIV Meds that cause peripheral neuropathy

- Stavudine, d4T (Zerit) = 30% neuropathy
- Didanosine, ddI (Videx) = 5% neuropathy
- **PEARL:** 2 meds above with Lamivudine, 3TC, (Epivir) all cause pancreatitis

NORMAL PRESSURE HYDROCEPHALUS - TRIAD

Mnemonic - (Wet - Wacky Wobbly)

Wet	Urinary incontinence)
Wacky	Mental confusion
Wobbly	Ataxia

- *HA and papilledema* are **ABSENT**. Drop attacks may occur. Normal pressure hydrocephalus may follow SAH, meningitis or head trauma, although the cause is usually *unknown*
- Caused by abnormal absorption of CSF by the arachnoid villa
- NPH is reversible
- Treatment: ventriculoperitoneal shunt
- **PEARL:** Most common cause of obstruction in CSF production and drainage pathway = SAH

PSEUDOTUMOR CEREBRI (IDIOPATHIC INTRACRANIAL HYPERTENSION)

- Most frequently in young, overweight women between the ages of 20 and 45
- Headache is the most common presenting complaint; papilledema on exam with normal MS
- Causes: pregnancy, medications (OCPs, steroids, vitamin A, tetracyclines)
- May see CN VI (Abducens) Palsy: (diplopia with lateral gaze); Loss of peripheral visual fields
- Elevated opening pressure on LP (opening pressure > 20 cm H2O in non-obese patients, and > 25 cm H2O in obese patients)
- **PEARL:** Normal opening pressure: 6–20 cm H2O in the lateral decubitus position
- **Treatment:** Serial LPs, acetazolamide 250 mg BID, steroids, weight loss
- **Surgical Treatment:** VP shunt or optic nerve fenstration

MULTIPLE SCLEROSIS (MS)

- Most common immune-mediated inflammatory demyelinating diseases of the CNS; axonal myelin sheaths are damaged, leading to slowed nerve conduction
- Onset: 15 to 50 years
- **Signs & symptoms:**
  - Most common presenting symptom of Multiple Sclerosis = optic neuritis
  - Pain: Headache most common, neuropathic pain, back pain and **Lhermitte sign** (electric shock-like sensations down the back and/or limbs upon flexion of the neck)
  - Central vertigo (nystagmus is common), gait and balance problems, diplopia, internuclear ophthalmoplegia (adductor weakness),* **opsoclonus - myoclonus syndrome**, limb ataxia, acute transverse myelitis, symptoms consistent with a Brown-Séquard syndrome; fatigue / exhaustion; motor weakness lower (paraplegia) more common > upper extremity, sensory > motor, DTRs exaggerated
  - Isolated neuropathy in cranial nerves III, IV or VI
  - Heat sensitivity (**Uhthoff phenomenon**)
  - 50% report bowel dysfunction and up to 75%report bladder dysfunction
- MRI diagnosis: multiple areas of demyelination
- Treatment: during acute flares (relapse) = high dose steroids; plasma exchange

***Opsoclonus - myoclonus syndrome (very rare)** = spontaneous conjugate rapid eye movements in all directions of gaze & involuntary myoclonic muscular contractions; Peds Pearl: 50% have an underlying neuroblastoma; other causes = infectious, MS, toxin (serotonin syndrome), cancers

SEIZURES

- Simple partial seizure: no AMS, brief
- Complex partial seizure: partial seizure with AMS + post-ictal
- Generalized seizures: AMS with + post-ictal; average duration of a typical generalized tonic-clonic seizure = 1 to 2 minutes; confusion & fatigue can last several hours
- Most common cause of recurrent seizures = non-compliance with antiepileptic medications

Status Epilepticus

- Seizure lasting > 5 minutes or 2 or more seizures without recovery in between
- Status epilepticus has an associated mortality of up to 20%.
- Status epilepticus = seizure lasting > 5 minutes or 2 or more seizures without recovery in between

Status Epilepticus (Adults) - Treatment Approach

1st: Benzodiazepines (Lorazepam 0.1 mg/kg IV, Max 4 mg IV, may repeat in 5 minutes or Diazepam 5 mg IV, or 20 mg PR or Midazolam 10 mg IM once)

2nd: Fosphenytoin (20 mg PE//kg IV max 1,500 mg, max infusion rate 150 PE's / min) OR
Levetiracetam 60 mg/kg IV (max 4,500 mg) over 15 minutes

3rd: Phenobarbital 20mg/kg IV at 50mg/min OR
Pentobarbital (5-15 mg/kg IV load, 0.5-5 mg/kg/hour infusion OR
Propofol (2-5 mg/kg bolus, 2-10 mg/kg/hr infusion)

RSI PEARL: Induction: Propofol or Ketofol; paralytic: Recuronium if seizure duration > 25 minutes
PEARL: Nondepolarizing neruomuscular blocking drugs will stop the tonic-clonic movements, but will not affect abnormal neuronal firing. Patient will need an EEG.

TABES DORSALIS

Progressive demyelination of *Posterior Column* and *Dorsal Nerve Roots.* (Know how to distinguish **Tabes Dorsalis** from **Normal Pressure Hydrocephalus)**

1. Ataxia
2. Urinary incontinence and loss of sexual function
3. Leg pain (Lancinating - appearing suddenly, spreading rapidly, and disappearing) often is an early symptom

Other neurologic presentations: progressive loss of pain sensation, loss of peripheral reflexes, impairment of vibration and position senses

PERIPHERAL VERTIGO

- Peripheral vertigo is most often due to cranial nerve VIII or vestibular lesions
- Nystagmus: unidirectional and fatiguing (short-lived) and suppressed with fixation; nystagmus has long latency. Usually have hearing loss. N/V/diaphoresis common;
- Examples: Benign paroxysmal positional vertigo (BPPV), vestibular labyrinthitis, vestibular neuronitis & Meniere's disease

Benign paroxysmal positional vertigo (BPPV)

- Disorder of the semicircular canals; debris is free floating within the canals.
- It only affects the semicircular canals, therefore there is NO associated hearing deficit

Vestibular labyrinthitis
Inflammation along the vestibulocochlear nerve (CN VIII)
Most commonly occurs after a viral illness or otitis media, lasts for several days, then resolves
+/- hearing loss; +/- tinnitus
Second most common cause of peripheral vertigo behind benign paroxysmal positional vertigo (BPPV)

Vestibular neuritis (neuronitis)
Inflammation of the vestibular nerve (branch of CNVIII)
Severe vertigo for days: no auditory symptoms
BPPV and vestibular neuritis due NOT result in hearing loss

Meniere's Disease (Idiopathic Endolymphatic Hydrops)
1) Vertigo
2) Unilateral diminished sensorineural hearing loss
3) Tinnitus intermittent; long symptom-free intervals; attacks in clusters

Meniere's Disease differential diagnosis = acoustic neuroma
Meniere's = true vertigo vs acoustic neuroma where the patient describes imbalance and disequilibrium

Acoustic neuroma
Acoustic neuroma (Vestibular schwannoma): a peripheral cause that can become central
1. Vertigo: not true vertigo (imbalance & disequilibrium)
2. Hearing loss: fluctuates and is progressive (+/-)
3. Tinnitus +/-

Peripheral Vertigo treatment options: 1) Sedative: diazepam 2) Antiemetic: promethazine (Phenergan), metoclopramide (Reglan) 3) Anticholinergic: Scopolamine patch 4) Anti-histamines: Antivert, Benadryl 5) Calcium antagonists: Nimodipine, Cinnarizine, Flurarazine
Epley maneuver - https://www.youtube.com/watch?v=9SLm76jQg3g&vl=en;

CENTRAL VERTIGO

Most often due to CVA of the posterior cerebral circulation (cerebellum & brainstem CVAs); Other causes: Wallenberg Syndrome, MS, vertebral artery dissection; acoustic neuroma (peripheral cause that can become central)
Nystagmus: multidirectional and short latency; non-fatiguing and not suppressed with fixation
Associated N/V/diaphoresis is **rare** and hearing loss is **unlikely**

TRIGEMINAL NEURALGIA

- Unilateral severe facial pain in lips, gums, cheek or chin - maxillary (V2) and mandibular (V3) distribution of the trigeminal (V) nerve. Ophthalmic division (V1) rarely involved
- Sharp, lightening-like bursts; right side > left; triggers: chewing, brushing teeth, shaving, washing, exposure to heat/cold, talking; Usually > 40 y/o (if younger think MS or TMJ)
- **Treatment:** Carbamazepine (Tegeretol): first line, Gabapentin (Neurontin), Lamotrigine (Lamictal), Baclofen, Amitriptyline, Phenytoin; Surgical decompression of nerve roots
- CT or MRI done to rule out structural lesions mimicking or triggering trigeminal neuralgia

MYASTHENIA GRAVIS

- **Myasthenia gravis (MG)**: autoimmune disease - antibodies directed against the acetylcholine receptor at NMJ → diplopia and ptosis most common presenting symptom, also = dysphagia, dysarthria; proximal muscle weakness worse at the end of the day.
  Females > males; teens to early 30's; thymomas thought to ↑ acetylcholine receptor antibodies; relieved with rest; normal reflexes, normal sensation.
- **Diagnosis:** Endrophonium (Tensilon) test, EMG; Tensilon Test is rarely performed due to the potential of life threatening bradycardia.
- **Treatment of MG**: Anticholinesterase medications
  - Neostigmine (Prostigmin) and Pyridostigmine (Mestinon)
- **Treatment of Myasthenic Crisis**
  - Assess respiratory status: negative inspiratory force (NIF)
  - IVIG + steroids or Plasma Exchange

Lambert-Eaton syndrome is associated with small cell lung cancer in about 50% of cases, and symptoms improve with repetitive use

Nerve Agents (sarin, soman, tabun, GF, VX) are organophosphates which are potent inhibitors of acetylcholinesterase → SLUDGE BAM syndrome. Treatment: atropine and 2-PAM (pralidoxime)

BOTULISM

- Botulism: neurotoxins → block the release of acetylcholine → descending symmetrical paralysis, ptosis, generalized weakness UE >LE, proximal muscles > distal, dizziness, dry mouth, diplopia, dilated/fixed pupils & blurred vision, dysphonia, dysarthria, dysphagia, and respiratory failure.
- Acetylcholine blockade results in: Decreased salivation GI Ileus & Urinary retention
- ↓ DTR's on physical exam, no pain
- Normal CSF, normal nerve conduction
- **PEARL:** Most common cause of foodborne botulism = home canned foods and honey
- **Treatment:** antitoxin → binds circulating toxin only
  - Equine serum heptavalent botulism antitoxin (> 1year old)
  - Human-derived botulism immune globulin (<1 year old)
  - If associated with wound: antibiotic
  - Intubate if vital capacity <30%; saline enema to cleanse GI tract of residual toxin

GUILLAIN-BARRE SYNDROME (GBS)

- Progressive, acending, symmetric paralysis; without sensory deficits or a sensory level; urinary retention may occur (differential diagnosis with urinary retention: spinal cord lesion and cauda equina syndrome)
- **Acute immune-mediated polyneuropathy** response to a preceding infection: destroys myelin sheath of peripheral nerves → results in demyelination
- **Common causes of GBS**: infection: gastroenteritis with Campylobacter jejuni infection (most common); 33% = idiopathic. Other causes: CMV, EBV, HIV, and Zika virus

Clinical course

- More severe in elderly
- More rapid recovery in children
- Rapid onset of symptoms = a poorer prognosis

Guillain-Barré syndrome – Management

- IVIG or Plasmapharesis (not both)
- Assess respiratory status: negative inspiratory force (NIF)

Guillain-Barré syndrome – Spirometry

- Spirometry tests that can help predict the need to intubate a patient with Guillain-Barré syndrome = NIF
- MIP also referred to as Negative Inspiratory Force (NIF)
- Normal > 60 cm H2O. If NIF is dropping or nears 20 cm H2O = respiratory support

SPIROMETRY PEARLS

- **Maximal inspiratory pressure (MIP)** = the maximal negative pressure a patient can generate while inhaling through a blocked mouthpiece after a full exhalation
- Measures the strength of the inspiratory muscles, primarily the diaphragm
  Average MIP = 100 for men, 70 cm H2O for women
- MIP is also referred to as the Negative Inspiratory Force (NIF)
- **Maximal expiratory pressure (MEP)** is the maximal pressure measured during forced expiration (with cheeks bulging) through a blocked mouthpiece after a full inhalation
- Measures expiratory muscle strength - correlates with ability to cough and clear secretions
  Average MEP = + 170 for men, + 110 cm H2O for women

TICK PARALYSIS

- Mimics GBS (ascending paralysis; loss of deep tendon reflexes (↓ DTR's); mostly kids, ataxia, normal CSF, tick at hairline, normal EMG testing

PERIODIC PARALYSIS

- Rare neuromuscular disorder related to a defect in muscle ion channels
- Several types: hypokalemic, hyperkalemic, and thyrotoxic
- Hallmark of periodic paralysis = painless muscle weakness precipitated by heavy exercise, fasting, stress, high-carbohydrate meals, or in the case of hyperkalemic periodic paralysis, consumption of potassium rich foods

AMYOTROPHIC LATERAL SCLEROSIS

- Lou Gherig's Disease: Progressive neruodegenerative disease that affects nerve cells in the brain and the spinal cord. Most common presentation = asymptomatic limb weakness (80%)
- Muscle weakness that gets worse over weeks to months, muscle spasticity, fasciulations, cramps and muscle wasting. Bulbular dysfunction present in 20% of patients with ALS (dysarthria of dysphagia)
- Other bulbar findings:
  UMN = laryngospsasm
  LMN = hoarseness
- Clinical hallmark of ALS: combination of upper and lower neuron signs and symptoms
- Upper motor neurons (UMN) are responsible for motor movement
- Lower motor neurons (LMN) prevent excessive muscle movement

UPPER MOTOR NEURON LESION *VS* LOWER MOTOR NEURON LESION

Differences Mnemonic - **(STORM Baby G)**

		UMNL	LMNL
S	**Strength**	Little overt weakness; Slowness of movement; stiffness Incoordination of movement	Significant Weakness
T	**Tone**	Increased (spasticity)	Decreased (flaccid)
O	**Other**	Spontaneous Clonus Pseudobular affect (inappropriate laughing, crying or yawning - early manifestation of ALS)	Fasciculations Muscle cramps
R	**Reflexes**	DTR's increased	Decreased
M	**Muscle Mass**	Minimal Loss	Atrophy
Baby	**Babinski**	Positive (toe up)	Negative (toe down)

SUBARACHNOID HEMORRHAGE (SAH)

- **Presentation:** abrupt onset, "worst headache" of their life," or "thunder-clap" headache; neck pain/ stiffness, onset during exertion, syncope
  Most commonly caused by a ruptured aneurysm
- **Diagnosis:** non-contrast CT scan
  If imaging with higher generation CT scanners performed within 6 hours of onset of HA is normal → virtually 100% certain that SAH has been ruled out
  Within 24 hours clinician can be 92% sure that SAH is ruled out
  If CT negative, and suspicion high, or delayed/early presentations → consider lumbar puncture
- **Hunt Hess Grading Scale for SAH**
  Classify the severity of a SAH based on clinical condition at presentation
  Used as a predictor of outcome; higher grades = lower survival rates
- Grade I = Mild HA, normal MS, no nerve deficit → projected survival of 70%
- Grade II = Severe HA, normal MS, +/- CN deficit → projected survival of 60%
- Grade III = Confused, somnolent, +/- CN deficit or mild motor deficit → projected survival of 50%
- Grade IV = Stupor, moderate / severe motor deficit, intermittent posturing → projected survival of 20%
- Grade V = Coma, reflex posturing or flaccid → projected survival of 10%
- Other grading system: **World Federation of Neurological Surgeons (WFNS)**
  WFNS system incorporates the Glasgow Coma Scale combined with the presence of motor deficit (Grade I-V)
- **Treatment**
  - Supportive: Hypovolemia is a risk factor for ischemic complications and should be avoided; avoid fever and hyperglycemia = associated with poor outcome
  - Blood pressure = Optimal range not clear; SBP <160 mmHg or MAP <110 mmHg recommended by guidelines
  - Labetalol, nicardipine, or enalapril are preferred. The use of vasodilators such as nitroprusside or nitroglycerin should be avoided because of their propensity to increase cerebral blood volume and therefore ICP

- Nimodipine (decreases vasospasm), po or NGT, 60 mg every 4 hours for 21 days
- Aneurysm repair: surgical clipping or endovascular coiling = to prevent rebleeding; performed as early as feasible, preferably within 24 hours, and immediately if rebleeding occurs
- Ventriculostomy and intraventricular pressure monitor = direct measurement of ICP and allows treatment by drainage of CSF for patients with symptomatic hydrocephalus or other causes of elevated ICP
- Prophylactic antiseizure drug therapy is not required in all patients unless unsecured aneurysms, poor neurologic grade, and/or large concentrations of blood at the cortex
- Prophylactic antiseizure drug therapy should be discontinued after the aneurysm is secured
- **Complications are common after SAH**
  Rebleeding, vasospasm and delayed cerebral ischemia, elevated intracranial pressure (ICP) related to hydrocephalus or other causes, hyponatremia, and seizures

VENTRICULOPERITONEAL (VP) SHUNT MALFUNCTION

The most common cause of shunt malfunction = obstruction

- **Obstruction**
  a) Proximal tubing obstruction due to choroid plexus
  b) Increased protein within the CSF
- **Symptoms:** increased ICP (vomiting, irritability, bulging fontanelle in infants, "sundown eyes" (patient unable to look up), HA, N/V, lethargy, ataxia, and CN palsies in older children and adults)
- **Treatment: neurosurgical consultation** = tap shunt and measure opening pressure
  Determine whether the obstruction is proximal (choroid plexus or increased protein = most common) or distal (thrombus) to direct intervention needed

Other Causes of shunt malfunction

- **Abdominal pseudocysts**
  Pseudocysts form around the peritoneal catheter
  Asymptomatic until pseudocysts become large enough to cause abdominal pain
- **Ventricular loculations**
  Loculations can lead to non-communicating, non-draining CSF accumulations
  If present in the 4th ventricle, loculations can obstruct the Sylvian aqueduct, leading to increased ICP and symptoms of brainstem compression
- **Mechanical failure**
  a) Fracture disconnection
  (delayed complication from degradation of tubing or growth of patient)

  b) Migration or misplacement of a shunt
  (disconnection occurs shortly after surgery)

  Though all will present with signs and symptoms of increased ICP, they are less common than obstructive causes of shunt malfunction

Pearl #1

- Slit ventricle syndrome (5%)
- The ventricles are overdrained, resulting in occlusion of the proximal shunt orifice, which limits drainage and causes ICP to rise
- As fluid reaccumulates in the ventricle, the occlusion is relieved, allowing drainage to resume
- Presentation = cyclical, episodic symptoms of raised ICP

Pearl#2

- Most common bacterial cause of external shunt infection = Staphylococcus epidermidis

CEREBRAL VENOUS THROMBOSIS (CVT)

- Headache, gradual onset or sudden and severe ("thunderclap")
- AMS
- CN VI palsy, focal neurologic deficit or seizures
- More common in women > men
- **Risk Factors**
  - Oral contraceptives - very strong risk factor (risk increases if women has prothrombotic condition or is obese)
  - Pregnancy and the puerperium (period of about 6 weeks after childbirth); ~25% of cases occurring during the postpartum period
  - Prothrombotic conditions (genetic or acquired)
  - Malignancy
  - Inflammatory diseases: SLE, Behçet disease, granulomatosis with polyangiitis (GPA) (formerly Wegener's), thromboangiitis obliterans, IBD, sarcoidosis
  - Infection 6 to 12% (orbital cellulitis, sinusitis)
  - Head injury and mechanical precipitants - less common
  - No identified cause (over 65 years old, 37% of time there is no identified cause)
- **Diagnosis**
  - MRI brain with MR venography imaging of choice
  - Head CT with CT venography (alternate option)
  - If diagnostic studies inconclusive and suspicion is high = angiography
- CT head non-contrast = delta sign
- CT head with contrast = empty delta sign
- **Treatment:** anticoagulation

NEUROLOGY PEARLS

- SLE CNS manifestations = seizures, CVA, psychosis, migraines and peripheral neuropathy
- Initial work-up of CSF shunt malfunction = CT head and shunt series (consider in any patient with shunt and decreased LOC)
- Back pain with neuro symptoms consider: Malignancy or Hematoma
  ↑ hyperreflexia, sensory > weakness, clonus and Babinski ddx = MS (consider adding brain MRI)
- Common etiologies of spinal subarachnoid hemorrhage = AVM, tumors and anticoagulation

- **DeCORticate** posturing: hyperextension of legs with flexion of the arms; remember arms are in flexion with hands over the heart ("**cor**") in de "**cor**"ticate posturing – results from damage to the descending motor pathways above the central midbrain
- **Decerebrate** posturing: hyperextension of both upper and lower extremities – refers to damage to the midbrain and upper pons; is a grave sign
- The most common cause of **delirium** in the elderly = medications, 22-39% of cases.
  Delirium symptom onset acute vs **dementia** progressive over months. Alterations in sleep-wake cycles are common
  Delirium = various hallucinations (visual, auditory, olfactory, tactile, gustatory) vs
  Functional Psychosis patient who only experience auditory hallucinations
  EEG = abnormal; bilateral diffuse symmetric abnormalities; relative generalized slowing with or without superimposed fast activity
- One of the hallmarks of **Acute Delirium** = short-term memory impairment; remote memory preserved
- **Post-traumatic seizures:** more common PEDS > adults; if dura disrupted the incidence of seizures with neuro deficits ↑; incidence of seizures ↑ than general population

CAUSES OF MICROCYTIC HYPOCHROMIC ANEMIAS

Mnemonic - (TAILS) [ANK, provided by Dr. Matt Jordan]

T	**T**halassemia
A	**A**nemia of chronic disease
I	**I**ron deficiency
L	**L**ead Poisoning
S	**S**ideroblastic

PEARL: Major cause of anemia worldwide = hookworm infection (Necator americanus); infective flatworm larva penetrate skin → adult worms penetrate into intestinal mucosa and feed → luminal blood loss - iron deficiency anemia due to ongoing loss of blood

CAUSES OF MACROCYTIC ANEMIA

Mnemonic - (FAB 5 Non-SHAM) (please do not call U. of Michigan's Fab 5 a Sham)

F	**F**olate deficiency
A	**A**lcohol abuse
B	**B**12 (cobalamin) deficiency
5	**5** other causes (Non-SHAM)

NON	**Non**-alcoholic fatty liver disease
S	**S**plenectomy
H	**H**ypothyroidism
A	***A**dverse medication effects
M	**M**yelodyspasia

*Long list of medications: HIV medications, anticonvulsants (Valproic acid and Phenytoin), Trimethoprim/sulfamethoxazole (TMP/SMX), Methotrexate (folate antagonist), chemotherapeutics and Metformin (↓B12 absorption)

Other causes: renal disease, down syndrome and chronic obstructive pulmonary disease

CAUSES OF THROMBOCYTOSIS

Mnemonic (PCP PCP PCP HIM NUTI)

P	**P**ost trauma
C	**C**ML (Chronic myelogenous leukemia)
P	**P**ost hemorrhage

P	**P**ostpartum
C	**C**irrhosis
P	**P**ost-splenectomy

P	**P**ancreatitis
C	**C**ollagen vascular Disease
P	**P**olycythemia vera
H	**H**emolytic anemia
I	**I**nfections (TB, acute bacterial and viral)
M	**M**yocardial infarction

N	**N**eoplasm (GI)
U	**U**nder Fe (iron deficiency)
T	**T**hermal burns
I	**I**BD

M	**M**etastatic cancer
A	**A**llergic Reactions
N	**N**ephrotic syndrome

CAUSES OF EOSINOPHILIA

Mnemonic - (NAAACP)

N	**N**eoplasms
A	**A**llergy
A	**A**sthma
A	**A**ddison's
C	**C**ollagen vascular disease (CVD)*
P	**P**arasites

*CVDs: systemic lupus erythematosus (SLE), rheumatoid arthritis (RA), progressive systemic sclerosis (PSS) or scleroderma (SD), dermatomyositis (DM) and polymyositis (PM), ankylosing spondylitis (AS), Sjögren syndrome (SS), and mixed connective-tissue disease (MCTD)

Churg-Strauss syndrome (CSS), or allergic granulomatous angiitis = **Eosinophilia**
Granulomatosis with polyangitis (GPA) (Formerly called Wegener's), another ANCA vasculitic syndrome similar to CSS however, **eosinophilia is absent** in GPA

THROMBOTIC THROMBOCYTOPENIC PURPURA (TTP)

Mnemonic - (FAT RN)

F	**F**ever in 90%
A	**A**nemia – Microangiopathic hemolytic anemia (MAHA) – schistocytes on smear
T	**T**hrombocytopenia
R	**R**enal failure
N	**N**eurologic sequelae (HA, confusion, CN palsies, seizures and coma)

- **Causes**: Pregnancy, AIDS, Autoimmune diseases (SLE, Scleroderma, Sjogren Syndrome); Cyclosporin, quinidine, tacrolimus
- Women > Men
- Pentad only present in 40%
- ↑LDH, ↑IBIL, ↑Reticulocyte count, ↓haptoglobin, ↑Cr, normal DIC panel
- Abdominal pain
- Affect any age but majority 10 to 40 years
- Women 60% of cases
- 1/3 of patients who survive initial episode experience relapse within 10 years
- Survival rate = 80-90% with early diagnosis and treatment. 95% MR with no treatment
- **Treatment**: Intravenous (IV) plasma exchange, also called plasmapheresis and IV steroids

PRIMARY IMMUNE THROMBOCYTOPENIC PURPURA

Formerly Idiopathic Thrombocytopenic Purpura (ITP)

- Self-limiting pediatric variant and chronic adult variant
- Patients having antibodies to platelet membrane glycoproteins
- Most often in children (usually 2 to 6 yrs); male = female; follows viral infection
- Usually **isolated** thrombocytopenia; M&M low; recovery may take weeks
- **Treatment** is supportive as the course is self limited with 90% spontaneous remission
- Platelet count < 20,000μL require treatment steroids + IV gamma globulin (IVIG) or Anti-D immunoglobulin
- Asymptomatic patients with platelets > 20,000/μl = Observation
- Platelet count < 50,000 μL with bleeding *or* risk factors for bleeding require treatment
- Add conjugated estrogen 25 mg IV x once if uterine bleeding
- Splenectomy in refractory cases (rarely needed)
- **Treatment option in Chronic Immune Thrombocytopenia (ITP):** colony -stimulating factor medication Romiplostim (Nplate)

HEMOLYTIC UREMIC SYNDROME (HUS)

Pediatric variant of TTP with bloody diarrhea and AKI as the predominant findings.
Use TTP Mnemonic with Pearls below:

- Can occur at any age however majority of cases < 5 years old
- Low grade fever 5-20%; abdominal pain, vomiting and bloody diarrhea, seizures, lethargy
- Renal manifestations more prominent than neurologic ones in HUS vs TTP
- 15% children vs 5% adults infected with *E. coli* O157:H7 go on to develop HUS
- Infection with *E. coli* O157:H7 should *not* be treated w/ antimotility drugs or antibiotics → ↑risk HUS
- E. Coli 0157:H7 produces Shiga-like toxin → toxin damages endothelial cells in the colon and kidney
- Other causes: Salmonela, Shigella, Step pneumonias, HIV, drug toxicity
- If CNS Involvement severe = Eculizumab (Soliris) monoclonal antibody therapy; otherwise treatment is supportive. No evidence that early dialysis affects clinical outcome. Indications for dialysis affects clinical outcome. Indications for dialysis in children with HUS are similar to those in children withother forms of AKI
- **TRIAD**
  1. MAHA (abnormal RBCs: schistocytes, spherocytes, segmented RBCs, burr cells and helmet cells)
  2. Thrombocytopenia (result of extensive microthromboses)
  3. Kidney failure (Most common cause of AKI in children)

3 CATEGORIES OF TRANSPLANT REJECTION

- **Hyperacute:** Occurs minutes to hours post-transplant; irreversible graft destruction, due to preformed antibodies
- **Acute**: Occurs 1-12 weeks post-transplant; humoral/T-cell mediated
- **Chronic:** Progressive with an insidious rejection: months-years post-transplant

TRANSPLANT PROBLEM PEARLS

- Cyclosporine toxicity: hyperkalemia, nephrotoxicity
- Azathioprine toxicity: BM suppression, hepatotoxicity, pancreatitis
- Graft Versus Host Disease (GVHD): Post allogeneic BMT, rash, diarrhea
- Renal transplant rejection: increased creatinine, tenderness over graft site, decreased urine output, fever
- Lung transplant rejection: cough, chest tightness
- Heart transplant rejection: fatigue, HF, no angina/CP
- Liver transplant rejection: fever, abnormal LFTs, RUQ pain
- Transplant rejection treatment: steroids

METS TO BONE

Mnemonic - (Many Kinds of Tumors Leaping Promptly To Bone)

Many	**M**ultiple **M**yelomas
Kinds	**K**idney
Of	**O**vary
Tumors	**T**esticular
Leaping	**L**ung **L**ymphoma
Promptly	**P**rostate
To	**T**hyroid
Bone	**B**reast

METASTATIC SPINAL CORD COMPRESSION

- Most common malignancies associated with spinal cord compression = Multiple myeloma, lung, breast and prostate
- Most common site of malignant spinal cord compression = thoracic vertebrae 70% > Cervical > lumbar; Most common site of metastasis on thoracic vertebrae = pedicles
- Most common symptom of spinal cord compression = pain; Back pain present in 90%; worse at night and worse recumbent position
- Most common early finding of spinal cord compression = motor weakness. Motor deficits > sensory deficits
- Urinary retention more common than bowel dysfunction
- Check CT, MRI or myelogram; Treatment options = steroids, radiation and surgery
- Emergent MRI = Gold standard for diagnosis; metastatic lesion can be seen on x-ray 50-70% of the time
- **PEARL**: In traumatic spinal cord injury - ATLS does not endorse steroids

HEME /ONC PEARLS

- **CANCER WITH JVD & DYSPNEA**
  - **Superior vena cava syndrome** = facial plethora, dilated veins chest/arms (caput medusae), HA
  - Most common cause = Small (oat) cell lung CA > bronchogenic (squamous) cell lung CA > lymphoma; CXR: right sided mass; consider: radiation, steroids, lasix, endovascular shunts, and thrombolytics if thrombotic etiology
  - **Cardiac tamponade;** Neoplasm is the most common cause of cardiac tamponade; Beck's Triad: JVD, hypotension, distant heart sounds
  - **Massive PE** → acute cor pulmonale; also ↓BP

- **CANCER WITH BACK PAIN**
  - **Spinal cord compression**
  - Most common: Prostate, thyroid, breast, lung, renal CA, multiple myeloma and lymphoma; Best prognosis with multiple myelemoa and lymphoma
  - If ambulatory prior to treatment 70% will remain ambulatory
  - If paralyzed prior to treatment <10% will walk again
  - **Treatment**: Decadron 10mg IV, radiation

- **CANCER WITH PARANEOPLASTIC SYNDROMES**
  - ↓Na+ → SIADH (euvolemic hyponatremia); small cell Lung CA
  - ↓Ca2+ → Calcitonin
  - ↑Ca2+ → Parathormone → "Stones (kidney), Abdominal groans (constipation, N/V, anorexia, pancreatitis), Psychic moans (mental status changes, seizures, coma) Bones (pain)"
  - ↑ACTH → Cushing syndrome (↑ cortisol), ↑Na+, ↓K+, (small cell Lung CA)
  - ↑ACTH → Gonadotropins / gynecomastia
  - ↑Serotonin → Carcinoid syndrome
  - Thymoma → ↑ acetylcholine receptor antibodies → Myasthenia gravis
  - Lambert-Eaton myasthenic syndrome (LEMS) → autoimmune attack on pre-synaptic motor nerve voltage-gated calcium channels (VGCC) → decrease in amount of acetylcholine in synapse → proximal muscle weakness, ↓DTR's & autonomic changes → (small cell Lung CA)
  - If ambulatory prior to treatment 70% will remain ambulatory
  - If paralyzed prior to treatment < 10% will walk again

- **Fever of unknown origin (FUO) consider malignancy** → lymphomas, acute leukemias, sarcomas, renal cell carcinomas, GI malignancies
  - FUO requires:
    - Temperature > 38.3° C (101° F) on several occasions
    - More than 3 weeks duration of illness
    - Failure to reach diagnosis despite 1 week of inpatient investigation
    -

HYPERVISCOSITY SYNDROME

- Hyperviscosity syndrome leads to end organ ischemia (stroke, mesenteric), blurred vision, HA, CHF; Retinal changes in hyperviscosity syndrome = "sausage-link" or "boxcar" segmentation
- **Polycythemia Vera** is a myeloproliferative neoplastic disease = elevated red blood cell mass; facial plethora (ruddy cyanosis), gouty arthritis, thrombosis, CRVO, fatigue, Aquagenic Pruitus (pruritius after warm bath or shower); HTN, splenomegaly
  - **Emergent treatment** of hyperviscosity syndrome secondary to symptomatic Polycythemia Vera: phlebotomy, (not more than 500 ml of blood is removed and the volume is replaced with an equal volume of normal saline), ASA and Hydroxyurea
- **Hyperviscosity Syndromes with Blast Crisis:** Multiple Myeloma (Increase IgG or IgA) and Waldenstrom's Macroglobulinemia (Increase IgM) (sludge immunoglobulins) and Leukemia (sludge WBC's)
  - **Treatment options:** Hydration is critical; dysproteinemias: plasmaphoresis; Blast transformations: leukaphoresis
- **PEARL:** Waldenstrom's macroglobulinemia (increased IgM) = most common cause of hyperviscosity syndrome

TUMOR LYSIS SYNDROME (TLS)

- Oncological emergency
- Massive tumor cell lysis and subsequent release of intracellular contents during the initiation of chemotherapy (Onset = 1 to 5 days after chemotherapy)
- The most common malignancies involved are:
  Aggressive lymphomas (especially Burkitt lymphoma)
  Leukemias = most common

Hallmark of TLS

a) Protein dreakdown = HYPER-**phosphatemia** → leads to HYPO-**calcemia** (calcium-phosphate precipitation) → muscle cramps and tetany and acute kidney injury (AKI)
b) DNA breakdown = HYPER-**uricemia** → leads to AKI
c) Cytosol breakdown = HYPER-**kalemia** → leads cardiac dysrhythmias and arrest

PEARL: Renal failure = strongest predictor of mortality
PEARL: Renal failure = secondary to deposition of uric acid and/or calcium phosphate crystals

TUMOR LYSIS SYNDROME (TLS)

Treatment

a) Aggressive hydration (consider diuretics if urine output not maintained or fluid overload occurs)
b) Hyperuricemia management: Rasburicase; consider allopurinol only in patients with contraindications to rasburicase such as G6PD deficiency
c) Treat hyperkalemia (caution with calcium - avoid calcium-phosphate precipitation and worsen AKI)
d) Early dialysis improves prognosis for AKI (rapidly reduce serum uric acid phosphate)
e) Urine alkalinization not routinely recommended
f) Symptomatic hypocalcemia: calcium gluconate; aysmptomatic hypocalcemia - no treatment

VON WILLEBRAND'S DISEASE (VWD)

von Willebrand factor is a glycoprotein that when activated plays an important role in hemostasis by:

- Forming adhesive bridges between platelets
- Forming adhesive bridges with subendothelial structures
- Contributes to fibrin clot formation (carries Factor VIII)
- Most common inherited bleeding disorder (autosomal dominant)

von Willebrand Disease results from:

- Type 1 - Decrease production of normal quantity of vWF (will also have low Factor VIII)
- Type 2 - From the production of dysfunctional vWF
- Type 3 - No production of of vWF (will also have low Factor VIII)
- Clinical: easy bleeding, skin bleeding, prolonged bleeding from mucosal surfaces (gums, GI, uterine)
- **PEARL:** Most common cause of vaginal bleeding related to primary coagulation disorder von Willebrand's disease

von Willebrand Disease Lab Findings

- Bleeding time = Increased
- vWF activity = Decreased
- Factor VIII activity = Decreased
- Platelet count = Normal
- PT/INR = Normal
- PTT = Normal (unless very low Factor VIII (Type 3) then → Increased)

Treatment

- Treatment of mild bleeding in von Willebrand's disease: Desmoprssin (DDAVP)
- Treatment of severe bleeding in von Willebrand's disease Cryoprecipitate Factor VIII 25 to 50 units /kg; + DDAVP

SICKLE CELL

ACUTE CHEST SYNDROME

- Infiltrate/infarcts, fever, cough, dyspnea, wheezing, hypoxia and chest pain
- Most common cause of death in sickle cell patient in U.S. (12% mortality)
- Most common cause of Acute Chest Syndrome = Mycoplasma and Chlamydia pneumonia
- Previously Strep pneumonia was the most common cause, however with pneumococcal vaccines and PCN prophylaxis *S. pneumo* rarely cause
- **Treatment**
  - Antibiotics - cover typical & atypical organisms (*Chlamydia pneumoniae*)
  - Fluid, pain management
  - Oxygenation
  - Exchange transfusion

ACUTE ISCHEMIC STROKE

- **Treatment**
  - Exchange transfusion (may also decrease stroke recurrence)

APLASTIC CRISIS

- Decrease in RBC production, rapid decline in hemoglobin
- Most common cause = Parvovirus B19, single stranded DNA virus, spread = respiratory droplets
- 30-60% patients with SCD get infected causing aplastic crisis
- **Diagnosis**
  - Pallor, fatigue, lethargy, SOB
  - Low hemoglobin level
  - Reticulocyte count = 0
- **Treatment**
  - Usually self limiting
  - Resolves after a week
  - Supportive care
  - +/- PRBC transfusion

SICKLE CELL VASO-OCCLUSIVE PAIN CRISIS

- Sickled cells lead to tissue infarcts and vascular occlusion
- **Treatment**: Determine source, pain control, hydration, hydroxyurea correcting hypoxemia

SPLENIC SEQUESTRATION

- Abdominal pain, splenomegaly, pallor and shock; 6months to 6 years
- Very low hemoglobin Reticulocytosis
- **Treatment**: Supportive; PRBC transfusion; Splenectomy

OTHER SICKLE CELL COMPLICATIONS

- **SEPSIS**
  - Antibiotics to cover encapsulated organisms

- **CHOLECYSTITIS**
  - Biliary stones from increased hemolysis
  - Cholecystectomy

- **PRIAPISM**
  - Aspiration; Exchange transfusion

- **AVASCULAR NECROSIS**
  - Most commonly occurs in femoral head followed by head of the humerus, knee, and small joints of the hands and feet
  - 40%-80% of cases of hip avascular necrosis are bilateral
  - Conservative management 4 to 6 months
  - Surgical options
  - a) Core decompression
  - b) Arthroplasty

EXCHANGE TRANSFUSION IN SICKLE CELL DISEASE

- Retinal infarction
- Stroke
- Priapism
- Pulmonary infarction

MASSIVE TRANSFUSION PROTOCOLS (MTP)

- Single unit of packed red blood cells (PRBC's) will increase hemoglobin 1g/dl and hematocrit 3%
- Blood:FFP:Platelet ratio
  - 1:1:1 probably best but 2:1:1 also ok
- Massive transfusions complications
  - Hypothermiaa
  - Hyperkalemia
  - Hypocalcemia
  - DIC
  - TRALI (transfusion related acute lung injury)
- Consider tranexamic acid to stabilize clots in massive transfusions
- Tranexamic acid (TXA): synthetic analog of the amino acid lysine
  Antifibrinolytic that reversibly binds to lysine receptor sites on plasminogen. This reduces conversion of plasminogen → plasmin → prevents fibrin degradation

TRANSFUSION COMPLICATIONS

1. **Acute hemolytic reaction:** due to ABO incompatibility; Immediate fever, chills, HA, back pain, hypotension, oliguria, dark urine and DIC; most commonly due to clerical errors. Stop transfusion, vigorous crystalloid infusion, diuretic therapy to maintain urine output
   PEARL: Most common cause of acute hemolytic transfusion reactions = transfuse wrong blood due to clerical error

2. **Febrile nonhemolytic transfusion reaction (FNHTR):** antibodies to donor WBCs and plasma proteins; fever, chills and malaise during or within a few hours of a blood transfusion.Use of leukocyte reduced packed red blood cells (PRBC) can reduce the incidence of recurrence; pretreatment with antipyretics. Most common transfusion reaction

3. **Allergic Reaction:** IgE mediated, urticaria or hives; treatment supportive antihistamines; antibody mediated response to donor's plasma

4. **Transfusion-related acute lung injury (TRALI):** Indistinguishable from ARDS; stop transfusion, supportive care; no evidence for diuretics or steroids

5. **Transfusion-associated graft vs host disease (GVHD):** immunocompromised patients, rash, pancytopenia, increased LFTs; stop transfusion, supportive care
   Prevention = use irradiated blood products in immunocompromised patients

6. **Disease transmission**
   Yersinia more stable in refrigerated blood
   HIV 1 per 2 million units
   HCV 1 per 1 million units
   HBV 1 per 350,000 units
   Chagas problem in South America
   West Nile Virus

HEME/ONC PEARLS

- Vitamin K dependent factors = II, VII, IX, X
- Extrinsic pathway and Common Pathways = Measured by PT/INR
- Intrinsic Pathway = Measured by PTT
- Extrinsic Pathway Coagulation factor = Factor VII
- Common Pathway Coagulation Factors I, II, V, and X (remember 1 x 2 x 5 = 10)
- **Fresh Frozen Plasma (FFP)**: Is the fluid portion of a unit of whole blood that is frozen in a designated time frame, usually within 8 hours. FFP contains all cogulation factors, fibrinogen, albumin, protein C, protein S, antithrombin
- **Cryoprecipitate contains**: vWF, Fibrinogen, Factor VIII and Factor XIII and fibronectin. Reserved for conditions with increased consumption and/or loss of fibrinogen: DIC or massive hemorrhage (trauma, OB, GI bleed); also used in the management of uremia-induced platelet dysfunction **PEARL**: Risk of transmission of infectious diseases (HIV, HBV or HCV) is significantly less with cryopercipitate vs. FFP
- **Prothrombin Complex Concentrate (PCC)** (trade name Kcentra Beriplex or Octaplex) contains: Vitamin K dependant coagulation factors II, VII, IX and X as well as protein C and S
- **PEARL:** PCC4 (Kcentra) contains heparin - screen for heparin allergy or history of heparin-induced thrombocytopenia before administration
- **Desmopressin (DDAVP)** = synthetic analog of vasopressin — DDAVP causes the release of stored von Willebrand factor and factor VIII from enothelial cells and platelets
  - vWF can inrease factor VIII by 3-5x (onset 30 minutes)
  - Dose: 0.3 mcg/kg/dose IV
  - vWF is also required for normal platelet adhesion
- **Hemophilia A** = **most common cause of hemophilia** in the US; 1 in 5,000 male births; Genetic deficiency in clotting Factor VIII: (↑ PTT)
- **Hemophilia B** = Christmas disease; Factor IX deficiency; 1 in 30,000 male births; (↑ PTT)
- Hemophilia A and B = X-linked recessive disorder – therefore a disease of men
- Intracranial hemorrhage is the most common noninfectious cause of death in hemophiliacs
- **Treatment of non-traumatic hemarthrosis in Hemophilia A patient**
  - Desmoprssin (DDAVP) or if N/A give Factor VIII 12.5 U/kg
  - Most patients will require 25 U/kg every 24 hours x 2-3 days for most bleeds
  - If severe bleeding, Factor VIII 50 U/kg
  - **PEARL**: 1 unit/kg of Factor VIII leads to a rise in plasma factor VIII of approximately 2%. EXAMPLE: 50 units/kg will increase factor VIII level by approximately 100%
- **Treatment of uremia-induced platelet dysfunction (missed dialysis = hyper-uremia)**
  - Desmopressin (DDAVP) and cryoprecipitate
  - 1 unit of platelets will increase platelet count 5-10,000 in adults
  - Ask for **single-donor platelets** when possible (contain the equivalent of 6 units of random donor platelet concentrates)
  - Pediatric patients: 5 ml/kg body weight of a random donor platelet concentration should increase the platelet count by 5,000/uL
  - When platelet levels decrease < 20,000/uL = concerned about risk of spontaneous bleeding
  - Pediatric patients: FFP 10-15 mL/kg of body weight will increase factor levels by 15-25%

PLATELET FUNCTION

Mnemonic - AAA - A

A	Adhere
A	Activate
A	Aggregate

A	Arterial clot formation (platelet plug results in arterial clot)

PEARL: Fibrin strands, end product from coagulation cascade, serve as the mesh that stabilize the platelet plug in an arterial clot

DISSEMINATED INTRAVASCULAR COAGULATION (DIC)

- Massive release of tissue factor (TF) into the circulation → widespread inappropriate activation of the coagulation system → small vessel thrombosis, consumption of clotting factors & platelets → hemorrhage
- Most common cause of DIC = Infection
- Other causes: amniotic fluid embolism, placental abruption, metastatic malignancy, sepsis, trauma, snake envenomation
- DIC Labs
  - PT, PTT, FDPs bleeding time = INCREASED
  - Platelets and fibrinogen = DECREASED
  - Peripheral smear = Schistocytes, helmet cells (MAHA)
- **Management**
  - Management priority: treat the underlying cause
  - FFP (elevated PT or aPTT > 1.5 or fibrinogen < 100 mg/dL)
  - Cryoprecipitate for the replacement fibrinogen
  - Platelets (if < 50,000/mm3 and active bleeding)
  - Packed red blood cells to maintain hemodynamics
  - Heparin or LMWH has selective use in DIC when fibrin deposits and thrombosis predominate; TXA should be considered in trauma related DIC

NEUTROPENIA

- Neutropenia absolute neutrophil count (ANC) < 500 cells/mcL
  - ANC = WBC count x % Total Neutrophils
  - Neutropenic Fever = neutropenia + Fever
  - Fever
    - Single oral temperature > 38.3°C (100.9°F)
    - Temperature > 38.0°C (100.4°F) sustained for > 1 hour
  - Greatest risk for developing neutropenic fever = 7 to 14 days after last chemotherapy session (corresponds to nadir in white blood cells after chemo treatment)
  - Most common cause of infectious neutropenic fever = bacteria, particularly gram-positive organisms
  - **Treatment**
    - Broad-spectrum antibiotics: cefepime, meropenem, imipenem-cilastatin, ceftazidime, or piperacillin-tazobactam + Vancomycin

LEUKEMIA

- Most common childhood cancer
- Can present with symptoms similar to other more common pediatric viral or bacterial illnesses
- FUO, petechiae, organomegaly (liver/spleen),
- Acute lymphoblastic leukemia (ALL) is the most common type of leukemia

MULTIPLE MYELOMA

Mnemonic - CRA(B)3

- Neoplastic proliferation of plasma cells in the bone marrow resulting in a monoclonal immunoglobulin
- Most common symptom = bone pain (from proliferation of plasma cells in the bone marrow)

C	**C**alcium elevated: (moans (AMS), groans (GI symptoms), stones (kidney), bones (pain - mainly back and ribs)
R	**R**enal insufficiency: deposition of monoclonal light chains (Bence Jones proteins) & hypercalcemia
A	**A**nemia: normochromic, normocytic; fatigue, pallor, generalized weakness; bleeding
B	**B**one lesions; lytic lesions ("punched out" lesions); pathologic fractures
B	**B**one pain
B	**B**ence Jones proteins (seen on protein electrophoresis urine analysis)

- **Electrolyte abnormalities**
  - HyperCalcemia
  - HyperUricemia
  - HypoKalemia
  - Peripheral blood smear: Rouleaux formations
  - **Treatment**: chemotherapy and autologous hematopoietic cell transplantation

ANTIPHOSPHOLIPID ANTIBODY SYNDROME

- Acquired
- Autoimmune
- Causes a hypercoagulable state
- Patient with a history of systemic lupus erythematosus (SLE) or other rheumatic diseases
- "1 in 5 rule"
  - 1 in 5 patients = younger than age 45 with stroke
  - 1 in 5 patients = deep vein thromboses (DVT)
  - 1 in 5 patients with recurrent pregnancy loss will test positive for antiphospholipid antibodies
- Recurrent DVTs
- Recurrent spontaneous abortions
- Recurrent cerebrovascular events, particularly in young people
- Thrombocytopenia
- 1% of patients with antiphospholipid antibody syndrome develop a rapidly progressive life-threatening form = **catastrophic antiphospholipid antibody syndrome**; Despite treatment, the mortality of catastrophic antiphospholpid antibody syndrome (CAPS) = 50%
- **Treatment:** anticoagulation

SYSTEMIC LUPUS ERYTHEMATOSUS (SLE)

Diagnosed when 4 of the SOAP BRAIN MD criteria are met

S	**S**erositis (Pleuritis more common > pericarditis; least common = peritonitis)
O	**O**ropharyngeal ulcers
A	**A**rthralgias (most common symptom) at least 2 peripheral joints
P	**P**hotosensitivity
B	**B**lood disorders (leukopenia, thrombocytopenia, and hemolysis)
R	**R**enal disorders (proteinuria or kidney injury)
A	**A**nti-nuclear antibody (ANA) positive
I	**I**mmuno-serology testing (anti-dsDNA, anti-Smith, anti-histone antibodies positive)
N	**N**eurological symptoms (Seizures, CVA, psychosis, migraines and peripheral neuropathy; psychiatric abnormalities)

M	**M**alar ("butterfly") rash
D	**D**iscoid rash

- African American more common; present with fever, lymphadenopathy, weight loss,malaise or arthritis
- Recurrent miscarriages
- Chronic arthralgias
- **Treatment:** NSAIDs, steroids, immunosuppressants, hydroxychloroquine

GLUCOSE-6-PHOSPHATE DEHYDROGENASE (G6PD) DEFICIENCY

- Most common human enzyme defect = deficiency of RBC enzyme Glucose-6-phosphate dehydrogenase (G-6-PD)
- Most common enzymatic disorder of red blood cells
- Enzyme found on X-chromosome; X-linked recessive
- Affects > 400 million people worldwide
- Common in Kurdish Jews (60-70%) > Sardinians (4-35%) > Nigerians (22%) > Thai (17%) > African Americans (12%) and Greeks (6%); lowest Japanese/Koreans (0-1%)
- G6PD catalyzes the initial step in the hexose monophosphate (HMP) shunt (also called pentose phosphate shunt)
- The main function of the HMP shunt is to protect RBCs against oxidative injury via the production of NADPH (HMP shunt is the only RBC source of NADPH)
- NADPH is an important cofactor in glutathione metabolism
- Deficiency in G6PD leads to less NADH production → leads to decrease in glutathione (destroyer of free radicals) → Hemolytic anemia once exposed to oxidative stressors
- Oxidant stress → hemolytic anemia, renal failure, low platelets

- **"Oxidant stressors"**
  - Antimalarials (primaquine), dapsone and anti-uricemic drugs rasburicase (Elitek) and pegloticase (Krystexxa) = most common
  - Naphthalene (mothballs, lavatory deodorant), nitrofurantoin, amyl nitrate, phenazopyridine (Pyridium), methylene blue (Methylthioninium chloride), chlorpropamide (Diabinese), dabrafenib (Tafinlar); fava beans ("favism"); infections; metabolic acidosis (DKA), sulfas
- **Presentation:** HA / N / F / C /, abdominal pain, back pain, dark urine, pallor, hemoglobinuria and jaundice; present within 24 hours
- **Labs:**
  - Anemia (could be remarkably severe or mild) and hemoglobinuria; **"bite cells", "blister cells"** and **Heinz bodies** (denatured globin chains attached RBC membrane) on peripheral smear; elevated LDH; elevated indirect bilirubin, reticulocyte count elevated, haptoglobin decreased
  - Direct or indirect demonstration of reduced G6PD activity in erythrocytes
- Self limited because only the older RBC's hemolyze

PORPHYRIAS

- Porphyrias are metabolic disorders caused by altered activities of enzymes within the heme biosynthetic pathway
- Altered enzyme activity is due to an inherited mutation in the gene for that enzyme (there are 8 enzymes that can be affected)
- The most notable exception is the most common of the porphyrias, porphyria cutanea tarda (PCT), which is caused by acquired inhibition of uroporphyrinogen decarboxylase (UROD)

Three most common Porphyrias can be divided into 3 categories based on symptoms

1. Type of Porphyria: **Acute Intermittent Porphyria (AIP)**
   - Clinical Category: Acute neurovisceral
   - Symptoms: abdominal pain, CP, back pain, N/V/ constipation; Weakness, motor and sensory peripheral neuropathy, psychiatric changes

2. Type of Porphyria: **Porphyria Cutanea Tarda (PCT)** = Most common porphyria in adults
   - Clinical Category: Chronic blistering cutaneous
   - Symptoms: Cutaneous photosensitivity - blistering, scarring and altered pigmentation

3. Type of Porphyria: **Erythropoietic ProtoPorphyria (EPP)** = Most common porphyria in children; third most common porphyria in adults
   - Clinical Category: Acute NON-blistering cutaneous
   - Symptoms: Pain with sun exposed skin, within minutes of sun exposure, erythema/swelling, no blisters or scarring

CONGENITAL HEART DISEASE - CYANOTIC

Most common indicators of a Congenital Heart Disease (CHD)

- Poor feeding
- Sweating with feeds
- Irritability
- Unexplained HTN
- Hepatomegaly
- Pathologic murmur

Right-to-left shunt

Deoxygenated blood from the right side of the heart enters the systemic circulation; An anatomic shunt (i.e., congenital cyanotic heart disease), allows deoxygenated blood to bypass the lungs and directly enters the systemic circulation. The hallmark of right-to-left shunt is that supplemental oxygen fails to increase arterial oxygen levels

Uncorrected left-to-right shunt

VSD, ASD or patent ductus arteriosus (PDA), can eventually become a right-to-left shunt, a phenomenon known as Eisenmenger's syndrome. This occurs when increased pulmonary blood flow from a left-to-right shunt leads to pulmonary hypertension and compensatory right ventricular hypertrophy, and, over time, right ventricular pressures surpass left ventricular pressures, resulting in a change in direction of the shunt

Mnemonic - (5 Terrible T's)

Right to left shunts causing early cyanosis

The hallmark of right-to-left shunt is that supplemental oxygen fails to increase arterial oxygen levels

T	**T**runcus Arteriosus (single arterial trunk exits ventricular portion of heart)
T	**T**ransposition of the Great Vessels Most common cause of cyanosis or CHF within the first **3 days** of life Aorta originates from RV and pulmonary artery from the LV TGA = aorta rises from the RV and the PA LA. Therefore, the two sides of the heart work in parallel rather than in series. The defect is incompatible with life unless there is a coexisting ASD, VSD or PDA) that creates life-saving left-to-right shunt. Most common cause of cyanosis in the first week of life and is more common in males and children of diabetic mothers
T	**T**ricuspid Valve Atresia Absence of TV, hypoplastic RV and VSD Small VSD's are dependent on the Ductus Arteriosus for Pulmonary blood flow Prostaglandin E1 (PGE1) can be life saving Side effects of PGE = apnea, bradycardia and hypotension
T	**T**etralogy of Fallot (Most common cyanotic congenital heart disease in kids > **4y/o**)
T	**T**otal Anomalous Pulmonary Venous Return (T-A-P V-R)

When trying to remember the 5 T's think of counting the fingers on your hand
[ANK from Drs. Lisa McQueen, Nathan Allen] From Nicole Colucci

1 finger	One arterial trunk exits the ventricle (Truncus Arteriosus)
2 fingers	Cross middle finger over index finger) = 2 vessels transposed Transposition of the Great Vessels
3 fingers	Tricuspid Valve Atresia (3 = Tri)
4 fingers	Tetralogy of Fallot (4 = Tetra)
5 fingers	Palm open all (total) fingers up = Total Anomalous Pulmonary Venous Return Also, 5 = 5 words (T-A-P V-R)

TETRALOGY OF FALLOT

Mnemonic - (POSH

P	**P**ulmonary stenosis (RV outflow tract obstruction - RVOTO)
O	**O**verriding aorta (Dextroposition of the aorta); the aortic valve is situated above the VSD with biventricular connection (connected to both the RV and LV)
S	**S**eptal defect - VSD
H	**H**ypertrophy – RV

- CXR = boot-shaped heart (caused by right ventricular hypertrophy (RVH) and an upturned cardiac apex ECG - Right axis deviation
- Unrepaired cyanosis congenital heart disease, antibiotic prophylaxis is administered to prevent bacterial endocarditis until surgical correction is performed.
- **PEARL:** VSD = Most Common Congenital Heart lesion
- Smaller VSD = worse; Bigger VSD = more blood mixing
- Murmur = harsh SEM , with single second heart sound

MANAGEMENT OF HYPERCYANOTIC OR TET SPELL

Mnemonic - (4P's) [ANK from Dr. Angela McCormick]

- **P**osition - Knees to chest or squatting → ↑ venous return to heart and ↑ SVR
- Increases SVR → promotes movement of blood from the right ventricle into the pulmonary circulation rather then the Aorta. The increase in venous return → increase in preload → improves RV filling → improves pulmonary flow
- **P**ain control - O2 and Morphine 0.2 mg/kg SQ or IM per dose → calms the child
- Propranolol 0.05 to 0.1 mg/kg IV or Esmolol (with consultation) Relaxes infundibular muscle spasm that causes RVOTO → Improves pulmonary blood flow
- **P**henylephrine 10 μg /kg bolus followed by infusion 2 to 5 μg/kg/min
 → ↑ SVR → ↑ BP Increases afterload which promotes RV flow into the pulmonary circulation rather than the aorta
- Oxygen = pulmonary vasodialator, systemic vasoconstrictor
- Bicarbonate 1mEq/kg → reverses the acidosis → decreases RR and cardiac effort
- Fluid boluses

If hypercyanotic episode is not recognized and treated early it may be fatal. Other complications = seizures, cerebral thrombosis, profound lactic acidosis and cardiac dysrhythmias

CONGENITAL DISORDER	CV MANIFESTATIONS
Downs	Atrial Septal Defect (ASD) SEM at left sternal border *Left to right* intra-cardiac shunt; present > 6 month = CHF
Turners	Coarctation of the aorta (↓pulse LEs, HTN UEs, SEM at cardiac base radiates → interscapula) = CHF Harsh SEM, radiates from left axilla (cardiac base) to the back
Rubella	Patient ductus arteriosus (PDA) *Left to right* intra-cardiac shunt; present < 6 months = CHF

TRICUSPID VALVE ATRESIA

- Absence of TV, hypoplastic RV and VSD
- Small VSD's are dependent on the Ductus Arteriosus for Pulmonary blood flow
- Prostaglandin E1 (PGE1) can be life saving
- Side effects of PGE = apnea, bradycardia and hypotension
- TGA = aorta rises from the RV and the PA LA. Sherry add this to Congenital HD Box
- Therefore, the two sides of the heart work in parallel rather than in series
- The defect is incompatible with life unless there is a coexisting ASD, VSD or PDA) that creates life-saving left-to-right shunt
- Most common cause of cyanosis in the first week of life and is more common in males and children of diabetic mothers

CONGESTIVE HEART FAILURE

- Neonatal period = Birth to 1 month
- Infants present with poor feeding, labored breathing and sweating, = CHF presentations
- Most common cause of CHF < **1 day** = non-cardiac (↓H/H, ↓glucose, ↓O2, ↓Ca2+, sepsis, acidosis) or premature neonate with PDA
- Most common cause of cyanosis or CHF within the first **3 days of life of life** =
- Transposition of the Great Vessels (TGV)
- Most common cause of CHF 1st **week** of life in full-term newborns = Hypoplastic LV (HPLV)
- Most common cause of CHF 2nd **week** of life in full-term newborns = Coarctation of the aorta
- VSD = CHF **4 to 12 weeks** of life, unless complicated by other cardiac disease then earlier

TREATMENT OF CHF

- Lasix 1 to 2 mg/kg IV
- Digoxin 0.05 mg/kg per day, in infants up to 2 y/o. Give first digitalizing dose in ED (50% daily dose), followed by one-fourth of the daily dose IV at 6 to 8 hour intervals
- Cardiogenic shock → inotropic agents
  - Dopamine or
  - Dobutamine
  - If Inotropic Support Fails
  - Combination of Nitroprusside or NTG + Dopamine

- Blue baby = Terrible T's
- Mottled or gray baby = Coarctation of the aorta or aortic stenosis
- Pink baby = VSD, PDA

COMMON CAUSES OF NEONATAL SEPSIS / MENINGITIS (< 1 MONTH)

Mnemonic: GEL

G	**G**roup B Strep. *(Strep. agalactiae)* Most common cause 49%
E	***E****. coli* 18%
L	**L**isteria 7%

TREATMENT OF NEONATAL MENINGITIS

- Ampicillin (will cover Listeria) 50 mg/kg q 6 hrs (max dose 2 grams) + Cefotaxime (Claforan) 200 mg/kg/day divided q 6-8 hrs (max dose 2 grams) or Ampicillin + Gentamycin
- If CSF pleocytosis and negative gram stain consider adding Acyclovir empirically for HSV

MOST COMMON CAUSES OF BACTERIAL MENINGITIS > 1 MONTH TO 50 YRS

- Streptococcus pneumoniae and Neisseria meningitidis. Less common cause H. Influenzae
- N. meningitidis = the most common cause of meningitis in young adults age 16 to 21
- Sensorineural hearing loss is a complication of herpes and Haemophilus influenzae meningitis and less common with meningococcal meningitis

TREATMENT OF MENINGITIS > 1 MONTH TO 50 YEARS

- Dexamethasone + Ceftriaxone or Cefotaxime + Vancomycin
- Ceftriaxone = 100 mg/kg (2 gm IV max) q 12 hrs
- Dexamethasone = 0.15 mg/kg IV q 6 hrs x 2 to 4 days; give 15 min prior or con-comitant with first dose of antibiotic to prevent neurologic complications.
- Vancomycin = 15 mg/kg IV q 6 hours; Adults max dose of 2-3 gm/day is suggested: 500 to 750mg IV q 6 hours
- Regimens are most effective in started as early as possible.

FEBRILE SEIZURES

- History of febrile seizure in first degree relative = most consistently identified risk factor for febrile seizure

- **Febrile Seizure Criteria**
    - Ages 6 months to 5 years
    - temperature > 38°C (100.4°)
    - Lack of CNS infection or inflammation or any metabolic condition that may result in seizure
    - No prior history of afebrile seizures
    - **PEARL:** 3% of all children

- **Simple Febrile Seizures** = < 15 minutes, generalized tonic-clonic, no focal neuro deficits, occurs once in 24 hours. You need all four elements to diagnose

- **Complex Febrile Seizures** = prolonged (>15 minutes), are focal, or multiple seizures occur during the same febrile illness
- Need only one element to diagnose; prolonged alteration in mental status (post-ictal) vs. simple febrile seizure that has a mild post-ictal period

- **Risk factors for recurrence:**
    - Young age of onset < 18 months old (strongest and most consistent risk factor for recurrence)
    - The younger the age of onset, of a febrile seizure, the more likelihood of recurrence
    - History of febrile seizure in first degree relative
    - Low grade temperature in ED
    - Brief duration between fever and seizure

- **Recurrent febrile seizure**
    - 50% of children < 12 months
    - 30% of children > 12 months

- **Risk of epilepsy > general population**
    - Children with simple febrile seizures have a 2% to 3% chance of developing epilepsy compared with a 1% rate of epilepsy in the general population
    - The younger the age at onset of a febrile seizure, the more likelihood of recurrence

- Simple vs. complex is NOT predictive of the risk of recurrence
- Viral infections are common causes: influenza, adenovirus and parainfluenza. **Human herpes 6** (HHV-6) infection is a particular risk for febrile seizures
- Neither a decline in IQ, academic performance or neurocognitive inattention nor behavioral abnormalities have been shown to be a consequence of recurrent simple febrile seizures
- Treatment with long-term anticonvulsants does not affect the long-term risk of developing epilepsy and is rarely warranted
- In situations in which parental anxiety associated with febrile seizures is severe, intermittent oral diazepam at the onset of febrile illness may be effective in preventing recurrence
- Antipyretics may improve comfort of the child, they will **not** prevent febrile seizures

2011 AAP Guidelines on Febrile Seizure

- Recommend LP
  1. If history or exam suggests meningitis
  2. Complex seizure
  3. Prolonged "post-ictal" period after brief seizure
- LP "is an option"
  1. Infants 6 to 12 months and under-immunized
  2. Pretreated with antibiotics
  3. Febrile status epileptics (FSE)
  4. Seizures that occur after the second day of a febrile illness

Patients at greatest risk for meningitis with febrile seizures

- < 18 moths
- Focal seizure
- Prolonged seizure
- Seizure in the ED
- Seen by a physician within the prior 48 hours

NEONATAL SEIZURES

- If benzodiazepines do not resolve neonatal seizure consider Pyridoxine Deficiency
- Pyridoxine Deficiency = autosomal recessive (two copies of an abnormal gene
- must be present in order for the disease or trait to develop - one from each parent)
- Treatment = Pyridoxine (B6)
- Check glucose, electrolytes, glucose, trauma - in neonates not as cause, but as an effect of seizure

Neonatal Status Epilepticus (< 1 year old) Status Epilepticus Treatment

1. Benzodiazepines
2. Phenobarbital (adults and non-neonatal option #2 = phosphenytoin)

STREPTOCOCCUS IDENTIFICATION

Alpha-hemolytic

- Streptococci from a GREEN zone around their colonies as a result of incomplete lysis of red blood cells (RBC's) in the agar
- *Streptococcus pneumoniae (Non-grouped)*
- *Strep viridans* (eg, *Strep mitis* and *Strep mutants)*

Beta-hemolytic

- Streptococci form a CLEAR zone around their colonies as a result of complete lysis of RBC's. Beta-hemolysis is due to the production of enzymes called hemolysins
- *Streptococcus pyogenes (Group A)*
- *Streptococcus agalactiae (Group B)*

Group (Lancefield Groups A-U)

- Streptococci are determined by antigenetic differences in C carbohydrate in the cell wall
- *Group A Streptococcus Pyogenes*
- *Group B Strep*tococcus agalactiae
- *Group D Enterococci* (eg. *Streptococcus faecalis*) → causes urinary, biliary/abdominal and cardiovascular infections
- Group D Non-enterococci (eg. *Streptococcus bovis*, alpha hemolytic) → Gastric CA association Group D hemolytic reaction is variable. Some are beta, alpha or non-hemolytic
- Non-group = *Streptococcus pneumoniae* and *Strep viridans*
- Groups C, E, F, G,H and K-U streptococci infrequently cause human disease

M protein

- Associated with virulence and determines the type of Group A β-hemolytic Strep. It interferes with ingestion by phagocytes

Anaerobic /microaerophilic Strep

- Peptostreptococci, variable hemolysis, cause mixed GI infections

STREPTOCOCCUS PNEUMONIAE "PNEUMOCOCCUS"

Mnemonics - (COMMONPLACES)

C	**C**onjunctivitis
O	**O**titis
M	**M**edia

M	**M**eningitis
O	**O**ptochin sensitive Strep viridans eg, Strep mitis and Strep mutants – both alpha hemolytic, are NOT inhibited by **O**ptochin
N	**N**asal Sinusitis

P	**P**enicillin (Drug of choice)
L	**L**obar pneumonia
A	**A**lpha hemolytic (Non-Grouped)
C	**C**apsule
E	**E**lderly are candidates for vaccination
S	**S**putum-rusty

STREPTOCOCCUS PYOGENES

Mnemonic - (PIECES)

Group A, beta-hemolytic Strep, Gram + spherical cocci in pairs or chains

P	Pharyngitis (get circumoral pallor) Penicillin = drug of choice If PCN allergy you can use Zithromax Zithromax Dose = 12mg/kg/day x 5 days – not the traditional 10mg/kg day #1 than 5mg/kg days #2 to 5 **PEARL:** Most common bacterial cause of pharyngitis
I	Impetigo (strep pyogenes = distant second; Staphlococcus Aureus = most common
E	Erysipelas
C	Cellulitis
E	Erythrogenic Toxin → Scarlet Fever (Type IV Hypersensitivity reaction)
S	Sequelae: 1) Rheumatic Fever (most common after pharyngitis) 2) Poststreptococcal GN (most common after skin infection-impetigo)

- Rheumatic Fever (RF) is a NON-infectious autoimmune disease typically occurring 2-4 weeks after Group A Strep pharyngitis. The immunologic reaction results from cross-reactions between streptococcal antigens and antigens of joint and heart tissue
- RF is prevented if strep infection treated within 8 days after onset
- Early antibiotic treatment = earlier resolution of symptoms & shortens course of illness by 1 day
- Not common < 2 y/o
- Occurs winter, spring
- Responsible for < 15% of pharyngitis in patients > 15 years old
- "Doughnut lesions" = erythematous papules with a pale center located on both the soft and hard palates, pathognomonic for Group A Strep pharyngitis

ACUTE GLOMERULONEPHRITIS (AGN)

- Triad: 1) Lower extremity and facial edema, 2) Microscopic hematuria, 3) HTN "smoky" urine. May be prevented if strep treated early, however cannot be prevented with PCN after onset of symptoms. Diagnosis: positive antistreptolysin test
- AGN occurs within 1 to 2 weeks following streptococcal throat infection and 3 to 6 weeks after streptococcal skin infection
- Type III Hypersensitivity
- **Treatment:** Furosemide (Lasix); nicardipine (Cardene) or nifedipine (Procardia) for BP control
- Avoid angiotensin-converting enzyme (ACE) inhibitors in BP control = cause hyperkalemia
- Reinfection with strep rarely leads to recurrence of AGN

5 MAJOR MODIFIED JONES CRITERIA FOR RHEUMATIC FEVER

Mnemonic - (EM Physicians Can Snuggle Continuously)

EM	**E**rythema **M**arginatum (pink rings on the trunk and inner surfaces of the arms and legs) Face is spared; non-pruitic
Physicians	**P**olyarthritis (symmetric, migratory-see mnemonic on migratory arthritis) Present in 75% of patients, large joints, most common symptom. Treat arthritis with ASA
CAn	**CA**rditis (steroids may be helpful) Carditis = tachycardia, CHF, now murmur, cardiomegaly, myocarditis, pericarditis, poses greatest rick for death, 30 to 50%
SNuggle	**S**ubcutaneous **N**odules (Painless and firm)
COntinuously	**C**h**O**rea (Sydenham's chorea = "Saint Vitus' Dance") Abrupt purposeless movement

Clinical diagnosis of Rheumatic Fever is made if 2 Major or 1 Major and 2 Minor criteria are present in patient with preceding Strep infection evidenced by:

1) ↑ ASO titer
2) Positive throat culture
3) Recent Scarlet Fever

Minor Criteria

- Fever
- Arthralgia
- ↑ PR interval
- ↑ ESR or CRP
- Previous rheumatic fever

Treat all children with ARF with PCN, eythromycin if PCN allergy for strep regardless of the culture results

CAUSES OF MIGRATORY ARTHRITIS

Mnemonic - (RF HSP LSD)

A tough one to remember, Try "if you had rheumatic fever, or HSP, you would want LSD."

RF	**R**heumatic **F**ever

H	HSP
S	**S**epsis (Strep, Staph, GC, Meningococcal)
P	**P**ulmonary Infection (Mycoplasma, Histo, Coccidia)

L	**L**yme disease
S	**S**BEndocarditis
D	**D**rugs (Ceclor)

SINUSES PRESENT AT BIRTH

Mnemonic - (ME)

M	**M**axillary
E	**E**thmoid

- Frontal sinuses develop at age 6 to 8 years old
- **PEARL:** adult patients →
  - Leaning forward exacerbates maxillary sinusitis
  - Supine position exacerbates ehtmoid sinusitis.
  - CT scan is the gold standard for diagnosis of sinusitis.
- Pott's puffy tumor = compliations of fronal sinusitis - subperiosteal abcess with soft tissue swelling causes pitting edema over the frontal bone; Although it can affect all ages, it is mostly found among teenagers and adolescents

PERITONSILLAR ABSCESS (PTA)

- Most common deep infection of the head and neck; develops primarily in adolescents and young adults; sore throat, fever, odynophagia, dysphagia, and referred otalgia; inferior and medial displacement of the affected tonsil with deviation of the uvula to the contralateral side; muffled, "hot potato" voice and trismus which can limit the examination. Most common = unilateral (peritonsillar cellulitis = bilateral). Treatment = Needle aspiration which is easier to perform, less painful for patients than I&D and is effective in 90% of patients + antibiotics to cover both Streptococci and oral anaerobe. Needle aspiration risk = injury to carotid artery

RETROPHARYNGEAL ABSCESS

- Commonly seen in children < 5 year old (most common 3 to 5); the retropharyngeal nodes atrophy with age; history of URI or posterior pharynx trauma
- Febrile, ill-appearing; cervical lymphadenopathy, dysphonia, drooling, dysphagia, neck held in extension, trismus, stridor, sorethroat, +/- bulge in posterior pharyngeal; nuchal rigidity; muffled voice

- Diagnosis: Lateral soft tissue neck (film should be taken during inspiration with the neck in slight extension) = retropharyngeal space at C2 = 2x diameter of the vertebral body or > one half the width of the vertebral body of C4
- Contrast enhanced CT can aid in defining the extent of the abscess formation
- Treatment in the Emergency Department: stabilization of the airway, intravenous antibiotics (ampicillin-sulbactam) and emergency consultation with ENT for I&D
- **PEARL:** Tracheal "rock" sign = tenderness with side-to-side movement of the larynx and trachea (commonly present in patients with a retropharyngeal abscess)

BACTERIAL TRACHEITIS

- 3 months to 6 years of age (usually 3 to 5 years old)
- URI symptoms, fever, barking cough, stridor
- Blood cultures rarely are positive
- Respiratory cultures are commonly polymicrobial with Staphylococcus aureus the most common isolated species
- Influenza A = increase the susceptibility to bacterial tracheitis

- **Clinical diagnosis**
  - The classic presentation is a child with suspected croup who continues to worsen despite treatment. High fever; develop increased risk for airway compromise
  - Treatment = broad-spectrum intravenous antibiotics, IVF, bronchoscopy, airway management in OR

LARYNGOTRACHEITIS (CROUP)

- Most common cause of croup = Parainfluenza virus; usually < 3 y/o
- Barking cough ("seal-like"), stridor, and retractions
- Symptoms worse at night
- CXR = "steeple sign" (subglottic tracheal narrowing)
- Treatment = Nebulized epinephrine (rapid local vasoconstriction of the subglottic mucosa reduces swelling) + steroids (dexamethasone)
- Accessory muscle use, bark-like cough and intercostal retractions can all be present in mild or in moderate and severe croup
- Stridor at rest = moderate and severe croup

PERTUSSIS

- **Catarrhal phase**
  - Earliest phase, lasts 1 to 2 weeks, viral syndrome-like presentation
  - **PEARL:** Two early clinical findings suggestive of pertussis = excessive lacrimation and conjunctival injection
  - Diagnostic tests are most accurate during this phase; however, the nonspecific clinical presentation rarely leads to suspicion of pertussis
- **Paroxysmal phase**
  - Second week of illness, lasts 2 to 6 weeks
  - Hallmark symptom = paroxysmal cough (severe, vigorous coughs that occur during a single expiration)
  - Paroxysms often occur in rapid succession
  - Following a prolonged cough paroxysm, a vigorous inspiration causes the "whooping" sound
  - Post-tussive syncope, emesis, abdominal wall hernias, rib fractures, lumbar strain and incontinence can occur during the paroxysmal phase

- **Convalescent phase** — Gradual reduction in the frequency and severity of cough. It usually lasts 1 to 2 weeks but may be prolonged
- Total duration of all 3 phases typically = 3 months but can last longer
- **Diagnosis:** CDC recommends use of PCR (nasopharynx) + culture for the diagnosis
- **Treatment:** macrolides - azithromycin (preferred in infants < 1 month), clarithromycin or erythromycin
- **Treatment:** Cough duration < 3 weeks = antibiotic therapy (this is the period of highest risk for transmission) = azithromycin or clarithromycin
- Primary goal of antibiotics = reduce infectivity not the duration of symptoms
- Postexposure antibiotic prophylaxis recommended = azithromycin or clarithromycin
- **PEARL:** Avoid contact until completion of at least five days of antibiotic therapy
- **PEARL:** Most common complication of *Bordetella pertussis* in infants = Apnea
- **PEARL:** Pneumonia is the most common cause of death

DIPHTHERIA

- *Corynebacterium diphtheriae*, club-shaped G+ aerobic rod, no capsule
- Spread person-person nasopharyngeal secretions (place patient in respiratory droplet isolation)
- Gray-green pseudomembrane, do not remove → ↑bleeding; "bull neck" appearance
- Exotoxin ¬→ disrupts protein synthesis → leads to cardiac and CNS disease
- Myocarditis → cardiomyopathy, CHF, Dysrhythmias
- CNS & PNS myelin sheath deterioration → peripheral neuropathy, muscle weakness (palate 1st)
- Diagnosis: by culture of pharynx and nose (alert lab as special media is needed)

Diphtheria Treatment

- Active immunization +
- Antitoxin (dose depends on site of infection and duration of symptoms) + Erythromycin or Penicillin x 7-14 days

OTITIS MEDIA (OM)

- Most common viral cause of otitis media = RSV
- Most common bacterial cause of otitis media = *Strep pneumoniae* 40% ; *Haemophilus Influenzae*, *M. catarrhalis*, *S. Aureas.* Treat all with High Dose Amoxicillin 90 mg/kg/day div q 12 or q 8 hours
- OM best confirmed = decreased mobility of TM and loss of normal landmarks
- Most common complication of otitis media = hearing (conductive) loss
  Another common complication of otitis media = perforation, which usually heals within 7 days
- Most common intracranial complication of otitis media = meningitis

OM "wait and see" before treatment criteria:

- Age =/ > 2 years old
- Unilateral infection
- Symptoms < 48 hours
- Temperature < 102.2 F
- Bullous myringitis = Most commonly caused by viruses; can also be seen with *Mycoplasma pneumoniae*

OTITIS EXTERNA

- Most common organism = *Pseudomonas aeruginosa; #2 = Staphylococcus aureus*

STAPHYLOCOCCAL SCALDED SKIN SYNDROME (SSSS)

- Most commonly affects children under 2 years of age (RARE > 6 years of age)
- Exotoxin-mediated
- Symptoms: fever, malaise, irritability, and pain
- Erythroderma (often starts around mouth) —> later flaccid, ill-defined, thin and fragile bullae (flexural areas, buttocks, hands and feet) and desquamation
- Conjunctivitis
- + Nickolsky
- Treated like a burn patient with aggressive wound care and intravenous fluid
- Anti-staphylococcal antibiotics: nafcillin or oxacillin (consider MRSA-coverage with vancomycin)
- Excellent prognosis when treated with appropriate antibiotics and supportive care

CONGENITAL TOXOPLASMOSIS (TOXOPLASMA GONDII)

Mnemonic - (THC3)

T	**T**oxoplasmosis
H	**H**ydrocephalus
C	**C**horioretinitis **C**erebral Calcification **C**at feces and raw meat sources

Note: The acquired form in adults may present as a mononucleosis-like syndrome.

KAWASAKI SYNDROME (MUCOCUTANEOUS LYMPH NODE SYNDROME)

Inflammatory vasculitis of unknown etiology; Peak incidence occurs in children 18-24 months old; almost all patients < 4 years old.

Diagnostic Criteria

- Fever for at least 5 days duration
- Illness that is not explained by other known disease process

AND 4 of the following 5 For Diagnosing Kawasaki Syndrome

1. Bilateral non-exudative conjunctivitis
2. Changes of lips and oral mucosa
   (strawberry tongue, red/fissured lips, oropharyngeal edema)
3. Changes of the extremities
   (erythema of the palms and soles, edema of the hands and feet, periungual desquamation)
4. Polymorphous rash
5. Cervical lymphadenopathy unilateral

PEARL: Complication = coronary artery aneurysm
PEARL: 2% to 4% develop coronary artery abnormalities despite prompt treatment
If high suspicion treatment: combination IVIG + high-dose aspirin (ASA); when initiated within 10 days decreases the progression to coronary artery dilation and aneurysm formation compared to ASA alone
PEARL: IVIG side effect = hypotension

KAWASAKI SYNDROME Mnemonic - (CREAM) [Mnemonic provided by Dr. Nicole Colucci]

C	**C**onjunctivitis – non exudative, bilateral
R	**R**ash, polymorphous; erythema to palms and soles
E	**E**dema (hands and feet, oropharyngeal edema; periungal desquamation)
A	**A**denopathy (unilateral, cervical)
M	**M**ucosal involvement (changes to lips and oral mucosa – strawberry tongue, red/fissured lips, oropharyngeal edema)

Labs: Leukocytosis, thrombocytosis, hypoalbuminemia, elevated CRP and ESR, WBCs in UA (sterile pyuria by inflammation of the urethra)
ECG: myocarditis and pericarditis
Myocarditis is the most common cause of death in the acute phase (first 10 days)
Myocarditis can lead to Dilated Cardiomyopathy (DCM)

IMMUNOGLOBULIN A VASCULITIS (IGAV)

formerly known as Henoch-Schönlein Purpura (HSP)

Mnemonic - (PANDAS) [ANK, mnemonic provided by Dr. Collucci]

P	**P**urpura, Palpable non-blanching, buttocks and lower legs Pathognomonic round, palpable purpura, NON-blanching, symmetrical rash on buttocks and legs; non-pruritic
A	**A**bdominal pain - colicky (50%); other GI symptoms include nausea, vomiting, transient paralytic ileus, GI hemorrhage bowel ischemia and necrosis, intussusception, and bowel perforation; GI symptoms usually present within eight (8) days of the appearance of the rash. Guaiac-positive stool (56%) may be present, but massive gastrointestinal hemorrhage is rare
N	**N**ephritis 25 – 50% (microscopic hematuria, proteinuria, elevated BUN/Cr)
D	**D**iarrhea (bloody)
A	**A**rthritis, polymigratory - The second most common manifestation (50-75%); arthritis is usually transient or migratory, oligoarticular (one to four joints) and usually affects the lower extremity large joints (hips, knees and ankles)
S	**S**crotal edema (2 – 35%) can mimic torsion

- IgA dominant immune complexes → systemic vasculitis - mainly arterioles and capillaries (Small vessel vasculitis)
- 75% cases 2 to 4 years (2 to 12 year old; boys > girls)
- Typically follows URI, in spring
- Intussusception = ileal ileal secondary to small bowel vasculitis
- **Treatment**
  - Supportive
  - Hydration, APAP, NSAIDs
  - Steroids for severe disease
  - Disease is typically self-limited
  - Most cases resolve within 6 to 8 weeks
  - Recurrence rate = 33%
  - Platelet count and coags are normal

REYE'S SYNDROME

- ↓ Glucose
- ↑ LFT's, except normal BILI, ↑ ammonia
- Mental Status changes with ↑ ICP and seizures

DUODENAL ATRESIA

- Usually diagnosed prenatally or first 1-2 days after birth
- Obstruction of the proximal small bowel → signs of obstruction → bilious vomiting and dehydration
- Double bubble sign on X-ray or prenatal ultrasound

HYPERTROPHIC PYLORIC STENOSIS

- 95% of cases between 3 -12 weeks; rare before 1 week and after 3 months
- Male > female 4:1; most common cause of gastric obstruction in infants
- More frequently in first born males
- NON-bilious projectile vomiting just after feeding; readily would want to refeed
- Pyloric olive = pathognomonic; 90% palpated in the epigastrium or RUQ; if + palpable mass = no imaging is indicated - get surgical consultation
- ↓ Cl-, ↓ K+; hypo-chloremic, hypo-kalemic metabolic alkalosis
- Diagnosis: Ultrasound is the gold standard; if US N/A then UGI.
  - US findings: target sign; pylorus thickened > 4mm and elongated > 14mm
- Treatment: fluid, correct electrolytes, surgery, consult, NPO, NGT

MALROTATION AND MIDGUT VOLVULUS

- Acute bilious emesis, 75% poor feeding, irritability and bloody stool in neonate and abdominal distention, toxic appearing
- Volvulus is a complication of malrotation
- Duodenal obstruction without volvulus
- Diagnosis: Upper GI = abnormal position of the duodenal C-loop and small bowel = "corkscrew" appearance
- Surgery is the only definitive treatment

INTUSSUSCEPTION

- Classic Triad: abdominal pain, vomiting, & bloody stools (hematochezia) =33%
- Most common cause of obstruction in children infants 6 months to 3 years of age, male > female
- Siblings of affected patients have a relative risk 20x > general population
- **PEARL:** Male > female also for Pyloric Stenosis, however PS presentation first few weeks of life
- Most common site ileo-cecum – 80%
- Causes: Most commonly caused by tumor or Meckels diverticulum, inverted appendix, polyps, duplication, lymphoma, HSP (if HSP site = ileal-ileal)
- 50% preceded by viral illness
- Colicky abdominal pain (acute pain, patient draws up legs) Severe pain → no pain → severe pain → no pain
- Bilious vomiting
- Check for "currant jelly" stools (late finding) only present in about 20% of cases
- Dance's Sign = RUQ sausage shaped mass (intussusception) & empty space in RLQ (cecum → RUQ) Dance's sign is pathognomonic for intussusception

- Diagnosis & Treatment = Air contrast or Barium enema; notify Peds surgery before enema (Air Contrast Enema advantages: better control of colonic pressure used for the reduction, safer, faster, less expensive and more effective than barium enema
- Ultrasound - see telescoping boweel, "target sign"
- Complications = 5 to 10% re-intussusception within 48 hours; severe sepsis or septic shock; bowel perforation

ANAL PRURITUS

- Most common cause of anal pruritus in kids = Pinworms (Enterobius vermicularis)
- Most prevalent parasite in the US = Enterobius vermicularis (pinworm); 20 to 30% kids infected
- Most common cause of perianal cellulitis in young children = *group A Streptococcus*

ANAL FISSURE

- The most common anorectal disorder in children and infants.
- Superficial tear in the anoderm that results when a hard piece of stool is forced through the anus. It is associated with constipation;
- Other causes peds/adults: local trauma, anal sex, vaginal delivery, diarrhea
- Sudden onset, searing pain during defecation
- Male = female
- Most common cause of minor rectal bleeding in children
- **Posterior midline** is the most common location because the skeletal muscle encircling the anus is the weakest at this location
- **Anterior midline** is second most common (most common in women)
- **Lateral Fissures** likely to be related to systemic illness include: leukemia, Crohn's disease, HIV, TB, and syphilis
- Acute fissures generally resolve in 2-4 weeks
- **Treatment** includes the WASH regimen (warm water, analgesic agents, stool softeners, high-fiber diet); Topical NTG or Nifedipine (CCB)

RECTAL PROLAPSE (PROCIDENTIA)

- Disease of the extremes of age; PEDS think Cystic Fibrosis; boys > girls;
- Elderly = history of excessive staining; women > men
- **PEARL:** Clues in elderly; constipation, fecal incontinence, abdominal discomfort, prolapsed anal mass
- **Treatment:** Non-emergent surgery; if incarcerated / strangulated = emergent surgery

MECKEL'S DIVERTICULUM – RULE OF 2'S

- Most common malformation of the GI tract
- TWO % of population is affected
- TWO% of affected patients ever become symptomatic
- TWO years of age = most will have presented
- TWO feet from terminal ileum = diverticulum location
- TWO x more common in male > female
- Most common cause of massive rectal bleeding = Meckel's (painless, brick or bright red bleeding)
- Most common cause of minor rectal bleeding (peds) = Anal fissures (painful)
- Child may be well appearing, or may have bilious vomiting & abdominal distention with rectal bleeding
- The bleeding occurs from ulcers in the diverticulum secondary to ectopic gastric mucosa → which is what takes up the Technetium (85% sensitivity and 95% specificity)
- May cause intussusception, volvulvus, hernia
- Diagnosis = technetium 99m scan (Meckels scan)
- Definitive treatment = surgery

NECROTIZING ENTEROCOLITIS

- Most common GI emergencies in neonates
- Presents within first few days of life (can be seen up to 6 months of age)
- **Risk factor** = premature ; others = congenital heart disease, rapid feeding, sepsis immunocompromised
- 10% cases occur in full term infants
- Most common cause on intestinal perforation in newborns
- Feeding intolerance, vomiting, abdominal distention, lethargy, bloody stools
- Emesis = bilious or coffee ground
- **Xray** = Pneumatosis intestinalis (air in bowel wall) = pathognomonic, seen in 75% of cases
- **Treatment** = antibiotics, fluid, NGT and surgery consult
- **PEARL:** Mimickers of blood appearing stools = red food, red dyes, Omnicef (Cefdinir), iron

GASTROSCHISIS AND OMPHALOCELE

- Gastroschisis = defect in abdominal wall → evisceration of abdominal structures without a sac
- Omphalocele = defect in umbilical ring → intestines protrude in a sac
- Gastroschisis 2x more common than Omphalocele
- ED Management = NGT and place plastic covering to prevent heat and water loss.

HIRSCHSPRUNG'S DISEASE

- Most common cause of obstruction in newborn (functional obstruction)
- Chronic constipation - or explosive bloody diarrhea
- 75% recto-sigmoid involvement
- Diagnosis made in nursery as there is no passage of meconium for 24-48 hours
- Bilious vomiting, tarry diarrhea, distended abdomen, poor feeding
- 5x more common in boys
- Associated with Down Syndrome
- Rectal Exam: increased rectal tone; empty rectal vault; sudden passage of stool upon withdrawal of the examiner's finger (i.e. blast or squirt sign)
- Diagnosis
    - Suspected on barium enema - normal segment of colon with proximal dilation (transition zone)
    - Confirmed by biopsy – congenital absence of parasympathetic ganglion cells
- Complication: Toxic Megacolon = progressive enlargement of proximal segment
- Complication: Enterocolitis (abdominal distension, fever , ↑WBC and bloody stool)
- Other complications; bowel obstruction, intestinal perforation
- Treatment is surgical; NGT, rectal tube; Surgical excision of aganglionic segment

NEONATAL JAUNDICE

Common = affects about 60%-80%

Physiologic Jaundice

- Results from physiologic hemolysis of fetal hemoglobin following birth → accumulation of unconjugated (indirect) bilirubin in the blood
- Within 2 to 3 days of birth; resolves within the first week after birth

Breastfeeding Failure Jaundice (Lactation Failure Jaundice)

- Results from inadequate milk production in a breastfeeding mom or difficulty breastfeeding an infant
- Presents within first week of life
- Nutritional deficiencies, weight loss, and dehydration
- **Treatment:** Lactation counseling and formula supplementation

Breast Milk Jaundice

- Common cause of unconjugated (indirect) hyperbilirubinemia
- Neonates > 1 week of age
- Due to the presence of glucuronyl transferase inhibiting substances in breast milk → results buildup of unconjugated (indirect) bilirubin in the blood
- Neonates are well appearing and gain weight appropriately
- Not typically associated with kernicterus
- **Treatment:** observation; if severe hyperbilirubinemia (total bilirubin > 25 mg/dL) = phototherapy

PEARL: Severe hyperbilirubinemia (TB > 25 mg/dL) = risk for developing **bilirubin-induced neurologic dysfunction (BIND)** - bilirubin crosses the blood-brain barrier and binds to brain tissue
Presenting acutely as acute bilirubin encephalopathy (ABE); if not adequately treated, long-term neurologic sequelae = kernicterus

Kernicterus

- Choreoathetoid cerebral palsy (CP; chorea, ballismus, tremor, and dystonia)
- Hearing loss due to auditory neuropathy
- Gaze abnormalities, especially upward gaze
- Dental enamel dysplasia

JAUNDICE PEARLS: Don't forget to consider

- Sepsis
- Glucose-6-phosphate dehydrogenase deficiency
- Crigler-Najjar syndromes (Type I = severe; significant hyperbilirubinemia develops 2 to 3 days after birth; treatment = lifelong phototherapy to avoid (BIND) or liver transplant)
- Type II = less severe, usually no treatment; if severe jaundice the hyperbilirubinemia responds to phenobarbital treatment
- Gilbert syndrome = most common inherited disorder of bilirubin glucuronidation; benign condition

PEDS - ORTHO PEARLS

SALTER-HARRIS CLASSIFICATION (S-A-L-TE-R)

Types I-V

I	S	Straight across growth plate
II	A	Above; across most of growth plate and Metaphysis (**M**) Most common growth plate fracture (75%)
III	L	Lower; across growth plate and extends down through the Epiphysis (**E**)
IV	TE	Through everything; fracture passes through Metaphysis growth plate and Epiphysis (**ME**)
V	cRush	Most common Salter-Harris fracture likely to result in bone-growth arrest; does not displace growth plate, however damages by direct compression

CAST - CHILDHOOD ACCIDENTAL SPIRAL TIBIA

- Spiral fractures of the distal 1/3 of the tibia (if mid-shaft suspect abuse); common in children who are walking, 9 months to 3 years; (Toddler Fractures)
- **Treatment:** Consult ortho for casting, long leg orthopedic cast for several weeks

TRANSIENT SYNOVITIS

- Most common cause of hip pain in children < 10 y/o = **transient tenosynovitis**; ↑ in boys; follows viral illness. Non-toxic, afebrile or low grade temperature, AP pelvis + Lateral hip films, + Frog-view lateral: CBC and ESR are both usually normal. Most common age = 3 to 6 years old; inflammation of synovium; self limiting; follows URI; affected hip held in flexion, abduction, and external rotation a the position of comfort respond to NSAIDs and rest; follow-up with PMD in 24 hours; excellent prognosis; associated with **Legg-Calve-Perthes**

LEGG-CALVE-PERTHES DISEASE

- Avascular necrosis of pediatric femoral head; age 2-10y/o; 5x ↑ in boys
  - Bilateral 15%
  - Non-toxic, afebrile, AP pelvis + Lateral hip films
  - Trendelenburg's sign = when the patient stands on the affected side the pelvis droops on the unaffected side due to weakened gluteal muscles

SLIPPED CAPITAL FEMORAL EPIPHYSIS

- Hip pain → knee in adolescent obese patient → **SCFE** (slipped capital femoral epiphysis); 2.5x ↑ in boys; ORIF
  - 10-14y/o
  - Non-toxic, afebrile, AP pelvis + Lateral

SUPRACONDYLAR FRACTURE

- Most common elbow fracture in childhood = **supracondylar fracture** of the distal humeral metaphysis – the distal fragment is most commonly displaced posteriorly
- Complication = Volkman's ischemic contracture (compartment syndrome)
- Type III supracondular fracture = most commonly associated with compartment syndrome: consider brachical artery injury

NURSEMAID'S ELBOW

- Common 1 to 5 years old – stretch annular ligament and subluxation of radial head
- History: child pulled by the wrist
- Injured arm held in slight flexion at the elbow & pronated

- **Nursemaid Elbow - Reduction**
  - a) Hyperpronation method: examiner supports the elbow with one hand with pressure on the radial head
    The examiners other hand is used to grasp the childs forearm and pronate it through a full range of motion. A clunk is felt as the radial head slips back into place
  - b) Spination-flexion method: examiner applies pressure over the radial head and then supinates and flexes the forearm in one smooth motion

SEPTIC JOINT

- Usually < 4 years old; male > female, toxic, febrile; order CBC, blood culture, CRP, ESR, synovial fluid, US
- Synovial Fluid: WBC cell count > 50,000 cells/mL, > 75% PMN predominance, glucose decreased, protein and lactate increased
- Kocher criteria can be used to determine the probability of pediatric septic joint Non-weight bearing highest risk of septic joint > ESR > Fever > WBC over 12,000
- IV Antibiotics, Ortho consult → surgical washout

OSGOOD-SCHLATTER DISEASE

- Pain and swelling over tibial tuberosity; adolescents; x-rays initially normal; Treatment = rest, avoidance of forced knee extension (running and jumping)

TORUS FRACTURE

- Cortical buckling of the distal radius, most commonly involving the metaphysis; axial force
- Children < 10 years old
- Prognosis is good, as cortical disruption and thus displacement and angulation does not occur
- Treatment:
- Distal radius torus fractures = splinted, and follow-up with primary care physician in 3 to 4 weeks
- Torus fractures of other bones should = splinted and follow-up with primary care physician or orthopedist in 1 week

SEVER'S DISEASE OR CALCANEAL APOPHYSITIS

- Most common cause of posterior heel pain in athletic 8 to 12-year olds
- Males > Females
- Apophysitis = inflammation of calcaneal growth plate (apophysis)
- Bilateral in 60% of the cases
- Exacerbated by running and jumping / relieved by rest
- Pain is elicited by squeezing the calcaneus and dorsiflexion of the heel is restricted secondary to tight heel cords = Positive Calcaneal Compression Test
- Radiographs: normal, but may show partial fragmentation and increased density of the calcaneal apophysis
- Treatment: conservative and supportive, Achilles tendon stretching exercises, NSAIDs, activity modifications

- **PEARL: PLANTAR FASCIITIS** = worse with the start of activity and improves with 10-15 minutes of continued activity; Sever's disease = worsens with activity

- Sever's disease is similar = Osgood-Schlatter disease
- **Greenstick fracture** = incomplete, angulated fractures of long bones; may need to complete fracture to achieve anatomic reduction
- Most common fractured bone in children = **clavicle**

CHILD ABUSE

1. Neglect 52%
2. Physical 24%
3. Sexual 12%
4. Emotional 6%

- Greatest risk factor = lower socioeconomic status
- Most common cause of death from child abuse = Head injury
- Head trauma is the most common cause of mortality
- Shaken Baby / Shaken-Impact Syndrome = Subdural hematomas, retinal hemorrhages, rib fractures, metaphyseal fractures of long bones

FRACTURES - PHYSICAL ABUSE

- Multiple fractures
- Fractures in different stages of healing
- Posterior rib
- Scapular
- Spinous process
- Sternum
- Metaphyseal lesions / corner / "bucket" handle = virtually pathognomonic for infant abuse
- PEARL: Order skeletal survey in any child with suspected abuse

MANDATED REPORTERS

- Physicians in all states are mandated reporters of child abuse and neglect
- All child abuse statutes provide immunity from liability for physicians who report suspected abuse
- May be liable for medical malpractice if child sustains injury due to failure to report

CLINICAL FINDINGS ASSOCIATED WITH SEXUAL ASSAULT

- A laceration to the posterior hymen is is concerning for a penetrating vaginal injury
- Acute lacerations, transections, and bruising of the hymen
- Diameter of the hymenal opening is not useful in diagnosing sexual abuse
- The most common exam finding in prepubertal girls that are victims of penetrating sexual abuse = a normal physical exam
- Molluscum contagiosum in a child should raise concern for = SEXUAL ASSAULT

SUDDEN UNEXPECTED DEATH OF INFANCY (SUDI)

- Most common cause of death in US for children between 1 month and 1 year of age; The term has largely replaced sudden infant death syndrome (SIDS)
- Risk factors: male sex, prone sleeping, sleeping on a soft surface, overheating from heavy bedding or clothing, prematurity, low birth weight; 2-3x higher in black and Native American; maternal drug use; family history of SUDI; Maternal smoking, particularly during pregnancy, is the strongest maternal risk factor
- Safe to Sleep campaign, formerly known as the Back to Sleep campaign, encourages parents to have their infants sleep on their backs (supine position) to reduce the risk of Sudden Unexpected Death of Infancy (SUDI)
- **PEARL:** Pacifier use, breast feeding and supine sleeping position = decreased risk of Sudden Unexpected Death of Infancy (SUDI)

- Most common cause of death 1 month to 1 year = SIDS (RARE before 1 month, risk factors for SIDS = winter, male > female if infectious etiology otherwise, male=female, if mom < 20 y/o, smokes, drugs, no pre-natal care and lower socioeconomic group)

WHY IS THIS BABY STILL CRYING *(From Pediatric EM Morsels)*

MNEMONIC IT CRIES

I	**I**nfectious: meningitis, UTI, sepsis
T	**T**rauma: intracranial bleed, fracture, non-accidental trauma

C	**C**ardiac: arrhythmia
R	**R**eaction to medication, reflux, rectal or anal fissure
I	**I**ntussusception
E	**E**yes: corneal abrasion, foreign body, glaucoma
S	**S**trangulation (torsion, hernia, hair tourniquet)

PEDS CARDIOLOGY / PALS

- Most common pediatric dysrhythmia = PSVT heart rate usually > 220, in adults less
  Treatment: Adenosine (Adenocard) 0.1 mg/kg (max 6mg) → 0.2 mg/kg (max 12 mg), may repeat x 1
  Unstable SVT Cardioversion: 0.5 to 1.0 J/kg → 2 J
- Carotid massage is not recommended in infants or children
- Hemodynamically stable child in SVT: Application of ice to the face = effective method of converting a to NSR; do not occlude the nose or mouth, → apply ice only over the patient's forehead, eyes, and bridge of the nose for 10–15 seconds

BLS GUIDELINE FOR A LONE RESCUER - SLIGHTLY DIFFERENT THEN ADULT

- Before calling for help
- 2 minutes of CPR in infants and children (1 to 8 years old)
- More likely to have respiratory arrest
- Exception if child has witnessed sudden cardiac arrest (rare) - in which case you call for help first and then start CPR

ENDOTRACHEAL TUBE (ETT) DIAMETER SIZE (MM)

- Uncuffed = (Age / 4) + 4
- Cuffed = (Age / 4) + 3.5
- 5th digit fingernail diameter
- C = Catheter size, foley / NGT = ETT x 2
- D = Depth of ETT insertion = ETT x 3
- C - Chest tube size= ETT x 4
- ETTs cuff pressures should be kept to < 20 cm H2O

SHOCK - FLUID BOLUS

- Cardiogenic 10 mL/kg
- Hypovolemic 20 mL/kg
- DKA 20 mL/Kg
- Septic 60 mL/kg

SHOCK - VASOPRESSORS

- If patient remains hypotensive after fluid bolus → start vasopressors
- Epinephrine for septic shock
- Norepinephrine for spinal shock
- Dobutamine for cardiogenic shock

PEARLS - PALS

- Verapamil is contraindicated in infants
- Pediatric arrest is most commonly respiratory in arrest
- Most common pre-arrest rhythm disturbance = bradycardia
- VT or VF usually occurs with congenital heart disease
- Bradycardia is most commonly an indicator of hypoxemia in the newborn
- First line drug for bradycardic arrest = Epinephrine 0.01 mg/kg of 1:100,000 IV/IO; ETT = 0.1 mg/kg 1:1,000; Repeat Epinephrine every 3 to 5 minutes
  If ↑ vagal tone or AV Block → Atropine 0.02 mg/kg (minimum dose 0.1mg; max total dose for child = 1 mg) → consider pacing
- Vfib/ Pulseless VT = 2 J /kg Biphasic → CPR 5 cycles → 4 J/kg biphasic
  Epinephrine 0.01 mg/kg; Amiodarone 5mg/kg
- Most common category of shock in the pediatric population = hypovolemic; fluid = 20cc/kg 0.9 NS
- Peds Post-arrest - the drug of choice in treating hypotension → epinephrine infusion
- Position of the ET tube at the lips (in cm's) should = 3 x size of ETT
- Anesthesia literature, as well as Pediatric Advanced Life Support (PALS) Guidelines, now supports that, beyond the newborn period, cuffed endotracheal (ET) tubes are equally as safe as uncuffed tubes, and are favored in some clinical circumstances such as:
  - Children at risk for aspiration
  - Burn victims
  - Children with severe lung disease who may require high ventilator pressures (eg, bronchiolitis, status asthmaticus, chronic lung disease)
- Pretreatment with atropine in RSI for children < 10 years old has fallen out of favor (lack of evidence to support)

TREATMENT OF HYPOGLYCEMIA

- Neonate = D10 5 to 10 mL/kg
- Child = D25 2 to 4 mL/kg
- Upper limit of **SBP** = (Age x 2) + 80
- **Weight in kilograms** = (Age x 2) + 8
  Newborn = 3 kg
  1 y/o = 10 kg
  5 y/o = 20 kg
  10 y/o = 30 kg
- BP least helpful VS ... kids can compensate; hypotension is a late ominous finding
- Bulb and tracheal suctioning NOT routinely recommended anymore

PEDIATRIC ASSESSMENT TRIANGLE - APLS (PROVIDED BY DR COLUCCI)

- Appearance
- Work of Breathing
- Circulation

APPEARANCE
MNEUMONIC - (TICLS)

T	Tone
I	Interaction
C	Consolability
L	Look and gaze
S	Speech and cry

- Breathing - ominous finding
  - RR > 60
  - RR <12
- Circulation: color, skin temp and perfusion

LOCATIONS FOR INTRAOSSEOUS (IO) LINE PLACEMENT

- Child
  - Proximal tibia
  - Distal tibia
  - Distal femur

- Adults: add
  - Sternum, which has the highest flow rate > proximal humerus > tibia
  - Iliac spine, humeral head, distal radius or ulna
  - Any medication given through a PIV can be given through an IO line
  - Diagnostic studies for glucose, HgB, pH, and Cr correlate well to IV samples

- **PEARL:** Central venous catheter placement & risk of local and bloodstream infection
  - HIGHEST RISK OF INFECTION = Femoral Vein
  - Internal jugular (IJ) line placement = Second highest
  - LOWEST RISK OF INFECTION = Subclavian (SC) venous access
  - IJ vein = DOUBLE → the risk of infection compared to SC vein

PEDIATRIC ONCOLOGY

- Leukemia is by far the most common childhood cancer (33%); brain tumors represent about 25%, lymphomas represent about 8%, and bone cancers (osteosarcoma and Ewing sarcoma) represent about 4%
- Cancers that are exclusive to children include Neuroblastoma, Wilms tumor, Rhabdomysarcoma and Retinoblastoma

NEUROBLASTOMA IN CHILDREN

- Most common site = adrenal glands
- More common in boys
- 3rd most common childhood cancer, after **leukemia** and **brain tumors**; most common solid extra-cranial tumor in children along with Wilms' tumor
- In the abdomen: non-tender abdominal mass, constipation, weight loss, anorexia; lower extremity edema, and enuresis from bladder compression (lead to UTIs)
- In the thorax: presents as a mediastinal mass, Horner syndrome, raccoon eyes (metastases) or superior vena cava syndrome
- In the spine: spinal cord compression, scoliosis, and enuresis (involuntary urination) or encopresis (involuntary defecation)
- 50% of patients will present late → Metastatic spread to: bone/bone marrow (common presentation = bone pain/limp), skin, liver, eye = periorbital ecchymosis ("raccoon's sign") and fevers
- Opsoclonus-myoclonus syndrome = spontaneous conjugate rapid eye movements in all directions of gaze & involuntary myoclonic muscular contractions
- 50% have an underlying neuroblastoma, however this is very rare and only a very small % of patients with neuroblastoma will develop opsoclonus-myoclonus syndrome
- **PEARL:** Infectious origin of Opsoclonus-myoclonus = HCV, EBV and HIV
- Irritability, tachycardia, HTN and diarrhea = catecholamine excess
- **Diagnosis:**
  - Elevation urine vanillylmandelic acid (VMA) and homovanillic acid (HVA) = breakdown products of epinephrine and norepinephrine
  - MRI of the chest, abdomen, and pelvis
- < 1 year old diagnosis = Excellent prognosis
- > 1 year old diagnosis = Poor prognosis

WILMS' TUMOR (NEPHROBLASTOMA)

- Malignant tumor of the kidney in young children
- With current therapies = 80-90% children survive
- 80% present with asymptomatic mass; abdominal pain or hematuria; varicocele less common; hypotension, anemia; renal US initial study
- **Treatment:** nephrectomy followed by chemotherapy, +/- radiation

MALIGNANT NECK MASSES

- Five Features Associated with Malignancy in Neck Masses
  1) Skin Ulcer
  2) Onset of the mass when the patient is a neonate
  3) Non-mobile, fixed to skin or fascia
  4) Progressive enlargement
  5) Size > 3cm and hard
- If a neck mass can be moved around and compressed it is NOT likely to by malignant

NON-MALIGNANT NECK MASSES

- **Branchial cleft cyst** (20% of pediatric neck masses)
  - Location: lateral, anterior to the border of the sternocleidomastoid near the angle of the mandible.
  - Non-tender (unless infected); fluctuant
  - Cyst may spontaneously rupture, leading to an external sinus
  - **Diagnosis**: Clinical Ultrasound: thin-walled, anechoic fluid-filled cyst
  - **Treatment**: surgical excision
  - Infected cyst: antibiotics prior to surgery
- **Thyroglossal duct cyst**: congenital mass resulting from the persistence of the thyroglossal duct
  - Location: midline, painless, soft, round, freely-movable mass

PEDIATRIC ID PEARLS

- **FEVER PEARLS**
  - For the purpose of investigating for a occult serious bacterial infection (SBI) in well appearing children, fever is defined as:
  - For infants < 90 days: temperature > 38.0°C (100.4°F) taken rectally
  - For infants 3 to 6 months temperature > 39.0°C (102.2°F)
  - Fever without source (FWS) = no source apparent after careful history and physical examination
  - Fever of unknown origin (FUO) requires:
    - Temperature > 38.3°C (101°F) on several occasions
    - More than 3 weeks' duration of illness

- **Neonatal Conjunctivitis (Ophthalmia Neonatorum)** - First month of life:
  - Day 1-2 = Chemical
  - Day 3 = *Gonorrhea*
  - Day 6 to first month of life = *Chlamydia trachomatis*
- Most common viral cause of conjunctivitis = Adenovirus
- "Previous" most common cause of epiglottitis = *H. influenzae* now the most common cause of epiglottitis = *S. pneumoniae* & *S. pyogenes*
- Most common cause of bronchiolitis = RSV; bronchodilators & steroids - no proven benefit; x-ray rarely helpful
- Hand-foot-mouth = Coxsackie; summer / fall
- Febrile infants < 90 days have an 8% chance of having a serious bacterial illness (SBI)
- Most common source for SBI = UTI in children 3 to 36 months of age
- Caucasian girls < 2 years old with temperature > 39 C (102.2 F) and no other source of infection have a 17% chance of having a UTI
- Jaundice (especially direct hyperbilirubuinemia) may be a presenting symptom of sepsis in neonates
- **Monospot** is positive in 30% of children 0 to 20 months with mononucleosis; Monospot may be negative the first week of illness
- **Roseola infantum (exanthem subitum)**: human herpes 6-infection → febrile 3-5 days →↓ fever →↑ macular rash. Most common exanthem in children < 2 year of age
- **Rubella (German measles)**: maculopapular rash spreads in a centrifugal pattern (head to feet); lymphadenopathy typical → posterior auricular and suboccipital; **"blueberry muffin"** skin rash; transmitted by respiratory droplets; **Forchheimer spots** = pinpoint petechia on the soft palate that coalesce

- Most common cause of cataracts in newborn
- Rubella and EBV are the most common viral cause of arthritis
- Rubella congenital infection and lead to major birth defects and death

- **Rubeola (Measles):** maculopapular rash spreads in a centrifugal pattern (head to feet); 3-4 day prodrome; **C x 3** = **C**ough, **C**oryza, **C**onjunctivitis and Koplik's spots (white lesions on buccal mucosa = pathognomonic)
- **Erythema Infectiosum:** fifth disease → parovirus B 19 → "**slapped cheek**" disease; school age kids; patients with sickle cell disease who are infected with Parvovirus B19 are at risk for developing aplastic crisis (**PEARL**: Aplastic crisis is defined as having a reticulocyte count of less than 1%; pallor, weakness, lethargy)
- **Mumps**: 5-15 y/o; infective 3 days before → 7 days after salivary gland swelling; 70-80% bilateral; spread = respiratory droplets; complications: meningitis. encephalitis, orchitis 15-25% post-pubertal men (sterility uncommon; 70% unilateral); uncommon complications include: GBS, transverse myelitis, oophoritis, mastitis, myocarditis, pancreatitis
- Most common cause of **acute cerebellar ataxia** = post-infection (especially varicella); occurs about 2 weeks after viral illness; rule out toxicologic causes, cerebellar tumors, trauma or infection (Coxsackie B, echovirus 6, EBV, influenza, mumps)

PEDIATRIC GI PEARLS

- Most common cause of **infantile diarrhea** = Rotavirus (ROTA = Right Out The Anus)
- Infants < 1 year are often colonized with **C. diff.** Avoid testing/treating C. diff in this age group
- **Mimickers of blood appearing stools** = red food, red dyes, Omnicef (Cefdinir), iron
- Most common cause of home accidental death < 6 y/o = **FB aspiration** (usually in right mainstem bronchus)
- Age Group most likely to **aspirate a FB** = 1 to 3 years with peak incidence at age 2
- Most common foods aspirated = nuts
- Common cause of **pediatric fatal aspiration** = food (especially hot dogs) and toy balloons
- Most common **esophageal impaction** → kids = coins; adults = food (meat/bones)
- If **button battery** has passed esophagus and patient is asymptomatic → no retrieval. If cell has not passed pylorus in 48 hours = endoscopic retrieval

MORE PEDS PEARLS

- Most common cause of **metabolic acidosis** in kids = prolonged diarrhea
- **Congenital adrenal hyperplasia** = adrenal insufficiency → ↓ Aldosterone →↓Na+ more common > K+ and ↓ cortisol; Refractory ↓BP: Girls = ambiguous genitalia (look both male and female) → treatment = Hydrocortisone 2 mg/kg IV/IO bolus (max 100mg)
    - Decrease in steroid synthesis
    - Presents between week #2 and 5 of life or childhood during precocious puberty
    - The most common form of CAH = 21-hydroxylase deficiency (90%)
- Most common cause of dysuria in school age girls = **non-specific vulvovaginitis**
- **Contact vulvovaginitis** = exposure of the vulvar epithelium and vaginal mucosa to an allergen or chemical irritant; local swelling, redness, itching and burnin
- 4-10% premenarchal children presenting with vaginal discharge will have a **vaginal foreign body;** malodorous, bloody or dark brown and occurs daily; small pieces of toilet paper and small objects or toys

SMALL BOWEL OBSTRUCTION - HISTORY

Mnemonic - (VODKA)

V	Vomiting
O	*Obstipation - Old Scar
D	Distension
K	(K) Crampy
A	Abdominal Pain

*Obstipation = 1) the act or condition of obstructing 2) extreme constipation due to obstruction

CAUSES OF SMALL BOWEL OBSTRUCTION

Mnemonic - (BEN VIP)

B	**B**ands (adhesions) = 60% (postoperative adhesions are the most common cause of SBOs)
E	**E**xternal Hernias = 10% (incarcerated hernias = third most common cause of SBO)
N	**N**eoplasm 20% (cancer second most common cause of SBO and most common cause of LBO)

V	**V**olvulus
I	**I**ntussusception
P	**P**ackets (swallowed FBs, bezoars, etc)

SBO PEARLS

- SBO → ↑ intraluminal pressure → capillary and lymphatic obstruction → ↑bowel wall edema
- Aggressive treatment has ↓Mortality Rate from 60% in 1900 to less than 5% today
- 35 to 50% of patients with complete SBO → resolution without surgical intervention
- Presentation: Diffuse crampy, colicky abdominal pain, abdominal distention, and vomiting
- Xray = multiple air-fluid levels, distended loops of small bowel, "string of pearls" (small round pockets of air line up & look like a string of pearls); paucity of stool and gas distal to obstruction
- Treatment: supportive, fluid surgery consult
- Postoperative adhesions are the most common cause of SBOs (60%), followed by cancer (20%), and then incarcerated hernias (10%)

CAUSES OF LARGE BOWEL OBSTRUCTION

Mnemonic - (CAtch VD)

CAtch	**CA**ncer = most common cause (50-70%) Most common cancer = adenocarcinoma
V	**V**olvulus = 2nd most common cause of LBO (10-25%) Most common site = sigmoid (70%) and cecum (30%)
D	**D**iverticulitis = 3rd most common cause of LBO (10-15%) secondary to scarring

- Other causes of LBO:
  Inflammatory disorders, benign tumors, foreign bodies, radiation and fecal impaction
- **Ogilvie syndrome**: enormous dilation of the RIGHT colon without mechanical obstruction (pseudo obstruction)
- History of LBO: diffuse colicky pain, obstipation; vomiting LATE or ABSENT; distension most common and prominent physical finding

CECAL VOLVULUS

- Results from incomplete embryologic fixation of the cecum, ascending colon, and terminal ileum to the posterior abdominal wall
- Cecal Volvulus occurs in all ages, but most common in 25 to 35 years of age vs Sigmoid Volvulus mean age 60 to 70 years of age
- Sigmoid Volvulus typically seen in debilitated or NH patient vs Cecal Volvulus seen in pregnancy, marathon runners and increased in GI malignancy
- Not associated with chronic constipation (unlike Sigmoid); onset of pain is acute in cecal volvulus vs more gradual onset in sigmoid volvulus
- **Diagnosis of Cecal Volvulus**
  - X-ray: “Kidney bean” / “coffee-bean sign
  - CT Abdomen: 90%; “Whirl sign”
- **Treatment:** Surgical exploration

SIGMOID VOLVULUS

- Mortality rate for Sigmoid Volvulus = 20% and is > 50% if gangrenous bowel
- **X-ray:** “Coffee bean sign” or a shape resembling a bent inner tube
- **Treatment** of non-strangulated Sigmoid Volvulus: decompression and detorsion using a rectal tube via the sigmoidscope = 85-95% Success

CAUSES OF ILEUS

Mnemonic - (Nurses (RN) and Physician Assistants (PA) FiX MI Burn GAP)

R	**R**etroperitoneal hematoma
N	**N**ephrolithiasis

P	**P**yelonephritis or Pneumonia
A	**A**bdominal Surgery

FiX	**Fx** (fractures – lumbar, rib)
MI	**M**yocardial Infarction
Burn	**Burn**s, especially if > 20%

G	**G**allstone ileus or Gastroenteritis
A	**A**ppendicitis
P	**P**ancreatitis

PEARL: Adynamic (paralytic) ileus is the most common cause of ileus overall

ILEUS	**SBO**
Minimal abdominal pain	Crampy abdominal pain
↓ or absent bowel sounds	↑ or normal bowel sounds
Gas in SI & colon on x-ray	Gas in SI only on x-ray
Nausea & vomiting	Nausea & vomiting
Obstipation & failure to pass flatus	Obstipation & failure to pass flatus
Abdominal distention	Abdominal distension

HERNIAS

1. Reducible
2. Incarcerated = irreducible
3. Strangulated = vascular compromise

DIRECT INGUINAL HERNIAS

- Intraabdominal contents bulge through an area of abdominal weakness at Hesselbach's triangle, medial to the inferior epigastric artery (IEA)

INDIRECT INGUINAL HERNIAS

- Intraabdominal contents traverse the inguinal canal, lateral to the IEA
- Most Common type
- Strangulation risk: indirect inguinal > direct inguinal hernias
- Age = Bimodal < 1 and > 40 years old
- **PEARL**: Inguinal hernias = most common type of hernia (75%)

UMBILICAL HERNIAS

- Common in children and usually close spontaneously; rarely becoming incarcerated

SPIGELIAN HERNIAS

- Occur at an area of abdominal muscle weakness at the lateral edge of the rectus abdominus muscle
- Right side > left
- Rare however high risk of strangulation
- Age 30 to 60 years old

FEMORAL HERNIA

Elderly female

APPENDICITIS

Mnemonic - (PAVEL'S P'S)

P	**P**ain-periumbilical → RLQ
A	**A**norexia
V	**V**omiting
E	**E**levated temperature, mild/normal. If elevated, think perforation
L	**L**eukocytosis – may be normal
S	**S**igns Rovsing's = palpate LLQ → RLQ pain Obturator = patient supine, flex knee and internally rotate right hip → RLQ pain (pelvic or retrocecal appendix) Iliopsoas = patient asked to extend right hip → RLQ pain (retrocecal appendix)

P	1) Perforation (high rate in kids, elderly and pregnancy) 2) Phlegmon (suppurative inflammation of SQ connective tissue) 3) Periappendiceal abscess 4) Peritonitis

- Appendicitis is the most common cause of abdominal pain requiring surgery (37%)
- 7% of population will develop appendicitis
- More common in men > women
- Tenderness at McBurney's point = 2/3 the way from the umbilicus to the Anterior Superior Iliac Spine (ASIS)
- Duration of pain > 48 hours, previous episodes of similar pain, lack of migration and RLQ pain, and presence of vomiting before the onset of pain = **lower risk of appendicitis**

Historical features that have a high positive likelihood ratio for acute appendicitis include

a) Migration of pain from periumbilical area → RLQ
b) Presence of RLQ tenderness
c) Abdominal wall rigidity

High Perforation rates in:

1. Children < 6y/o (65%) - atypical presentation and inability to communicate
2. Elderly (45-70% vs 10-15% in patients under < 60 y/o) - thin appendix wall and poor blood supply to the appendix
3. Pregnancy

Most common cause of surgical abdomen in children = appendicitis

> 66% cases are in patients < 30y/o (peak incidence = 11 to 20 y/o)

Condition most commonly mistaken for acute appendicitis in children = **mesenteric adenitis** and gastroenteritis

Most common surgical emergency in pregnancy = appendicitis
Higher perforation rate in pregnancy
Fetal loss 20% with perforated appy
Pain may be in RUQ
Most patients with appendicitis will have pain in RLQ, even in 3rd Trimester

Threshold for human teratogenesis = 10 rad; fetus most vulnerable 8 to 15 weeks gestation
CT abdomen = 3.5 rad

APPENDICITIS PATHOPHYSIOLOGY

- Lumen obstruction (fecaliths –most common, lymphoid hyperplasia, dietary matter, worms, tumors, granulomatous disease, adhesions) → increased edema as mucus continues to be secreted → edema and vascular compromise → followed by bacterial invasion

APPENDICITIS - ULTRASOUND FINDINGS

- Diameter > 6 mm
- Wall thickness > 3 mm
- Target sign
- Appendicolith
- Noncompressible appendix (perforated appendicitis may be compressible).

APPENDICITIS COMPUTED TOMOGRAPHY (CT) FINDINGS

- Enlarged appendiceal diameter > 6mm with an occluded lumen
- Appendiceal wall thickening (>2mm)
- Periappendiceal fat stranding
- Appendiceal wall enhancement
- Appendicolith (25% of patients)

APPENDICITIS TREATMENT

- Acute nonperforated appendicitis: appendectomy should be performed within 12hours of diagnosis
- Antibiotics to cover: enteric gram-negative bacilli, anaerobes, enterococci
- Piperacillin-tazobactam or Quinolone + Metronidazole

CAUSES OF PANCREATITIS

Mnemonic - (ABCDEF SHIP LIST)

A	**A**lcohol
B	**B**iliary (Gall Stones) Most common cause 45%, alcohol #2; endoscopic retrograde cholangiopancreatography (ERCP) removal of gallstones decreases mortality and morbidity especially in severe pancreatitis
C	**C**ancer – pancreatic
D	**D**rugs (see below)
E	**E**RCP (3% post procedure)
F	**F**amilial

S	**S**corpion stings

H	↑Hyper-calcemia (rare)
I	Idiopathic = 3rd most common cause (thought to be a form of microlithiasis)
P	Posterior duodenal ulcer erosion (Anterior erode into peritoneum)
P	Pancreas divisum

L	Lipids ↑TG > 1,000 mg/dL
I	Infection (mumps, coxsackie, HBV, EBV, influenza, legionella, mycoplasma, West Nile Virus)
S	Surgery – post op
T	Trauma

DRUGS THAT CAUSE PANCREATITIS

Mnemonic - (PAST DATE) 2

P	Pentamidine	Propofol
A	Azathioprine (Imuran) common cause	Amiodarone
S	Sulfa	Steroids
T	Thiazides	Tylenol

D	Depakote (valproic acid)	Diphenoxylate (lomotil)
A	ASA and NSAIDs	Amlodipine
T	Tetracyclines	Tamoxifen
E	Ethacrynic acid	Estrogen

HIV MEDICATIONS THE CAUSE PANCREATITIS

Mnemonic - (Z-LSD)

Drug, abbreviations (Brand Name in the US)

Z	Zalcitabine	(ddc) (also 30% neuropathy)
L	Lamivudine	3TC (Epivir)
S	Stavudine	d4T (Zerit); also 30% neuropathy
D	Didanosine	ddI (Videx); also 15% neuropathy; Dilated cardiomyopathy (DCM)

- All three HIV medications are Nucleoside analog Reverse Transcriptase Inhibitors (NRTIs)
- NRTIs are also associated with Lactic Acidosis, if lactate > 2.5 NRTI should be stopped
- NRTI and non-NRTIs bind to HIVs reverse transcriptase → block DNA polymerase → preventing the production fo a DNA copy of viral RNA)

PANCREATITIS - RANSON'S CRITERIA

Mnemonic - (All Wild Girls Like Soccer)

On admission

All	Age > 55
Wild	WBC > 16,000
Girls	Glucose > 200
Like	LDH > 350
Soccer	SGOT (AST) > 250

Within 48 hours

- Hct ↓ > 10%
- BUN ↑ > 5
- Ca2+ < 8
- PO2 < 60
- Base deficit > 4
- Fluid sequestration > 61

Ranson Criteria help gauge bad prognosis, however they have poor predictive value.

- **Amylase** rises within 6 to 24 hours however returns to normal in 3 to 7 days
- **Lipase** rises within 4 to 8 hours and stays elevated for 7 to 14 days
- ↑lipase > 3x upper limit of normal with history c/w pancreatitis to make the diagnosis
- The absolute level of serum amylase and lipase do not correlate with for disease severity and have **no prognostic** value
- Lipase and amylase both exist in other tissues
- Experts recommend lipase over amylase when seeking diagnosis of pancreatitis
- **Overall mortality rate** (MR) = 5%
- **Mortality rate of severe pancreatitis** (see complications below) = 14 - 25%
- **Complications of acute pancreatitis:** pleural effusions (left), ARDS, myocardial depression, DIC, renal failure, shock, phlegmons, abscesses, pseudocysts and necrosis
- **Signs of Hemorrhagic Pancreatitis** are uncommon (3%), but if present MR = 37%

  Cullen sign = periumbilical ecchymosis
  Turner sign = flank ecchymosis
- **Treatment**: aggressive fluid management, analgesia, oxygen administration and early nutrition
- **Pancreatitis diagnostic strategy:**
  - US to evaluate for biliary disease
  - CT Scan = when gallstones are not suspected, in severe pancreatitis, acute deterioration, lack of improvement within 72 hours, the diagnosis is uncertain

BILIARY PATHOLOGY DEFINITIONS

- **Cholelithiasis**: gallstones in the gallbladder
- Biliary colic: pain caused by a stone temporarily obstructing the cystic duct
- **Cholecystitis**: inflammation of the gallbladder from obstruction of the cystic duct
  Choledocholithiasis: stone in the common bile duct
- **Cholangitis**: bacterial infection superimposed on an obstruction of the biliary tree gallstone, neoplasm or stricture

GALLSTONES

Mnemonic - (4 F's)

F	**F**emale
F	**F**at
F	>**F**orty
F	**F**ertile

- Gall stones < 20% picked up on KUB, cholesterol GS = 80% and these are radiolucent
- PEARL: Kidney stones > 90% picked up on KUB

ACUTE CHOLECYSTITIS

- Most common cause of pancreatitis 45%; Alcohol #2
- Most common surgical emergency in elderly with abdominal pain
- **Most common organisms:** *E. coli* (27%), Klebsiella species (16%), Enterococcus species (15%), *Streptococcus* species (8%), Enterobacter species (7%) and P. aeruginosa (7%)
- **Murphy's Sign:** inspiratory arrest, due to pain, with palpation of RUQ / over GB
  - Tender RUQ → radiates to the right scapula
- **Boas sign:** hyperaesthesia (increased or altered sensitivity) below the right scapula
- **Labs:** leukocytosis with or without a left shift, ↑ or normal aminotransferases; bilirubin usually within normal limits
- **Diagnosis:** Ultrasound is the procedure of choice for investigating the gallbladder

GALLBLADDER ULTRASOUND

- The most sensitive sonographic finding in acute cholecystitis =sonographic Murphy sign; Other findings: Cholelithiasis - look for shadowing; Gallbladder wall thickening > 3mm abnormal; Pericholecystic fluid; Sludge
- Most sensitive and specific test for cholecystitis = Hepatobiliary iminodiacetic acid **(HIDA) scan**
- **PEARL**: **Acalculous cholecystitis** due to biliary stasis and obstruction has an atypical presentation and higher morbidity and mortality than calculous cholecystitis; 5 to 10% of cholecystitis
- **PEARL**: **Emphysematous Cholecystitis** associated with air in the biliary tree and gallstone ileus

CHOLANGITIS

- Patients have a higher fever, appear more ill and have abnormal labs compared to the patient with cholecystitis
- **Frequent Causes of Acute Ascending Cholangitis:** biliary calculi (up to 70%), malignancy (biliary, duodenal and pancreatic cancers) or biliary strictures
- **Biliary Stricture examples:** congenital, post-infectious (AIDS cholangiopathy) or inflammatory (primary sclerosing cholangitis (PSC)
- **Frequent organisms:** Gram-negative: Escherichia coli (most common) > Klebsiella > Enterobacter cloacae; Bacteroides. Gram-positive most common = Enterococcus

- **Charcot's Triad:** present in only 25% patients with cholangitis
  1) Fever
  2) RUQ pain
  3) Jaundice
- **Reynolds's Pentad: Charcot's triad *plus***
  4) Mental status changes 5) Hypotension
- **Labs:** Leukocytosis, elevated alkaline phosphatase, and conjugated ("direct") bilirubin; aminotransferases may be as high as 2000 IU/L (similar pattern with hepatic necrosis)
- **Imaging**
  - **Ultrasound (US):** evaluate for common bile duct dilatation or stones
  - **Computed tomography (CT):** identify malignancy or sclerosing cholangitis
- **Endoscopic retrograde cholangiopancreatography (ERCP):** diagnostic and therapeutic
- Most patients with mild to moderate cholangitis will respond to antibiotic treatment, and biliary drainage can be performed within 24–48 hours
- **Severe cholangitis:** urgent biliary decompression within 24 hours
- **PEARL**: Antibiotic coverage MUST include Enterococcus
  Piperacillin-tazobactam or cefepime + metronidazole

PORCELAIN GALLBLADDER

- Uncommon manifestation of chronic cholecystitis, characterized by intramural calcification of the gallbladder wall
- The diagnosis is suggested by an abdominal radiograph revealing an incidental calcified gallbladder.
- Patients with a porcelain gallbladder are often asymptomatic, but are at increased risk for the development of gallbladder carcinoma (poor prognosis)

NONALCOHOLIC FATTY LIVER (NAFL) DISEASE

- Most common cause of liver disease in the US and other Western industrialized countries (result of increase in weight gain & obesity)
- A benign condition

HEPATITIS PEARLS

- Aspartate aminotransferase (AST)
- Alanine aminotransferase (ALT)
- ALT is more specific to the liver then AST
- **Hepatocellular necrosis:** AST (GOT) / ALT (GPT) < 2
- **Alcoholic Hepatitis:** AST (GOT) > 2x ALT (GPT); ratio AST /ALT > 2
  Alcoholic hepatitis can present with liver enzymes as high as the 500's
- **Viral hepatitis:** ALT generally >> AST; can present with liver enzyme elevation > 25x normal
- Highest elevation in liver enzymes: **acute toxic hepatitis** (acetaminophen) *or* in **ischemic hepatitis (shock liver);** may also be elevated in cholangitis
- **Ischemic hepatitis (shock liver):** misnomer since the injury is not mediated by an inflammatory process; usually from blood loss in trauma

- **PEARL:** Amanita phalloides mushroom consumption can lead to fulminant liver failure
- Scleral icterus when serum BILI > 2.5
- Elevated PT / INR: reflects hepatic synthetic function; if elevated = clue for complicated course
- **Transmission**
  - HAV: RNA virus, spread: fecal → oral route
  - HBV: DNA virus, transmitted hematogenously and sexually
  - HCV: RNA virus, transmitted hematogenously
- **Incubation period**
  - HAV is 15-45 days
  - HBV is 60-90 days
  - HCV is 30-90 days

HBV PEARLS

- **IgM anti-HBc:** antibody to core antigen (cAg); indicates acute infection
- **Anti-HBc IgG:** prior infection (best maker for prior HBV infection)
- **Anti-HBs:** Hepatitis B surface antibody to surface Antigen (sAg)
  Immune due to vaccination or
  Immunity/recovery from natural HBV infection
- **Anti-HBe:** antibody to eAg: resolving infection and decreased infectivity; (recovery from hepatitis B or chronic hepatitis with LOW infectivity)
- **Anti-HBc IgM:** Total hepatitis B core antibody; + very early in acute hepatitis B infection and persists for life; Positive = previous or ongoing infection with HBV in an undefined time frame
- **HBsAg:** surface antigen indicates acute or chronic infection; person is infectious; HBsAg is the antigen used to make the hepatitis B vaccine
- **Hb eAg** antigen associated with acute or chronic infection and indicates high infectivity
- 10% of adults and 90% of neonates infected with HBV develop chronic hepatitis
  In addition to chronic hepatitis & cirrhosis, HBV is associated with hepatocellular CA

MORE HEPATITIS PEARLS

- **HDV**: DEpendent on HBV coinfection
- **HEV**: fecal-oral (Enteric) high mortality rate among pregnant (Expectant) patients, Epidemics
- **HAV** and **HEV** are fecal-oral: "The vowels hit your bowels"
- Fecal excretion of **HAV** usually occurs prior to symptoms of acute HAV infection
- **IgM** antibody to **HAV** → indicates acute infection; no chronic carrier state
- **Hepatitis C** = the most common form of viral hepatitis in the United States
  HCV is the most common cause of liver cancer and liver transplants
- HCV: IVDA, Chronic hepatitis, Cirrhosis, Carcinoma, Carrier
  50% HCV develop chronic hepatitis, 20% of this group develop cirrhosis within 10 years

Treatment options for Chronic HCV (genotype 1 or 3)

- Daclatasvir (Daklinza) + Sofosbuvir (Sovaldi) with or without ribavirin
- Anti-HCV = antibody that defines infection with HCV, acute or past
  Risk of HCV = 0.03% per unit of blood transfused

HEPATITIS PROPHYLAXIS

- **Hepatitis A:** Immune Serum Globulin (ISG): 0.02 ml/kg IM within 14 days of exposure; Vaccine is available
- **Hepatitis B** if previously unvaccinated: HBIG 0.06 ml/kg IM, simultaneously with HBV vaccine series with first shot in the deltoid

HEPATITIS VACCINE

- HAV and HBV have preventative vaccines available

HEPATORENAL SYNDROME

- Cause of acute kidney injury (AKI) in patients with end-stage liver disease
- Portal congestion and hypertension → arterial vasodilation in the splanchnic circulation → overall reduction in systemic vascular resistance (SVR) → decline in renal perfusion → renin is released in an attempt to increase BP, but this further compromises the glomerular filtration rate
- Using vasopressors (vasopressin (preferred), norepinephrine, or midodrine) to cause splanchnic vasoconstriction corrects the systemic and renal hemodynamic abnormalities
- There are two types of hepatorenal syndrome
    - **Type I** is more severe and is defined as a 2-fold rise in serum Cr to a level above 2.5 mg/dL over a period of < 2 weeks
    - **Type II** is less severe and presents as ascites that is resistant to diuretics
- A frequent precipitant of hepatorenal syndrome is **acute bacterial infection** or **gastrointestinal bleeding**
- The overall approach to treatment of hepatorenal syndrome is to treat the underlying liver disease, but when this is not possible in the short term, medical therapy with vasopressors and concomitant albumin is recommended.

END-STAGE LIVER DISEASE

- **King's College Criteria** are the most widely used for selecting patients for liver transplantation
- The **Model for End-Stage Liver Disease (MELD)** score is used to predict mortality in patients with chronic liver disease, has also been applied as a prognostic model in patients with acute liver failure
- Tests that reflect hepatocyte synthetic function = prothrombin time (PT) and albumin. A significant elevation in PT, or significant decrease in serum albumin of a patient suggests the synthetic function is compromised and that the patient's liver is failing.

HEPATOTOXINS

- Hepatotoxins lead to hepatocellular necrosis
- AST : ALT < 1

Acetominophen	NSAIDS
Amphotericin	Ketoconazole
INH	Amiodarone
Phenytoin	Valproic acid
Iron	Halothane
Cocaine	Ecstasy (MDMA)
Mushrooms	Carbon tetrachloride
White Phosphorus	Inorganic arsenicals, thallium & borates

Reye Syndrome: resembles fulminant liver failure, but microvesicular fatty infiltration occurs without hepatocellular necrosis

Medications that may have **Cholestatic picture** chlorpromazine, haldol, anabolic or oral contraceptive steroids and erythromycin estolate

LIVER ABSCESS

- Usually polymicrobial; *Escherichia coli* and *Klebsiella pneumonia* = 2 most frequently isolated pathogens; other pathogens: anaerobes, *Bacteroides, Fusobacterium*, microaerophilic/anaerobic *Strep (Peptostreptococcus*); aerobic *Strep* (*Strep. faecalis*) and *Pseudomonas*
- A colonic source usually initial source of infection (diverticulits > biliary disease > appendicitis)
- If hematagenous spread = *Staphylococcus aureus*
- Patients with Crohn's disease = *Staphylococcus milleri*
- Most common test question = *Entamoeba histolytica* (causes 10% of liver abscess cases)
- **Treatment**: Flagyl; IR drainage

CAUSES OF FECAL LEUKOCYTES

Mnemonic - (I Can SEEE Leukocytes In Your SHample)

Inflammatory diarrhea typically refers to grossly bloody diarrhea and fever, suggesting invasion and breakdown of the intestinal epithelium barrier

I	**I**schemic colitis
Can	**Cam**pylobacter, Guillain Barre Syndrome; poultry, eggs
S	**S**almonella Rose spots, fever with relative bradycardia; sickle cell or asplenic patients; pet turtle or inguana; after eating poultry, eggs; hemolytic-uremic syndrome (HUS)
E	***E.*** *coli* 0157:H7 (EHEC: enterohemorrhagic *E.coli*) HUS → microthrombi → renal failure; antibiotics and anti-motility agents should be avoided with Shiga-toxin producing E. Coli O157:H7 - risk of developing HUS
E	***E.*** *coli* (EIEC: enteroinvasive *E. coli*)
E	**E**ntamoeba histolytica Mimics appendicitis - similar to Yersinia

LEUKOCYTES

In	**IN**flammatory bowel disease (IBD)
Your	**YER**sinia enterocolitica (mimics appendicitis; erythema nodosum)
Shample	**SH**igella (Seizures, Reactive Arthritis (formerly Reiter Syndrome) and HUS; mucoid bloody diarrhea + ↑ Fever) Reactive Arthritis (formerly Reiter Syndrome): can't see, can't pee, can't climb a tree: urethritis, iritis, arthritis

Organisms that produce **variable findings on microscopic stool examination**, depending on the invasive properties of the strain and the degree of colonic involvement include:

- *Clostridium difficile*
- *Aeromonas*
- *Vibrio parahaemolyticus* (most common cause of gastroenteritis in Japan)

- *Staph aureus, Bacillus cereus, and Clostridium botulinum* (botulism) exert toxic effects via a **preformed toxin**
- Toxins present in the food prior to ingestion cause rapid onset of symptoms, typically within 1-6 hours
- *Enterotoxigenic E. Coli* and *Vibrio cholerae* produce an **enterotoxin** produced after ingestion
- Viruses cause the majority of infectious diarrheas followed by bacteria
- Norovirus = the most common cause of acute infectious diarrhea
- Norovirus is *not* associated with a preformed toxin
- **PEARL**: Most common bacterial cause of infectious diarrhea = *Campylobacter jejuni*
- **PEARL**: Foodborne illness associated with premature delivery in pregnant women = *Listeria*

DIARRHEA PEARLS

- Most common cause of travelers diarrhea: ***Enterotoxigenic E. coli (ETEC)*** produces a toxin that acts on the intestinal lining (non-invasive / non-bloody diarrhea)
- ***Enteropathogenic E. coli (EPEC)*** attach to the intestinal mucosa, causing diarrhea in children and adults → exact mechanism unclear. Subtle changes in the microvillus surface have been noted in association with attached EPEC, and this damage may cause diarrhea
- ***Entamoeba histolytica*** (causes 10% of liver abscess cases); noninvasive colitis / fecal leukocyte negative, with bloody diarrhea; 10% of world population infected, however only 10% get clinical disease; infects colon → mimics UC;
  Treatment: Flagyl
- Most common causes of diarrhea in AIDS patients: ***Cryptosporidium*** and ***Cytomegalovirus***
- Most common cause of chronic diarrhea in AIDS patients: ***Cryptosporidium*** or ***Isospora belli***
- Most common symptom in AIDS patient: diarrhea
- Most common infection of GI tract in AIDS patient: oral **Candida**; May be asymptomatic, if severe may cause odynophagia; treatment: clotrimazole or nystatin
- ***Bacillus cereus:*** enteritis after eating fried rice

- **Ciguatera** fish poisoning: caused by consumption of reef fish that feed on dinoflagellates (algae); most common ciguatoxin carriers: red snapper, grouper, amberjack, sea bass, sturgeon, barracuda; symptoms: N/V/D, paresthesias, paradoxical temperature reversal, teeth feel loose, vertigo, ataxia and coma; treatment: supportive (amitriptyline, fluids); if bradycardic → atropine and dopamine; consider Mannitol in severe cases including neurological symptoms
- **Scombroid** fish poisoning: caused by consumption of dark meat fish (tuna, mackerel, skipjack, bonito, marlin); nonscombroid species (mahi-mahi sardine, yellowtail, herring, and bluefish); histamine-like reaction: flushing, palpitations, HA, N/V/D, diffuse, macular, blanching erythema, peppery bitter taste; onset within 60 minutes of eating fish; typically self-limited and will resolve within 6 hours. Treatment includes antihistamines and supportive care
- Diarrhea in patients with pet turtle or inguana, asplenic or with sickle cell: ***Salmonella***
- Diarrhea after eating potato salad or mayonnaise: ***Staph aureus***
- Diarrhea after eating raw oysters: ***Vibrio cholera***
- Most common water-borne diarrhea US: ***Giardia lamblia***; Parasite however no Eosinophilia; Best test to confirm diagnosis: Stool Antigen (not O&P); Most common protozoal infection in the US; Beaver is common reservoir - "Beaver Fever"
  PEARL: Beavers can cause rabies
- Most common symptom with **Giardiasis**: acute watery or pale explosive, offensive smelling diarrhea; 90%; abdominal colicky pain / distention /flatulence in 75% or asymptomatic; Risk for Giardiasis: hikers/campers, children at daycare, persons who engage in oral-anal contact
- Most common intestinal parasite in the US = ***Giardia lamblia;*** treatment: Metronidazole (Flagyl)

CAUSES OF POST-OP FEVERS

Mnemonic - (7 W's)

W	**W**ind (atelectasis or pneumonia) – first 24 hours
W	**W**ater (UTI) – days 3 to 5
W	**W**anes → veins → check IV sites – days 3 to 5
W	**W**alk (DVT/PE) > 5 days post-op
W	**W**ound > 5 days post-op
W	**W**onder drugs → drug fever
W	**W**omen → endometritis

ARTERIAL OCCLUSION

Mnemonic - (6 P's)

P	**P**ain
P	**P**ulselessness
P	**P**allor (limb initially white, with time cyanosis may appear indicating desaturation of blood with ongoing ischemia)
P	**P**olar (for cold, and rhymes with pallor)
P	**P**aresthesias (complete anesthesia = immediate surgical intervention)
P	**P**aralysis (last finding)

ARTERIAL OCCLUSION

- Most common cause of arterial occlusion = arterial embolism
- Arterial embolism originates from the heart (80%), specifically from the left ventricle 70%; Second most common cause = thrombosis (20%)
- Atrial fibrillation (AF) and Myocardial infarction (MI) are the two most common causes of thrombus within the heart → arterial emboli to LE's
- Afib is present in 60-75% of peripheral arterial embolic events
- Most common site of arterial embolism occlusion = bifurcation of common femoral artery; Other bifurcation sites: common iliac, and popliteal artery bifurcations

CAUSES OF ARTERIAL OCCLUSION - ARTERIAL EMBOLUS

- **Cardiac sources**
  - Atrial fibrillation (AF)
  - Myocardial infarction (MI)
  - Valvular disease, debris from prosthetic valves, endocarditis (septic emboli)
  - Atrial myxomas
- **Arterial sources**
  - AAA
  - Atherosclerotic plaque
- **Native Arterial Thrombus**
  - Atherosclerotic plaque
  - Arterial dissection
  - Low flow state
  - Thrombophilia (hypercoagulable)
- **Arterial Thrombus after intervention**
  - Angioplasty site
  - Stent/stent-graft site
  - Prosthetic bypass graft
  - Vein bypass graft
- **Arterial Injury**
  - Iatrogenic
  - Trauma
- **Diagnostical tools**
  - Duplex ultrasonography, computed tomography angiography (CTA), and magnetic resonance angiography (MRA)
  - CTA and MRA are used most often because the duplex ultrasonography, although non-invasive, is not precise in planning revascularization
- **Ankle Brachial Index**: normal > 90%, mild 70-90%, moderate 50-70% and severe arterial insufficiency < 50% (0.5) (inflate cuff above ankle, doppler → DP or PT, compare to brachial BP)

ARTERIAL OCCLUSION - TREATMENT

- NON-Limb threatening ischemia from embolism: vascular surgery referral for Fogarty catheter embolectomy
- NON-Limb threatening ischemia from thrombosis: Heparinization; consider intra-arterial thrombolysis
- Limb threatening ischemia from embolism: vascular surgery referral for Fogarty catheter embolectomy
- Limb threatening ischemia from thrombosis: vascular surgery referral for direct or Fogarty catheter embolectomy and vascular bypass grafting
- Limb threatening irreversible ischemia or very ill or lesion cannot be bypassed: amputation

THROMBOANGIITIS OBLITERANS (TAO) (BUERGER'S DISEASE)

- Nonatherosclerotic, segmental, inflammatory disease
- Most commonly affects the small to medium-sized arteries and veins of the extremities (upper and lower)
- Smokers
- Painful, tender, red/dark nodule over peripheral artery

LERICHE SYNDROME

- Aortoiliac Occlusive Disease
- Claudication / pain of the buttocks and thighs
- Absent /decreased femoral pulses
- Erectile Dysfunction

POST-OP COMPLICATIONS OF THYROIDECTOMY

Mnemonic - (THYROIDS)

T	**T**etany-hypoparathyroidism (hypercalcemia)
H	**H**emorrhage
Y	**Y**ell – recurrent laryngeal → stridor & superior laryngeal nerve → voice fatigue
R	**R**ecurrent hyperthyroidism
O	**O**esophageal damage
I	**I**nfection
D	**D**eaths
S	**S**torm-thyroid storm - tachypnea, tachycardia and fever

GASTROSTOMY TUBES

- Replace if clogged, fractured or ruptured balloon
- Most common cause for replacement = accidental removal
- Do NOT replace if tract is immature (created within 4 weeks)
- Premature removal could result in peritoneal contamination
- with gastric contents and peritonitis
- Abdominal pain or pain with manipulation of G-tube
  a) Administer antibiotics for presumed abscess or infection
  b) CT of the abdomen and pelvis
  c) Consult specialist who placed the tube

SURGERY / GI PEARLS

- Most common GI disease in the US = **gastroenteritis**
- Most common cause of **vomiting** in adults = medications
- Most common cause of **upper neuromuscular swallowing dysfunction** = CVA
  2nd = polymyositis or dermatomyositis
- Most common cause of **lower swallowing dysfunction** = intrinsic motility disorder (achalasia, spasm)
- **Diverticulitis**
  - Bugs: E. coli, Klebsiella pneumonia, Bacteroides, Enterococcus faecalis
  - Drugs - Outpatient: Amoxicilin-clavulanate 875/125 mg po bid; Ciprofloxacin 500 mg po bid + Metronidazole 500 mg po qid x 7 to 10 days
  - Drugs - Inpatient: Piperacillin-tazobactam or Ertapenem 1 gm IV q 24 hours
  - Drugs - Severe, life threatening: Meropenem 1 gm IV q 8 hours
- Most common cause of significant LGI bleed = **diverticulosis**; Painless; usually right side > left
- 10-15% of BRPR is from UGI source
- **Diagnose Bleeding Site:** Angiography requires a brisk bleeding rate (0.5-2 mL/min)
  Technetium-Labeled Tagged RBC Nuclear Scan or GI bleeding scan- is more sensitive and can detect bleeding sites of 0.1mL/min
- **Mallory-Weiss tears** = partial thickness esophageal tear with bleeding after vomiting
- **Boerhaave syndrome** = full thickness esophageal rupture can also occur after vomiting, during childbirth, forceful coughing; however the most common cause = IATROGENIC most common stie = distal, left posterolateral (Weakest portion)
- Classic triad presentation of **Boerhaave syndrome (Mackler Triad)** < 50% = vomiting, CP, and subcutaneous emphysema

  SOB may be secondary to pleuritic CP or left-sided pleural effusion (common), or pneumothorax
  Hamman's crunch = Pneumomediastinum; (20%), CXR = mediastinal air; could also have pneumothorax or left pleural effusion.
  Most common complication of Boerhaave Syndrome = Mediastinitis
  Esophagram helps confirm diagnosis; Gastrografin (water-soluble contrast) = 90% sensitivity
- Most common cause of esophageal perforations = Iatrogenic perforations (others: FBs, caustic burns, Boerhaave's)
- Most common site of **Iatrogenic perforations** = pharyngoesophageal junction or the esophagogastric junction
- > 90% of **spontaneous esophageal perforations** occur in the distal esophagus
- **Foreign Bodies** → Most common in kids = 80%; 18 to 48 months
- **Most common site for Esophageal foreign bodies to lodge**
  #1 = Level of cricopharyngeus muscle (C6)
  #2 = Aortic arch (T4)
  #3 = GE junction
- Most common **esophageal impaction** in kids = coins
- Most common **esophageal impaction** in adults = food (meat/bones); treatment = glucagon IV, NTG, procardia .... EGD

- **Glucagon** 1 to 2mgIV
  - Relaxes esophageal smooth muscle and the LES
  - Little effect on the motility of the proximal esophagus
  - Less effective in patients with structural abnormalities, such as strictures or rings
  - Success rate 15 to 50%
- NTG, Procardia (may cause hypotension)
- Only ancedotgal evidence that nitroglycerin 0.4mg sublingually helps relax the esophagus to allow passage of the food bolus
- Get EGD!
- Simethicone, carbonated beverages, tartaric acid, mixed with bicarbonate and papain (meat tenderizer) are NOT treatment options for esophageal food impation - possible **esophageal perforation**
- If perforation suspected → water-soluble contrast (Gastrograffin)
- CXR **esophageal foreign body** = frontal plane; tracheal = sagittal plane
- Most common **age group to aspirate FB** = 1 to 3 years
- **Button battery ingestion**: if in duodenum → observe; if in esophagus → immediate removal; if not removed in 8 hours there is a risk of esophageal perforation secondary to rapid erosion
- Most common **malignancy of esophagus** = adenocarcinoma, (no longer squamous cell); adenocarcinoma has continued to rise since 1970 and is now > 50% of all esophageal carcinomas
- **Barrett's esophagus** is a risk factor for adenocarcinoma; up to 10% of patients with Barrett's esophagus will develop adenocarcinoma
- Most common **benign stomach neoplasms** = Polyps (90% hyperplastic/inflammatory polyps, 10% adenomatous – single cauliflower-like malignant transformation risk)
- Most common **malignancy of stomach** = Adenocarcinoma; Check → CEA, Virchow supraclavicular-node; blacks > whites; lymphoma second most common stomach malignancy
- **Krukenberg tumor** → Primary stomach or breast CA metastasis to ovary (usually both ovaries; accounts for 5% of ovarian cancers)
- **Klatskin tumor** = cholangiocarcinoma – cancer of biliary tree
- Most common chronic infection in liver or kidney transplant = CMV
- Most common malignancy of small intestine in the US = Adenocarcinoma
- Most common malignancy of large intestine = Adenocarcinoma
- **Toxic megacolon** occurs in 5% of case of Ulcerative Colitis; cause unclear; transverse colon more common
- **Ulcerative Colitis lesions** = erythema nodosum, pyoderma gangrenosum and aphtous stomatitis
- **Crohn's** = peri-anal disease (fistulas and fissures), bowel malignancies 3x more common
- Most common **anorectal abscess** = perianal (may be first presentation of Crohn's)
- Most common **cause of SBP** = *E. coli* 50%, Enterococcus, Strep. Pneumo (Tx = Amp + Gent)

PEPTIC ULCER DISEASE

- Most common cause of UGI bleed = PUD; melena present in 33% of LGI bleeds (need 150-200cc of blood in GI tract for minimum of 8 hours for stool to turn black)
- Duodenal ulcers > more common than gastric ulcers
- Duodenal ulcers improve with food, gastric ulcers worsen with food
- Duodenlal ulcer pain awakens patient at night (50-58%); postprandial pain (1 to 2 hour delay)
- Gastric ulcers bleed more often than duodenal
- Most common location of gastric ulcer = lesser curvature of body and antrum
- **PEARL:** Most common cause of UGI bleeding in pregnancy = esophagitis
- Most common cause of peptic ulcer disease and gastritis = H. pylori
- 95% of patients with duodenal ulcers, and 70% of those with gastric ulcers, have evidence of H. pylori infection
- H. pylori = gram-negative, urease-producing, flagellated bacterium that lives on the mucosal lining of the stomach
- **Risk factors for PUD**
    - ETOH
    - Cigarettes
    - Caffeine
    - ASA
    - NSAIDs
    - Family HIstory
    - **H. Pylori** infection
- PUD - Associated with mucosa-associated lymphoid tissue lymphoma (**MALT lymphoma**); eradication of infection leads to remission in many patients with low-grade tumors
- Associated with an increased risk of gastric cancer
- **Diagnosis**: serologic tests or invasively at endoscopy
- **Treatment**: "triple therapy" (proton pump inhibitor, clarithromycin, and amoxicillin or metronidazole)
- Proton pump inhibitor (PPI) regimen shown to reduce length of hospital stay (LOS), rebleeding, and the need for blood transfusion in patients with bleeding peptic ulcer disease = Intermittent PPI boluses
- **Stress Ulcer PEARLS**
  Most common location of **stress ulcers** = body and fundus; examples = Curling's ulcers (burns); Cushing's ulcers (associated with ICP → head trauma and CNS tumors); sepsis and shock
- **Perforation PEARLS**
  Most common cause of **visceral perforation** = ulcers
  The most common cause of colonic perforation = diverticulitis
  Most common site of large bowel perforation = cecum

MANAGEMENT OF ESOPHAGEAL VARICES

- Octreotide (Sandostatin) - for the first 24 hours of hospitalization
- Protonix (Pantoprazole) - 80 mg IV bolus, 8 mg/hr drip
- IV fluids
- Blood products (PRBCs, FFP, platelets)
- Ceftriaxone 1 gm q 24 hours x 5 days; cirrhosis patients have increased risk of gut bacteria translocation in the settinng of acute bleeding; antibiotics decrease mortality rate (MR) and length of stay (LOS) in the hospital
- Vasopressin is the pressor of choice for reducing splanchnic blood flow and portal HTN in patients with severe UGI variceal bleeding
- EGD within 12 hours (banding, sclerotherapy)
- **PEARL:** No evidence that NGT placement aggravates hemorrhage from varices or Mallory-Weiss tears
- Octreotide (Sandostatin) mimics natural somatostatin (50 mcg IV bolus followed by 50 mcg/hr drip) → splanchnic vasoconstriction → ↓ variceal bleeding (similar to vasopressin without coronary vasoconstriction)
- Octreotide has been shown to reduce mortality and improve hemostasis in patients with variceal bleeding
- **TOX PEARL** → Octreotide is used in the treatment of refractory hypoglycemia from oral hypoglycemic agents
- **PEARL:** PPI Increases gastric pH to allow clot formation. PPI acts on the H + K + ATPase of the gastric parietal cell blocking the secretion of H+ ions
- Most common cause of esophageal varices in USA = ETOH abuse
- Most common cause of esophageal varices worldwide = Schistosomiasis

ASCITES AND SPONTANEOUS BACTERIAL PERITONITIS (SBP)

- **Diagnosis**
  - Total ascitic white blood cell count of > 1,000 mm3
  - or a PMN count >250 cells/mm3; pH < 7.34
  - is diagnostic for spontaneous bacterial peritonitis

- **Treatment**: 3rd generation Cephalosporin
  - Cefotaxime 2gm every 8 hours; consider albumin
  - Fluoroquinolone or Bactrim prophyaxis for patients with history of SBP might prevent future episodes of SBP and hepatorenal syndrome; IV albumin at the time of diagnosis of SBP may prevent hepatorenal syndrome
  - Antibiotic administration in SBP should be delayed until fluid is obtained for analysis; Most common organism = E. coli

ANAL FISSURE

- The most common anorectal disorder in children and infants. An anal fissure is a superficial tear in the anoderm that results when a hard piece of stool is forced through the anus. It is associated with constipation; other causes peds/adults: local trauma, anal sex, vaginal delivery, diarrhea
- Sudden onset, searing pain during defecation, minor GI bleed
- Male = female
- Acute fissures generally resolve in 2-4 weeks
- Most common cause of severe acute rectal pain in adults or peds
- **Posterior midline** = most common location because the skeletal muscle encircling the anus is the weakest at this location
- **Anterior midline** - second most common (most common in women)
- **Lateral Fissures** likely to be related to systemic illness include: leukemia, Crohn's disease, HIV, TB, and syphilis
- **Treatment**: Treatment Topical NTG or Nifedipine (CCB) and **WASH Regimen**

W	**W**arm water (Sitz baths)
A	**A**nalgesics
S	**S**tool softeners
H	**H**igh fiber diet

ANORECTAL ABSCESS

- Swelling, perianal fluctuant mass or drainage, skin changes (erythema) lateral to anus
- Managed in ED; Give antibiotic after I&D (Augmentin x 5 days), complications after I&D include fistula OR recurrent abscess formation
- **Dentate Line**
  - Fluctuance above the dentate line = surgical consultation
  - Abscess below the dentate line = treat in ED with I&D
- **Indications for packing an abscess**
  - Large size > 5 cm
  - Pilonidal abscess
  - Abscess in patients with DM immunocompromised
- **Antibiotic considerations**
  - Advised for a large abscess
  - Suspicion for cellulitis
  - Multiple lesions, and in high-risk patients
- **PERIRECTAL ABSCESS (intersphincteric, ischiorectal, or supralevator)**
  - Surgical consultation
  - If fever and urinary retention - think deeper more complicated perirectal abscess

PROCTITIS

- Tenesmus, if infectious rectal discharge
- Causes: Sexually transmitted > radiation, autoimmune
- STD causes: HSV-2, HIV, Syphilis, Chlamydia trachomatis, Neisseria gonorrhea
- Most common organism = N. gonorrhoeae
- Radiation Proctocolitis: consider infection or perforation
- If mild case: treat supportively with steroid enema or foam

IRRITABLE BOWEL SYNDROME

- Typically young women
- History of anxiety
- Episodic abdominal pain
- Undulating pattern of normal stools and diarrhea
- Mucous at times
- Chronic - normal labs/exam
- **Treatment**
  - Fiber, avoid lactulose, gluten or gas-producing foods exercise, hydration, treat anxiety symptoms
  - Allergy testing

CROHN'S

- Granulomatous lesions -affects anywhere from mouth to anus (Ulcerative colitis is typically limited to the colon)
- Involve all layers of intestinal wall
- Skip areas
- 75% involve the ileum
- Perianal disease is common
- Crohn's disease
- Both UC and Crohn's present with abdominal pain, fever, and bloody diarrhea
- Both UC and Crohn's can cause Toxic Megacolon
- Infliximab (Remicade)
  - Used to treat Crohn's disease & ulcerative colitis
- **PEARL**: Infliximab (Remicade) is also used in the treatment of other autoimmune diseases including: rheumatoid arthritis, ankylosing spondylitis, psoriasis, psoriatic arthritis, and Behçet's disease

MESENTERIC ISCHEMIA

- Most common cause of acute mesenteric ischemia = Cardiac emboli to the superior mesenteric artery (SMA) (Atrial fibrillation, atherosclerotic heart disease, valvular heart disease, recent MI)
- Other causes: SMA thrombus, venous thromosis, non-occlusive mesenteric ischemia (heart failure, vasoconstrictive medications)
- Sudden onset, poorly localized pain
- Abdominal pain out of proportion to that expected based on physical examination Guaic positive stool
- Lactic acidosis (late finding)
- Most common finding on abdominal CT in acute mesenteric ischemia = Bowel wall edema; thickened bowel wall; pneumatosis intestinalis; rarely see superior mesenteric artery or vein thrombosis
- **Diagnosis**
  - CT Angiogram (Angiography - gold standard)

URGENT ENDOSCOPY TO REMOVE A FOREIGN BODY

- Button battery in esophagus
- A long or sharp object
- Multiple objects
- FB ingested > 24 hours
- Airway compromise
- Evidence of perforation
  - Odynophagia = pain on swallowing
  - Dysphagia = difficulty swallowing

PLUMMER-VINSON SYNDROME

- Classic triad = glossitis, iron-deficiency anemia and esophageal webs
- Very rare, however important to recognize because patients at increased risk of squamous cell carcinoma of the pharynx and the esophagus

TRAUMA PEARLS - TRAUMATIC BRAIN INJURY

Failure to repair GALEA during scalp laceration can lead to:

- Loss of function of the frontalis muscle
- Subgaleal hematoma
- Poorer cosmetic outcomes
- Wider Scar
- Scar may be depressed

- Leading cause of traumatic death in adults and PEDS = severe **Traumatic Brain Injury (TBI);** #2 = thoracic trauma

- Severe Traumatic Brain Injury (**TBI**) = GCS < 8
  Most common cause of severe **TBI** = Falls 28% > MVC #2

FACTORS THAT INCREASE MORTALITY in TBI

- Hypotension = #1 (SBP < 100 mmHg)
- Hypoxia (PaO2 < 60mmHg)
- Fever and hyperglycemia should be avoided for their potential to exacerbate secondary neurologic injury
- Keep PaCO2 over 30 mmHg
- **PEARL**: A single episode of hypotension in patients with traumatic brain injury = double mortality

DECREASING INTRACRANIAL PRESSURE (ICP)

- Elevate HOB to 30 degrees, hyperventilation and osmotic therapy (hypertonic saline or mannitol)
- Hyperventilation to a PaCO2 of 30 to 35 mmHg is the fastest means to decrease ICP, but only lasts a short while; hyperventilation causes cerebral vasoconstriction and onset of effect < 30 seconds
- Hyperventilation should be avoided in the first 24 to 48 hrs and should not exceed PaCO2 <30 mmHg except as a temporizing measure in patients with impending cerebral herniation
- No evidence that corticosteroids decrease ICP

Seizure > 20 minutes after trauma = worse prognosis; ↑ possibility of internal injury and development of seizures later

SEIZURE PROPHYLAXIS

- Depressed skull fracture
- Penetrating brain injury
- Intracranial Hemorrhage
- Acute SDH or Epidural
- Prior history of seizures
- Seizure at time of injury or ED presentation
- Intubated and paralyzed head injury patient

BASILAR SKULL FRACTURE

Basilar skull fracture: petrous portion of the temporal bone is most commonly fractured; CN VII and VIII entrapmernt

1. Racoon eyes (periorbital ecchymosis)
2. Battle sign (mastoid ecchymosis)
3. Hemotympanum
4. CSF rhinorrhea /otorrhea (Blood + CSF = Halo sign → think of an egg → yolk = blood, egg white = CSF

3% incidence of traumatic carotid-cavernous fistula after basilar skull fracture

- Most common traumatic **herniation syndrome** = uncus of temporal lobe → transtentorial herniation; CN III compressed → ipsilateral, dilated, non-reactive pupil; ptosis; contralateral hemiparesis; ptosis; contralateral Babinski; as the herniation progresses → decerebrate posturing
- 2nd Most common **herniation syndrome** = central transtentorial herniation = decreased LOC, bilateral muscle weakness, Babinski reflexes, Cushing's

  PEARL: NORMAL DOLL'S EYE: When head is turned, eyes turn in opposite direction = intact brainstem
- Most common cause of post-traumatic coma = **Diffuse axonal injury**
- **Subdural**: crescent shape on CT; bridging veins much more common than epidural and ↑mortality vs epidural; occur in very young & very old & very intoxicated; Indications for emergent surgery in SDH = neurologic deterioration or midline shift > 5 mm
- **Epidural:** lens-shaped/ biconvex/ football shaped on CT; laceration of the middle meningeal artery; "lucid interval"; rare in very young and very old
- Trauma is the most common cause of **subarachnoid hemorrhage (SAH)**
  Most common CT abnormality after severe closed head injury = **traumatic SAH**
- **PEARL:** Most common location for intracerebral bleeds = frontal and temporal
- **PEARL:** Pinpoint pupils and brain injury = pontine lesion
- Most common bone fractured in children with **skull fractures** = parietal bone (60-70%)
- 15 to 30% of **linear skull fractures** in children have been associated with an intracranial injury
- **Growing Skull Fractures:** linear skull fractures in children that enlarge over time and produce a cranial defect. Result from tear in dura, present months to years following the initial injury, usually require surgical correction
- **Depressed skull fractures** > the full thickness of the skull = surgical elevation

Indications for Obtaining Head CT in Children with Head Trauma

- AMS
- Headache
- Loss of consciousness
- Amnesia
- Seizure
- Focal neurologic deficits
- Evidence of basilar or depressed skull fractures
- Irritability or behavior changes
- Scalp hematoma in children < 2 years old
- Persistent vomiting

Significant head or facial trauma have 5 to10% associated **C-spine injuries**

INTERPRETING C-SPINE PLAIN FILMS

HISTORY FOR C-SPINE

Mnemonic - (A MUST)

A	**A**ltered mental status
M	**M**echanism
U	**U**nderlying condition
S	**S**ymptoms
T	**T**iming (when symptoms began in relation to event)

Nexus Criteria for C-spine imaging

If any criteria present, cannot clear C-spine clinically

- Midline spinal tenderness
- Focal neurological deficit
- Altered level of consciousness
- Intoxication
- Distracting injury present
- The biggest difference between NEXUS criteria and Canadian C-spine rule:
  The addition of patients 65 years old and older = high risk of injury;
  Ability to move the neck

INTERPRETING C-SPINES

Mnemonic ABCs)

A	**A**lignment
B	**B**ones
C	**C**artilage
s	**S**oft-tissue

You need to visualize all 7 cervical vertebrae down to the top of T1

Alignment check 3 lines → smooth lordotic curves

1) Anterior aspect of vertebral bodies
2) Posterior aspect of vertebral bodies
3) Spinolaminar line

- **PEARL:** PEDS: 4% of kids < 8 years have pseudosubluxation of C2-C3
- **Bones** check vertebral bodies; ensure anterior and posterior heights are similar (> 3mm difference suggests fracture)
- **Cartilage** intervertebral joint spaces and facet joints
- **Soft-tissue**
  Prevertebral swelling, *6mm at C2 and 22mm at C6*
  Measure from anterior border of C2 to posterior wall of pharynx (6-at-2 and 22-at-6): PEARL:
  Pediatrics < 15 years old, same holds for C2, however at C6 <14mm
- **Predental space:** space from the anterior aspect of the odontoid process and the posterior aspect of the anterior ring of C1; normal predental space:
  < 3mm in adults
  < 5mm in children
  Widen predental space = C1-C2 injury

SPINAL CORD INJURY WITHOUT RADIOGRAPHIC ABNORMALITY (SCIWORA)

- More common in children - increased mobility of cervical spine, increased laxity of the ligaments of the spine and children have larger size heads
  Most common mechanism flexion and extension

CLAY-SHOVELER'S FRACTURE (FLEXION)

- Avulsion fracture of C7 spinous process due to sudden flexion

DENS, C2 (AXIS) FRACTURES

- Most commonly injured part of spine
- Type I - avulsion fracture of apex of dens (usually stable) - treated with cervical collar
- Type II - fracture through the base of the dens (unstable) - treated with halo vest or surgical fixation
- Type III - fracture extends into the body of the axis (unstable) - treated with halo vest or surgical fixation
- Most common level of C-spine injury in Elderly = C1 to C3 (higher than younger, non-peds patients)
- Type II - most common type of C2 fracture in the elderly
- Most common cervical fracture in kids = higher cervical (especially C2); more common in older kids

UNSTABLE C-SPINE FRACTURES

Mnemonic - (Jefferson Bit Off a Hangman's Thumb) [Dr. Morgan Barnell]

Jefferson	**Jefferson** fracture (C1, Atlas) "burst" fracture; Compression fracture; axial load injury
Bit	**B**ilateral facet dislocation (**Unilateral facet dislocations** most commonly occur at the level of C3-C7 - Stable; Flexion & rotation; **Bilateral facet dislocations** are more common in thoracic or lumbar spine and are unstable; Flexion injury
Off	**O**dontoid fracture (C2, Axis) C2 Fracture, odontoid process also called dens; Types II and III unstable; Hyperextension or flexion injury
A	**A**tlanto-occipital dislocation; pure flexion injury
Hangman's	**Hangman's** fracture C2 (Axis) Fracture of bilateral pars interarticularis (between the lamina and pedicle); Hyperextension up to 30% have other spine fracture; cord damage is minimal (neural foramen is greatest at C2)
Thumb	**T**eardrop fracture Flexion or extension Teardrop Fracture = unstable (flexion more unstable then extension)

- **PEARL:** Patients with spinal cord injury have 25% associated head injury
- **PEARL:** Spinal cord injury may result in spinal shock
  Spinal shock = hypotension, bradycardia and warm skin;
  diagnosis of exclusion

- Most common facial fracture: nasal (rule-out septal hematoma); #2 mandible
- Most common Mandible Fracture: Body 29% > Condyle 26% > Angle 25% > Symphysis 17%

Mayersak RJ. Initial evaluation and management of facial trauma in adults. Post TW, ed. UpToDate. Waltham, MA: UpToDate Inc. Accessed January 31, 2018.

- Jaw deviates towards fracture on maximal opening
- Most common side of mandibular fractues = left
- **PEARL**: Most common side of pelvic ring fractures = left
- **PEARL**: Subungal or buccal ecchymosis is *pathognomonic* for mandibular fracture
- Myth that mandible fractures must occur in pairs due to the U-shape of the bone
- > 40% of mandible fractures are isolated

- **Tongue-blade test** is performed by attempting to twist a tongue-blade that is held between a patient's molars. If the examiner is able to break the tongue-blade by twisting without causing the patient pain, mandibular fracture has been ruled out (100% Sn)- cost effective screening test for a mandibular fracture.

DENTAL FRACTURES

Classified according to the Ellis Classification

- **Ellis I fractures** = involve the enamel only
- Non-painful chips or worn edges
- No treatment is necessary; routine dental referral

- **Ellis II fractures** are through the enamel and the dentin
- The dentin is yellow and holds many nerve fibers. Fractures exposing the dentin cause pain and hypersensitivity to cold and hot temperatures
- Treatment: covering of the exposed dentin with
- calcium hydroxide or zinc oxide paste and routine dental referral

- **Ellis III fractures** are through all three layers of the tooth (enamel, dentin & pulp)
- Emergency **treatment**: cover pulp with calcium hydroxide or zinc oxide paste and urgent (< 48 h) dental referral for pulpotomy or pulpectomy to prevent infection

FACIAL AND DENTAL NERVE BLOCKS

- Supraorbital: Ipsilateral forehead and scalp
- Infraorbital: area between lower eyelid and upper lip
- Posterior superior alveolar: Ipsilateral maxillary molars
- Inferior alveolar: Ipsilateral mandibular teeth, lower lip, chin
- Mental: Ipsilateral lower lip and chin

LOCAL ANESTHESIA PEARLS

2 "i's" in generic denotes an amide; amide allergies are very rare

- Amides: Lidocaine, Bupivacaine, Prilocaine, Mepivacaine and Etidocaine
- Esters: benzocaine, procaine (Novocaine) and tetracaine more commonly cause allergic reactions; they are broken down into the compound PABA, a known allergen

- If allergic to amides (see above) and esthers → consider benadryl
- Benadryl dose = 1cc (50mg/ml) diluted in 9cc of NS

- Maximum dose of lidocaine of infiltration:
  - *Without* epinephrine = 5 mg/kg
  - *With* epinephrine = 7 mg/kg

- Avoid TAC (tetracaine, adrenaline, cocaine) or LET (lidocaine, epinephrine and tetracaine) on mucosal membranes, pinna of the ear, nose, penis, fingers and toes

- XAP = lidocaine, adrenaline (epinephrine) and pontocaine (tetracaine)

- LET = lidocaine, epinephrine and tetracaine
- Bupivacaine is not recommended for use in children < 12 y/o
- Systemic toxicity from local anesthetics (following inadvertent intravascular injection) = AMS, seizures, acidosis, dysrhythmias, hypotension, and cardiac arrest
- Bupivacaine = most cardiotoxic of all local anesthetics
- Benzocaine = methemoglobinemia
- Lidocaine = seizures, hypotension
- Antidote for treatment of systemic toxicity from local anesthetics:
- intralipid fat emulsion (lipid emulsion)

ALVEOLAR FRACTURES

- True fractures of the root which are part of the mandible
- Treatment = repositioning of the tooth if it is subluxed or dislocated and splinting; eat only soft foods and liquids; Urgent endodontist referral is recommended as treatment involves splinting with wire for six weeks

PRIMARY TEETH

- By age 12 you usually have permanent teeth; do not replace primary teeth
- Permanent tooth: replace intact avulsed permanent tooth into the socket as soon as possible; Survival drops 1% every 1 minute tooth remains out of socket

AVULSED PERMANENT TOOTH MANAGEMENT

- Transport in patients mouth or in milk
- Can be stored in Hank's solution
- Handle by crown
- Do not scrub = destroy periodontal ligaments
- If extra-oral time < 60 minutes = rinse with normal saline
- If extra-oral time > 60 minutes = soak in citric acid / fluoride & consult oral surgeon

LE FORTE FRACTURES

Le Forte classification system describes maxillary facial fractures - Four Classes

- **I = Horizontal** fracture involving only the maxilla at level of nasal fossa; if SQ air → sinus fracture; Upper teeth and hard palate are freely moveable, but not the nose; fractures involve the hard palate; "Speak no evil"
- **II = Pyramidal fracture** = vertical fractures through the maxilla, nasal bones, medial aspects of the orbits. Blood in nares, rhino or otorrhea; swollen mid-face; Freely movable midface - hard palate and nose, not the eyes; Fracture extends into the orbital floor; "See no evil"
- **III = Craniofacial disjunction;** "dishface"; entire face moves but not head; CSF rhinorrhea; Fracture involves zygoma; craniofacial disruption; "Hear no evil"
- **LeForte IV Fractures** are LeForte III fractures that also involve the frontal bone
- Manage airway (unstable facial structures or significant bleeding); ofter open fractures = require IV antibiotics; concomitant injuries, (ocular trauma, CNS involvement, and cervical spine fractures; early consultation with a facial surgeon

- **Orbital Blow-Out Fracture:** Vertical diplopia - entrapment of inferior rectus muscle → results in limited upgaze and may cause pain on attempted upgaze; endophthalmos; fractures along the floor usually affect the infraorbital nerve → hypoesthesia of the cheek and upper
- Weakest area of Orbit = floor (contents prolapse into maxillary sinus)
- **Retrobulbar hematoma**: eye pain, diplopia, visual loss, reduction of ocular motility, proptosis, ↑IOP, ecchymosis of eyelids, chemosis, ophthalmoplegia, APD; Treatment = lateral canthotomy
- **PEARL:** Monocular diplopia = lens dislocation

AURICULAR HEMATOMA

- Occur after blunt trauma to the ear (wrestlers)
- Without proper treatment, the cartilaginous structures of the ear can become permanently deformed (cauliflower ear)
- Treatment: Incision & drainage of the hematoma by making a small incision in the helix or antihelix, followed by application of a pressure dressing to maintain the contours of the ear
- If acute (< 48 hours) and small (<2cm) = needle aspiration

EAR LACERATIONS

- Need rapid repair to:
  1) cover the auricular cartilage to limit infection
  2) Prevention of auricular hematoma
- Next-day follow-up to ensure hematoma reaccumulation has not occurred

TRIPOD FRACTURE

- Zygomatico –**Maxillary** articulation - infraorbital rim fracture
- Zygomatico - **Temporal** articulation - at the arch; Zygomatic Arch
- Zygomatico - **Frontal** articulation; Lateral orbital rim
- Flat cheek, diplopia, anesthesia to cheek/upper lip, cheek or periorbital edema = **Tripod fracture**
- **PEARL:** Most common Zygomatic fracture = **arch** > tripod; both uncommon
- **PEARL:** Isolated arch fracture - ok for outpatient management/elective repair

ZONES OF THE NECK

- Zone I - (base of neck) extends superiorly from the sternal notch/clavicles → cricoid cartilage
- Zone II - (midneck) cricoid cartilage → angle of the mandible
- Zone III - (upper neck) angle of the mandible → base of skull
- **PEARL:** Penetrating violation of platysma (neck muscle) = concern for injury to the underlying neck structures

PENETRATING NECK TRAUMA - HARD SIGNS VS SOFT SIGNS

Hard signs

- Airway obstruction / stridor
- Cerebral ischemia
- Major hemoptysis / hematemesis
- Decreased or absent radial pulse
- Expanding, pulsatile hematoma
  Shock non-responsive to fluid
- Severe acute bleeding
- Vascular bruit or thrill
- Focal neurological deficit

Soft signs

- Chest tube leak
- Dysphasia / dysphonia
- Dyspnea
- Minor hemoptysis / hematemesis
- Mediastinal emphysema
- Subcutaneous emphysema
- Not expanding hematoma

- Hard signs = emergent intervention
- Soft signs = further investigation

EVALUATE FOR ESOPHAGEAL TRAUMA

- Esophogram + Esophagoscopy
- Risk of life-threatening mediastinitis with esophageal injury

BLUNT CHEST TRAUMA - CARDIAC EVALUATION

- Most common area of heart injured in blunt trauma = Right ventricle
- Most common rhythm disturbance = sinus tachycardia; other = atrial fibrillation
- Most common valvulopathy due to chest trauma = Aortic Regurgitation (AR)
- **Beck's Triad:** 1) Muffled heart tones 2) ↓BP 3) JVD (↑CVP) = cardiac tamponade
- Most common echocardiographic findings with cardiac tamponade = right ventricular diastolic collapse
- Electrical alternans on ECG is pathognomonic for cardiac tamponade
- Order troponins despite that they are not a sensitive indicator of blunt cardiac trauma

Dispostion after blunt chest trauma:

- No abnormalities on ECG or cardiac enzymes and stable vitals => patient can be observed 4-6 hours then sent home (effectively rules out myocardial contusion)
- If elevated troponins, dysrhythmias or ECG abnormalities, or unstable vital signs, the patient needs to be stabilized and monitored closely with admission to the hospital for monitoring and echocardiography
- **PEARL: Commotio cordis** (Latin, "agitation of the heart"): lethal disruption of heart rhythm that occurs as a result of a blow to the precordial region causing VF cardiac arrest

FLAIL CHEST

- Flail Chest: > 3 consecutive rib fractures in 2 or more places; produces a free-floating, unstable segment of chest wall → paradoxical chest wall movement
- Pathognomonic paradoxical inward movement of the broken chest wall segment during inspiration and outward movement during expiration
- Most common associated lung injury: **pulmonary contusions**
- Major cause of respiratory insufficiency: pulmonary contusion
- Management: early intubation with positive pressure ventilation reduces mortality
- Supportive care: aggressive pulmonary toilet, intercostal nerve blocks, indwelling epidural catheters; fluid administration; ↑ morbidity (pneumonia, sepsis, pneumothorax)

PULMONARY CONTUSIONS

- **Symptoms:** dyspnea, chest pain, tachypnea, tachycardia, cyanosis, hypotension, minor hemoptysis is common, if major - think pulmonary laceration
- **Exam**: Rales, decreased breath sounds
- **Diagnostic** *hallmark* on CXR: asymmetric opacities; may not develop until 24 hours after traumatic event; X-ray findings worsen over 72 hours; CT better then plain films at defining the extent of the contusion, but can fail to reveal the severity of the contusion initially
- **Management**: avoid intubation - higher complication rates; if alert try NIV
- Judicial use of fluids;
- **PEARL**: Most common significant chest injury in PEDS = pulmonary contusion; > 25% often require mech. ventilation
- **PEARL**: > 80% children with pulmonary contusion will have extrathoracic injuries
- **"Good lung"** positioned down (good to ground) = to improve V/Q matching and oxygenation
- **"Bad lung" positioned down** (dependent position) in conditions below:
  a) Massive hemoptysis (to prevent blood from filling the good lung)
  b) Large pulmonary abscesses (to prevent pus from filling the good lung)
  c) Unilateral emphysema (to prevent hyperinflation)
- **Chest wall injuries associated with an increased risk of intrathoracic or intraabdominal injuries**
  a) Sternal fractures
  b) Scapular fracture
  c) Posterior sternoclavicular dislocation
  d) Flail chest

STERNAL FRACTURES

- Isolated, non-displaced sternal fractures have low overall mortality rates
- 5% of blunt chest traumas
- Most are transverse; diagnosed on lateral CXR
- Associated with diagonal seatbelt strap and steering wheel
- No association of sternal fractures and aortic rupture
- CT Chest: Assess for anterior vs posterior displacement; Posterior displacement associated with more severe neurovascular injuries

BLUNT AORTIC INJURIES

- 90% occur in the descending aorta at the isthmus between left subclavian artery and the ligamentum arteriosum; 80% die at scene; 50% who survive die in 24 hours
- Traumatic aortic injuries that survive to ED presentation are typically contained by overlying adventitia but can rupture within 24 hours → get CT Chest angiogram

PNEUMOMEDIASTINUM CAUSES

- Esophageal perforation
- Tracheobronchial injury
- Interstitial pulmonary emphysema tracking into mediastinum
- **PEARL: Hamman's sign:** crunching sound, synchronous with each heartbeat, heard over the precordium; reflects the presence of air in the mediastinum
- **PEARL:** the esophagus is the most rapidly fatal perforation of the GI tract

TRACHEOBRONCHIAL INJURY

- Consider tracheobronchial injury in any of the following:
- Labored breathing
- Hemoptysis
- SQ emphysema
- Tension pneumothorax
- Persistent air leak from chest tube
- Confirm with Bronchoscopy

NEEDLE CRICOTHYROTOMY

Indications for Percutaneous Transtracheal Ventilation ("Needle Cric")

- Cannot control airway with standard interventions or LMA
- Severe maxillofacial trauma
- Obstructive processes

Contraindications for Percutaneous Transtracheal Ventilation ("Needle Cric")

- Damaged cricoid cartilage
- Tracheal rupture
- Caution with complete upper airway obstruction

SURGICAL AIRWAY OF CHOICE IN CHILDREN < 10-12

- Oxygenation = adequate; ventilation = inadequate
- Jet ventilation preferred to wall O2
- Initial I:E ratio = 1:4

Needle cricothyrotomy procedure options

a) 12 or 14-gauge angiocatheter is inserted into the cricothyroid membrane
b) Transtracheal ventilation using available commercial devices

3 options if commercial kits are not available

a) Attach a 3.0 or 3.5 ETT connector directly to angiocatheter; bag through connector
b) Attach a 3 mL syringe (plunger removed) to angiocatheter; attach a 7.0 or 7.5 ETT connector to open end of syringe; bag through connector
c) Attach a 3 mL syringe (plunger removed) to angiocatheter; insert 5.5 ETT directly into barrel of syringe; bag through the ETT

CRICOTHYROTOMY is contraindicated in children < 10 cricoid
Membrane is small and cannot accommodate insertion of a tracheostomy tube

CHEST TRAUMA PEARLS

INDICATIONS FOR TUBE THORACOSTOMY

- Pneumothorax - Open or closed (moderate to large) or Tension
- Respiratory symptoms regardless of size of pneumothorax
- Hemothorax, Hemopneumothorax, Hydrothorax, Chylothorax, Empyema, large Effusion
- Patients with pneumothorax who are intubated or about to be intubated
- Patients with pneumothorax about to undergo air transport
- Bilateral Pneumothoraces regardless of size

COMPLICATIONS OF TUBE THORACOSTOMY

- Pulmonary edema, contralateral pneumothorax, infection (cellulitis, empyema), bronchopleural fistula, pleural leak, formation of hemothorax (lung parenchyma, vs intercostal artery injury), placement (in abdomen, SQ tissue etc), intercostal vessel or nerve injury (avoid inferior margin of rib)

- **PEARL: Tension pneumothorax** = ↓ BP, distended neck veins, ↓ breath sounds and tracheal deviation
- **PEARL: Hemothorax** can be seen on upright CXR with 200 to 300cc of blood
- **PEARL: Communicating /open pneumothorax** ("sucking chest wound") = GSW to chest leaves defect (hole) in thoracic wall
- EMS Treatment = occlusive dressing taped on three sides;
- ED treatment = chest tube and occlusive dressing;

INDICATION FOR THORACOTOMY AFTER INITIAL CHEST TUBE DRAINAGE

- 20 mL/kg or 1,500 mL of blood
- Other indications:
- Unstable vital signs
- > 300 mL/hour (or 7 mL/kg/hr) x 4 hours
- Patient decompensates after initial response to resuscitation
- **PEARL**: Use a large chest tube (34 – 40F)

INDICATIONS FOR EMERGENCY DEPARTMENT THORACOTOMY (EDT)

1) Penetrating Traumatic Cardiac Arrest

a) Cardiac arrest in the ED
b) Cardiac arrest at any point with initial vital signs in the field
c) SBP < 50 mm HG after fluid resuscitation

2) Blunt Traumatic arrest

Cardiac arrest in the ED

3) Other:

a) Suspected air embolism
b) Large pericardial effusion with pericardial tamponade after Stab Wound (SW) → attempt emergent pericardiocentesis; aspiration of 5 to 10 mL of blood may result in clinical improvement; if pericardiocentesis is unsuccessful or clinical status deteriorates then → thoracotomy

PEARL: Pericardial incision is made at the apex of the diaphragm anterior and parallel to the left phrenic nerve. Survival rate for patients undergoing resuscitative thoracotomy after cardiac arrest from penetrating trauma is roughly 15%; survival rate with blunt trauma is much LESS

PEARL: AIR EMBOLISM

- **Durant maneuver:** place the patient in the left lateral decubitus, head low position and trendelenburg positions → decrease air leaving through RV outflow tract
  a) Could attempt direct removal of air from the venous circulation by aspiration from a central venous catheter in the right atrium
  b) Thoracotomy

ABDOMINAL TRAUMA PEARLS

- Most commonly injured intra-abdominal structure in pediatric patients = spleen; **Kehr's sign** (referred pain shoulder)
- Most commonly solid organ damaged after blunt trauma = spleen
- Most commonly solid organ damaged after penetrating trauma = liver

FAST SCAN

- Fluid (blood) will appear anechoic

FAST SCAN VIEWS

1) Hepatorenal recess (Morrison's Pouch) = 85% of positive FAST exams
2) Perisplenic (splenorenal) view
3) Subxiphoid pericardial window
4) Suprapubic window (Douglas pouch)

Extended FAST

(E-FAST) add
1) Bilateral hemithoraces
2) Upper anterior chest

FAST Positive (+)

- Patient Stable = to CT
- Patient Unstable = to OR

Unstable patient with Fast Negative (-)
- Repeat FAST or DPL

DIAPHRAGMATIC INJURIES

- Most common site of diaphragmatic injury = posterolateral;
- Left hemidiaphragm (70–80%) >> Right (liver protects on right); 5% bilateral
- **PEARL:** most common site herniated disks rupture, and almost all spinal hematomas = posterolateral location
- Diaphragmatic injuries are more common in penetrating trauma
- Blunt trauma causes larger tears vs penetrating
- Blunt trauma is associated with higher MR
- Symptoms: related to the degree of herniation of abdominal contents; SOB, postive Kehr's sign

Diagnostic options:
- CXR shows 20–34% of diaphragmatic injuries
- CT chest with abdomen
- Laparoscopy is both diagnostic and therapeutic for small diaphragmatic injuries
- **Disposition** = OR

BLAST INJURIES - PRIMARY, SECONDARY, TERTIARY & QUATERNARY

- 1°: Blast pressure wave → direct effect from shockwave → hollow organ injury, barotrauma (TM perforation > lung > bowel injury)
- 2°: Projectiles from explosion → flying objects striking victim (penetrating trauma, lacerations, amputations)
- 3°: Blunt trauma from explosion → victim flies through the air striking objects
- 4°: Environmental associated injuries / contamination from device → burns, radiation exposure, CO or CN exposure

Blast Pearls
- Most common blast injury = tympanic membrane rupture
- Blast lung = the most common fatal primary blast injury
- Any patient with blast injury = gets a CXR

MASS CASUALTY

- Simple Triage and Rapid Treatment (START) technique
- Perform rapid assessment of patient's respirations, perfusion and mental status (RPM)

- Walk = green tag (walking wounded)
- Remaining patient assessment = RPM and assign tags
- Red (immediate) tags
- Yellow (delayed) tags
- Black (deceased) tags
- First step = asses respirations; no spontaneous respirations → make one attempt to reposition the airway → no improvement → black tag
- RR > 30 breaths/minute = red tag
- RR < 30 breaths/minute → assess perfusion; Radial pulse is absent or capillary refill > 2 seconds = red tag
- If RR < 30 and + radial pulse or capillary refill less than 2 seconds → assess mental status
- If victim follows commands, RR < 30 and + radial pulse = yellow tag
- If they cannot follow commands = red tag

- **PEARL:** START assessment only airway management given = reposition the airway
  Intubation, bag-valve mask oxygenation or other means of oxygenation will take too much time away from other potentially salvageable patients
- **PEARL**: Difference between **START and JumpSTART** airway management protocol = apneic adults are given airway positioning and children are given 5 rescue breaths

BURN & PRESSURE ULCER PEARLS

- Thermal burns are classified by the depth of the injury and align fairly well with the stages of pressure ulcers

Superficial (First-Degree)

- Burns only injure the epidermis; red and painful skin but no blistering, similar to a mild sunburn
- Stage 1 pressure ulcers are also characterized by intact, painful, and discolored skin

Partial thickness (Second-degree)

- Burns involve the entire epidermis and part of the dermis
  - Superficial Partial
  - Partial Deep
- Blistering, pain; moist blanching skin beneath deroofed blisters
- Stage 2 pressure ulcers similarly present as painful blisters or ulcers

Full Partial Thickness (Third-Degree) Burns

- Involve the full depth of the dermis
- Deeper tissues such as subcutaneous tissues may be exposed
- White, leathery, and insensate due to damage of nerve endings in the dermis
- Stage 3 pressure ulcers are similarly full thickness and may expose subcutaneous fat but not tendon or bone

Fourth-degree burns

- Extend into bones and joints, charred and insensate
- Stage 4 pressure ulcers expose bone, tendon, or muscle

TRANSFER TO BURN CENTER

- Partial thickness burn >10% BSA
- Circumfrential
- Chemical
- Electrical
- Inhalation injury - airway
- CNS / Cardiac
- Very young/old
- Hands / feet / face / genitals / perineum or major joints
- Burns with trauma
- Burns in patients with complex pre-existing medical conditions that would complicate management

RULE OF 9S

ADULT		PEDIATRIC	
9%	Head and Neck	**18%**	Head and neck
18%	Anterior trunk	**18%**	Anterior trunk
18%	Posterior trunk	**18%**	Posterior trunk
18%	Right leg (including the foot)	**14%**	Right left (including the foot)
18%	Left leg (including the foot)	**14%**	Left leg (including the foot)
9%	Right arm (including the hand)	**9%**	Right arm (including the hand)
9%	Left arm (including the hand)	**9%**	Left arm (including the hand
1%	Genitalia		

Patients Palm = 1% of total body surface area

Parkland formula (Baxter Formula)

- Applies on to Partial (2cd degree) and Full Thickness (3rd degree) burns
- Lactated Ringers (LR)
- 4 mL x weight (kg) x % total BSA burned
- 3mL x weight (kg) x % total BSA burned
- 50% given in first 8 hours, remainder over 16 hours

Target urine output

- 0.5 - 1 mL/kg/h in adults
- 1 - 2 mL/kg/h in children

Alkalis = liquefaction necrosis = full thickness damage; alkalis burns much worse than acid burs

Acids = coagulation necrosis

HYDROFLUORIC ACID BURN

- Sources: Glass etching, home rust remover, metal cleaning and electronic manufacturing
- Deep penetration burns
- Treatment: 10% calcium gluconate gel
- Arterial catheter placed for arterial infusion of 10% calcium gluconate

OB TRAUMA PEARLS

- Gravid uterus displaces the chest cavity upwards (diaphragm is positioned 4 cm higher than in the non-pregnant state) and pelvic and abdominal organs are displaced cephalad
  a) Chest tubes should be placed in a higher location to avoid inadvertent abdominal placement of a chest tube
  b) Bowel injuries are less common following blunt abdominal trauma
- Hemorrhage risk is increased following bony or soft tissue injuries to the pelvis (pelvic venous system becomes engorged and total circulating blood volume is increased up to 45%)
- Transport pregnant trauma patients in left lateral tilt position to reduce compression of the inferior vena cava (IVC) by the uterus
- Cardiac output, blood volume, and heart rate all increase in pregnancy. The physiologic hypervolemia of pregnancy can mask acute blood loss, and hypotension may be a late finding

- Functional residual capacity (FRC) decreases by 20%
- Oxygen requirement is increased by 20%
- FRC and oxygen requirement changes in pregnancy results in ——> decreased pulmonary reserve
- Decreased pulmonary reserve puts the pregnant patient at a greater risk of desaturation during endotracheal intubation

- Risk of gastric aspiration during endotracheal intubation is higher
- (decreased gastro-esophageal sphincter tone and decreased gastric motility)

- Leading non-OB cause of **maternal death** = Blunt trauma
- Most common cause of the blunt injury = MVC > #2 domestic violence (abdomen most common site of trauma) and > #3 falls

- Primary cause of **fetal death** in trauma = maternal shock and death
- Second most common cause of fetal death in trauma = placental abruption;
- **PEARL**: 30% of placental abruptions after trauma will not have vaginal bleeding

Placental abruption is a clinical diagnosis: vaginal bleeding, abdominal pain, uterine tenderness, uterine contractions, and fetal distress

TRAUMATIC UTERINE RUPTURE

- Rare complication following blunt and penetrating abdominal trauma
- **Risk factors:** multiple C-sections, uterine scar, cocaine, prostaglandin use
- Using lap belt alone increases > the risk of developing uterine rupture and placental abruption
- **Signs:** maternal shock, abdominal pain, peritoneal signs, abnormal fetal lie, easily palpable fetal anatomy and fetal bradycardia, fetal demise
- **Treatment:** aggressive resuscitation and emergent surgical and obstetric consultation for repair

Most common obstetrical complication of abdominal trauma in pregnancy = **uterine contractions**

ORTHOPEDICS

DESCRIBING ORTHOPEDIC RADIOGRAPHS

Open vs. Closed

Fractures line

Relates to long axis of involved bone (spiral, oblique or transverse)
Simple vs. Comminuted (more than 2 fractures segment)

Location

Which bone is fractured, left vs. right, dominant vs. non-dominant hand, approximate location-proximal, middle or distal 1/3 for long bones, use standard reference points – humeral neck, tibial plateau or intertrochanteric region of femur, extra/intraarticular extension etc.

Position of bone fragments

- **Displacement:** describe the ***distal*** fragment in relation to the ***proximal*** one (describe in %)
- **Alignment:** describes relationships of longitude axis of one fragment to another
- **Angulation**: any deviation from normal alignment, describe by direction of the apex of the angle formed by the two fragments – give degree and direction (dorsal vs. volar or radial vs ulnar) of deformity. The angle is OPPOSITE the direction of displacement of the distal fragment.

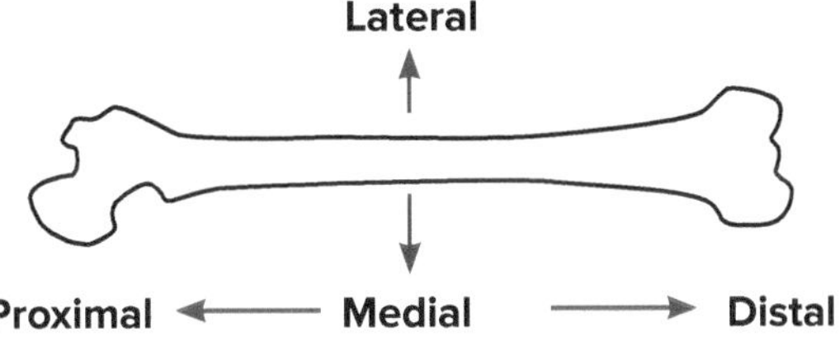

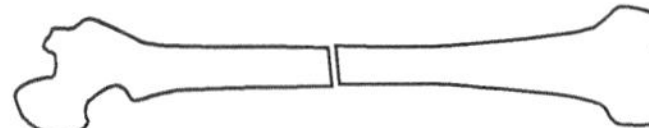

Distraction without displacement or angulation

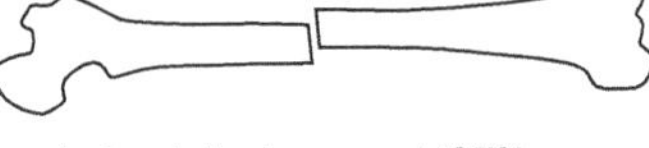

Lateral displacement (25% - 50%) without angulation

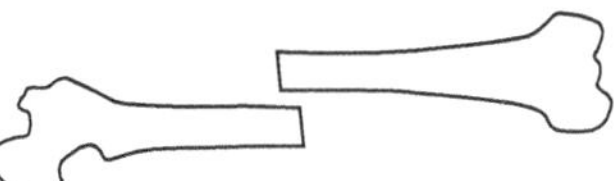

Complete 100% lateral displacement with shortening and without angulation

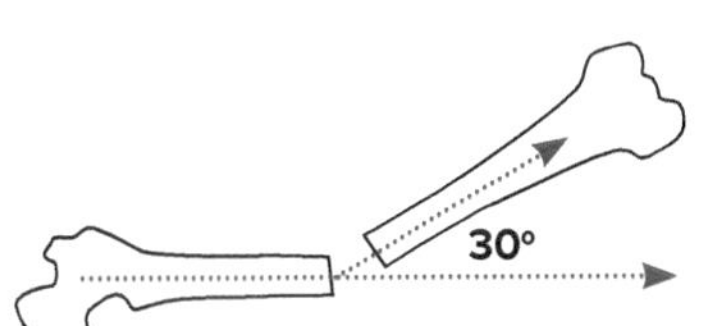

Lateral angulation (30°) without displacement

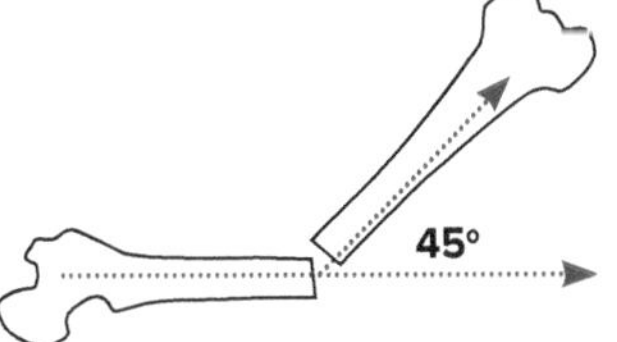

Lateral displacement about 50% and lateral angulation (45°)

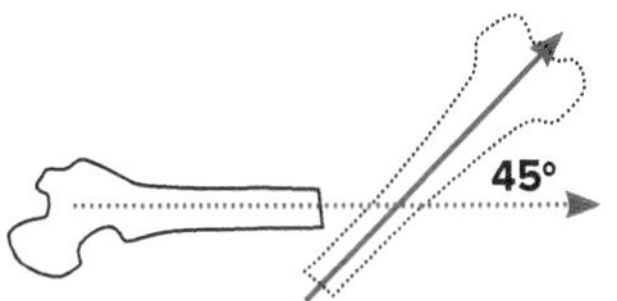

Complete medial displacement with shortening and lateral angulation (about 45°)

SUBUNGUAL HEMATOMAS

Nail Trephination Indications

- Hematoma > 50% of nail bed
- Painful hematomas regardless of size
- < 48 hours old

- Handheld electrocautery (preferred); heated paper clip; 18-gauge needle/syringe
- Clean and dry for 2 days

- **PEARL:** Acrylic nails are flammable: drill with large gauge needle
- **PEARL:** False nails: remove with acetone

- Distal phalanx fractures will be seen 25% of the time with hematomas > 50% and are not a contraindication to trephination

- **PEARL:** even though subungual hematomas associated with tuft fracture are considered "open fractures" prophylactic antibiotics are not indicated

Nail Trephination Contraindications

- Disrupted nail edge (suggests deep nail bed laceration that will require repair)
- Fingertip avulsions that requires subungal sutures for repair

RAYNAUD'S

Vasospasm with cold exposure

Three (3) Stages of a Raynaud Vasospasm

Mnemonic: (PCR)

P	**P**allor (vasoconstriction)
C	**C**yanosis (ischemia)
R	**R**ubor (from hyperemia and reperfusion)

Raynaud's Treatment

- Rewarming
- Nifedipine (Procardia, Adalat) is the initial drug of choice
- Other options: Topical nitroglycerin; topical iloprost (a prostaglandin analog); SSRIs Sildenafil (Viagra), tadalafil (Cialis)

BOUTONNIÈRE DEFORMITY

- Disruption of extensor hood near the PIP
- Central slip: inserts at base of the middle phalanx
- Lateral bands: insert in the distal phalanx (make up parts of the "extensor hood"; all aid in finger extension)
- Injury: central slip is disrupted and lateral bands slip volarly over the PIP joint
- **Exam**: PIP in flexion and DIP in extension
- Deformity develops 10–21 days after injury
- **Treatment**: PIP splinted in extension; DIP and MCP joints should have FROM; splint for 6 weeks
- Most common cause of central slip disruption = rheumatoid arthritis (RA)

SWAN NECK DEFORMITY

- Stretching or disruption of the volar plate of the proximal interphalangeal (PIP) joint
- **Exam**:
  - PIP joint = hyperextension
  - DIP joint = hyperflexion
- **PEARL**: Swan-neck deformity occurs in approximately 50% of patients with rheumatoid arthritis
- **Treatment** of acute injury: long-term splint device (double-ring splint) for six weeks
- If swan neck deformity is refractory to splint immobilization and physical therapy, surgery can be considered

MALLET FINGER

- Disruption of extensor tendon at the DIP
- **Exam:** DIP = flexion
- **Treatment:** splint DIP in extension; PIP should have FROM
- Immobilize in extension for 6 to 8 weeks
- If untreated → swan neck deformity

JERSEY FINGER

- Traumatic avulsion of the flexor digitorum profundus tendon from the distal interphalangeal (DIP) joint of a finger
- **Exam**: the affected digit will appear more extended than the other fingers; ring finger most commonly affected
- **Treatment:** Splint finger in slight flexion, immobilizing distal interphalangeal (DIP) and proximal interphalangeal (PIP) joints of the affected finger; early surgical repair (7-10 days)
- **PEARL**: Finger flexion is controlled by two tendons:
  - Flexor digitorum superficialis (FDS): inserts on the middle phalanx
  - Flexor digitorum profundus (FDP): inserts on the distal phalanx and courses deep to and between the FDS tendons

TRIGGER FINGER (STENOSING FLEXOR TENOSYNOVITIS)

- Prevalence 2%, most common among women in the 5th or 6th decade of life; painless; no injury. It can occur in one or more fingers in each hand and can be bilateral. Prevalence is higher among patients with DM, RA, or conditions that cause systemic deposition of protein (amyloidosis)
- **Treatment:** conservative - splint, NSAID's; if no improvement then steroid injection; if no improvement then surgery

FINGER AMPUTATION

- Wrap in moist gauze, store in plastic bag & place into ice water

Indications for non-operative management of fingertip amputations

- No bone exposed
- No tendon exposed
- Less than 2 cm of skin loss

BOXER'S FRACTURE

- Fracture of the 5th metacarpal neck, most common angle in volar direction
- Acceptable Metacarpal Angulation to avoid functional impairment
  < 10° Index finger
  < 20° Middle finger
  < 30° Ring finger
  < 40° Little finger
- Normal head-to-neck angle of the metacarpals = 15°
- Angulation references are based upon this baseline
- Thus, fracture angulation is = to the measured angle on the lateral x-ray minus 15°
- Most common sites 2cd - 5th metacarpal fractures = neck and shaft
- Most common site for first (thumb) MC fracture = base

BENNETT'S FRACTURE

- Fracture-dislocation or fracture-subluxation of the base of the 1st (thumb) metacarpal; unstable; often require surgery

ROLANDO'S FRACTURE

- Comminuted Bennett's fracture; fracture fragments may form a T or Y pattern at the metacarpal base; require surgery; worse prognosis then Bennett's

GAMEKEEPER'S THUMB (SKIER'S THUMB)

- Most common cause = skiing (not twisting the necks of hares)
- Forced abduction → **Ulnar collateral ligament (UCL)** ruptures 10x more often then radial collateral ligament (RCL)
- **Exam**: weak pincer grasp, valGus stress → causes > 35° of laxity, tenderness along ulnar aspect of joint
- UCL rupture if > 35% joint laxity or > 15% more laxity than is present in uninjured thumb; know Stenner's lesion (UCL is prevented from healing by the interposed adductor aponeurosis chronic instability)
- **Treat** complete rupture of UCL with surgery; treat incomplete tear with thumb spicca cast 4 weeks

DE QUERVAIN'S TENDONITIS

- Tenosynovitis of the 1st dorsal compartment (abductor pollicis longus and the extensor pollicis brevis) of the wrist
- Overuse syndrome that causes pain at the radial styloid
- **Finkelstein's test:** Cup the thumb, close the fist, and ulnar deviate the wrist => produce pain along the APL & EPB
- **Treatment:** NSAIDs and thumb spicca

CARPAL TUNNEL SYNDROME (CTS)

- **Median mononeuropathy;** most common entrapment neuropathy in the US
- Median nerve sensory distribution
- Paresthesias over the first 3 digits & radial aspect of 4th
- Most sensitive examination finding is alteration in sensation to the distal tuft of the index finger
- Can have weakened grip strength
- Sensory findings precede motor symptoms
- Symptoms worse at night
- Can be bilateral; Women > men
- Pregnancy, hypothyroidism, DM obese - worse

- Phalen Test 70% Sn, 70% Sp
- Tinel Sign 50% Sn, 75% Sp
- Manual carpal compression test 65% Sn, 85% Sp

- **Diagnosis:** Nerve conduction studies (electromyography) used to confirm the diagnosis with Sn 90%

- **Treatment:** Volar wrist splint in neutral position; severe symptoms: surgical decompression
- **PEARL:** Most sensitive bedside test for nerve injury in a finger = two-point discrimination
- **PEARL**: Normal two-point discrimination = between 2 and 5 mm at the volar fingertip

BONES OF THE WRIST

Mnemonic - (Some Lovers Try Positions That They Can't Handle) [ANK]

Some	Scaphoid
Lovers	Lunate
Try	Triquetrum
Positions	Pisiform
That	Trapezium
They	Trapezoid
Can't	Capitate
Handle	Hamate

Begin mnemonic:
1st row
→ RADIAL, proximal row → ULNARLY; scaphoid → pisiform

2nd Row
→ RADIAL, distal row → ULNARLY; trapezium → hamate

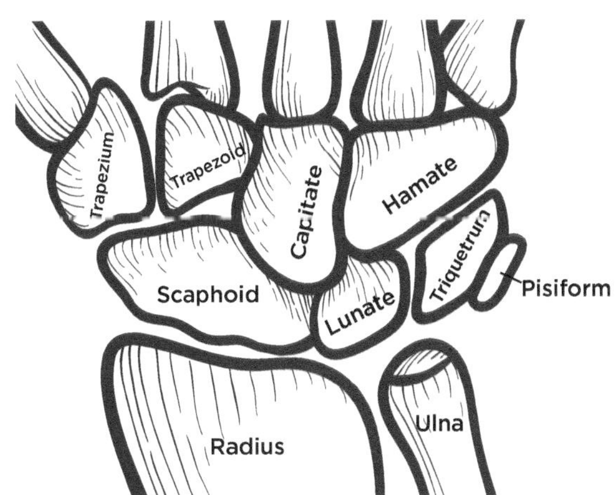

MOST COMMON CARPAL FRACTURES

- Scaphoid > 60-80% > triquetrum 5-10% > lunate 1-5%
- Proximal scaphoid fracture = worse prognosis
- 10-20% with scaphoid fractures will have normal x-ray
- If snuffbox tenderness → follow-up x-ray in 7-10 days
- Hamate fracture: golfers; uncommon 2-4%
- **Kienbocks Disease** = avascular necrosis of the lunate from repetitive microtrauma or undiagnosed lunate fracture

CARPAL DISLOCATIONS

- Most common dislocated carpal bone: **lunate dislocation**
- Lunate is displaced and rotated volarly = "**spilled teacup**" on lateral film
- Lunate overlaps the capitate = "**piece of pie**" appearance on the AP view

PERILUNATE DISLOCATION

- Lunate is aligned with the distal radius & the remaining carpal bones are dorsally displaced
- Significant ligamentous injury
- Mechanism: FOOSH
- If untreated: risk for developing: median nerve compression, vascular necrosis, compartment syndrome and long-term disability
- Ortho consult: urgent open dislocation reduction
- Most common nerve injury: Median Nerve
- **PEARL**: Perilunate dislocation is commonly associated with = scaphoid fracture

SCAPHOLUNATE DISSOCIATION

- Scapholunate gap > 3mm = **"Terry Thomas" sign**
- Treatment: immobilizing wrist in a thumb spica splint; orthopedic / hand surgeon follow up
- Prognosis: excellent with operative repair
- Complications: median nerve palsy; scapholunate advanced collapse (SLAC) – results in degenerative diease of the scaphoid and lunate; chronic pain and arthritis
- **PEARL**: Distal radius fracture in as many as 31% of cases

COLLES FRACTURE

(Remember Collie = Dog)

D	**D**istal Radial fracture
D	**D**orsal displacement of radial fragment
D	**D**inner-fork deformity

- 60% with Colles fractures have ulnar styloid fracture
- Most common nerve injured = median nerve
- Reduction using a hematoma block
- Immobilization: sugar tong splint (do not immobilize beyond the MCP joints to enable finger mobility)
- Orthopedic or hand surgery follow-up in 5-7 days

Smith Fracture = Reverse Colles fracture (volar displacement of distal fragment)

BARTON FRACTURE

- Dorsal or volar rim fracture of distal radius
- Often fracture / dislocations or subluxations of the radiocarpal joint
- The dislocation separates it from a Smith or Colles fracture
- Immobilization: sugar tong splint
- Orthopedic or hand surgery follow-up

HUTCHINSON FRACTURE (CHAUFFEUR'S OR BACKFIRE FRACTURE)

- Intra-articular radial styloid fracture
- Associated with carpal ligamentous injury or scaphoid fracture
- Immobilization: sugar tong splint
- Orthopedic or hand surgery follow-up

GANGLION CYSTS

- Most common soft tissue tumors of the hand and wrist
- Benign growths (herniation of degenerated connective tissue from tendon sheaths, ligaments, and bursae)
- Most often 2cd - 4th decades of life
- Women 3x more often > men
- Asymptomatic aside from gradual increase in size
- May become painful due to repetitive movement, cause limited ROM (tendon impingement), or cause sensory and motor nerve palsies as a result of nerve compression, particularly the median nerve with volar wrist ganglion cysts
- **Diagnosis:** clinical evaluation in combination with ultrasound or MRI
  Historically, ganglion cysts were managed with rapid external compression ("Bible bump" or "Gideon disease") - this technique is contraindicated
- **Treatment options:**
  For asymptomatic cysts: bracing and observation (50% of cysts will resolve on their own)
  Painful, cysts: needle aspirated (may require multiple drainages)
  If unsuccessful, surgical excision is the definitive management of recurrent symptomatic ganglion cysts (may require multiple procedures for total removal)

EVALUATION OF ELBOW RADIOGRAPHS IN KIDS

Mnemonic - (Careful Resurrection Medical Training Offers Learning) (CRITOE)

		Ossification Center	**First Appears (year/old)** *Note odd numbers*
Careful	**C**	**C**apitellum	1
Resurrection	**R**	**R**adial head	3
Medical	**I**	**M**edical epicondyle (**I**nternal epicondyle)	5
Training	**T**	**T**rochlea	7
Offers	**O**	**O**lecranon	9
Learning	**E**	**L**ateral epicondyle (**E**xternal epicondyle)	11

Other mnemonic = CRITOE → I = Internal (Medial) and E = External (Lateral epicondyle)
Comparison views are helpful for evaluating elbow radiographs in kids
PEARL: Posterior fat pad on x-ray = supracondylar fracture or radial head fracture

GALEAZZI'S FRACTURE

Mnemonic - (SURF-surf the sea of Galilee)

S	**S**ubluxated
U	**U**lna (distal radial-ulnar joint (DRUJ)
R	**R**adial shaft (middle/ distal junction)
F	**F**racture

MONTEGGIA FRACTURE

Mnemonic - (BURD)

B	**B**roken
U	**U**lna (proximal)
R	**R**adial head
D	**D**islocation (anterior in 60%)

√ Radial nerve → wrist extension; also → posterior interosseus branch → finger extension; and another branch of radial nerve, which is purely sensory → sensation dorsum of hand

- Treatment usually requires surgical fixation
- 80% of **scapular injuries** have associated lung, chest wall or shoulder girdle injury

RADIAL TUNNEL SYNDROME

- Compression of the posterior interosseous nerve in the radial tunnel of the forearm → causes pain just distal to the lateral epicondyle

CLAVICLE

- Most commonly fractured bone in the body
- S-shaped bone with middle third most common site of fracture 85%
- Most can be treated with sling only
- Most common complication of a clavicle fracture = non-union or malunion
- Vascular injuries are rare

ROTATOR CUFF MUSCLES

Mnemonic - (SITS)

S	**S**upraspinatus → ABDuction; most common rotator cuff muscle injured (85-90%) ("Empty Can Test")
I	**I**nfraspinatus → External rotation
T	**T**eres Minor → External rotation and ADDuction (ADD - Add to body)
S	**S**ubscapularis → Internal rotation

PEARL: All 4 muscles originate on the scapula, transverse the glenohumeral joint and insert on the proximal humerus

PEARL: Calcific tendonitis: Calcification along the rotator cuff tendons. Presents with subacute onset shoulder pain and decreased range of motion

SHOULDER IS MADE UP OF 3 JOINTS

Mnemonic - (GAS)

G	**G**lenohumeral
A	**A**cromioclavicular (AC)
S	**S**ternoclavicular

ACROMIOCLAVICULAR (AC) JOINT SEPARATION

Grades (I to VI)

I AC ligament sprain: most common
II AC ligament torn + coraco-clavicular (CC) ligament sprain; can see joint space widening on x-ray, with minimal upward displacement of the clavicle
III AC and CC torn; complete disruption of joint and more significant upward displacement of the clavicle
IV Clavicle displaced posteriorly
V Clavicle displaced superiorly and anteriorly
VI Clavicle displaced inferiorly (rare)

Treatment

Type I-II: sling, orthopedic referral within a couple weeks
Type III: sling, orthopedic referral, however more urgent orthopedic referral +/- surgery
Type IV-VI: sling, urgent orthopedic referral, surgery

ANTERIOR SHOULDER DISLOCATION

- Most common dislocation of shoulder
- Most common nerve injury: **axillary nerve** (test pinprick sensation over the skin of deltoid muscle)
- Exam: arm in slight ABduction and EXternal rotation
- Consider Rotator Cuff injury
- Scapular manipulation, Stimson method, and traction-countertraction method are all appropriate methods to reduce anterior shoulder dislocations
- Hippocratic technique not recommended due to axillary nerve damage

HILL-SACHS DEFORMITY

- The most common associated fracture with anterior shoulder dislocation Compression fracture of the posterolateral humeral head (10% to 50%)
- Hill-Sachs deformities are usually of limited clinical significance
- No additional treatment

BANKART FRACTURE

- Fracture of the inferior glenoid rim
- Seen in 5% of anterior shoulder dislocations

INFERIOR SHOULDER DISLOCATIONS (LUXATIO ERECTA)

- Arm is usually fully abducted and held above the head on presentation
- 1% of dislocations

POSTERIOR SHOULDER DISLOCATIONS

- Usually secondary to seizure or electric shock
- Subacromial being common type of posterior dislocations
- 50% of are missed on initial evaluation
- Most commonly mistaken for adhesive capsulitis
- **"Rim sign":** Increased distance between the humeral head and glenoid rim (diminished overlap of humeral head and glenoid fosssa)
- **"Light bulb" sign:** appearance of the humeral head due to fixed internal rotation

PROXIMAL HUMERUS FRACTURES

- Evaluate for axillary nerve injury
- Treatment: sling & swathe

HUMERAL SHAFT FRACTURE

- Most common nerve injury: radial nerve (wrist and finger extension, sensation dorsum of hand)
- Other injuries: brachial artery or vein, ulnar and median nerves

NERVE INJURIES SECONDARY TO HUMERUS FRACTURES

https://www.ezmedlearning.com/blog/upper-extremity-nerve-injuries (Reference provided by Dr. Adam Madej)

Mnemonic - (ARM)

A	**Axillary nerve**	Fracture to the head of the humerus (or shoulder dislocation)
R	**Radial nerve**	Fracture to the mid-shaft humerus
M	**Median nerve**	Fracture to the distal third of the humerus (supracondylar fracture)

BICEP TENDON RUPTURE

- Complete or partial disruption of the biceps brachii tendon from the radial tuberosity insertion site
- Mechanism: contraction against resistance
- Presentation: "Popeye" appearance of the upper arm muscles (distal retraction of the muscle)
- Diagnostics: X-ray - evaluate for avulsion fracture or dislocation; Ultrasound; MRI
- Management: immobilize the arm in a sling for comfort
- Outpatient operative repair can be considered for those with significant weakness, persistent symptoms after 3 months, or sooner in competitive athletes and manual laborers

ELBOW DISLOCATION

- Most common dislocation: posterior
- Most common nerve injured: ulnar nerve (test intrinsic muscles of hand and sensation over ulnar side of hand)
- Vascular injuries 5 to 13%, most common = brachial artery

RADIAL HEAD FRACTURE

- Most common elbow fracture
- Immobilization
  - Non-displaced involving < 1/3 of the articular surface: sling and early mobilization of the elbow
  - All others: posterior long arm splint
  - Open Reduction if fracture is: displaced > 1/3 of the articular surface or angulated > 30 degrees

OLECRANON FRACTURES

- Presentation: impairment of triceps function and frequently complicated by ulnar nerve injury
- 2%-12% of patients with olecranon fractures have associated ulnar nerve dysfunction
- Elbow stiffness and decreased flexion and extension range of motion (75%)
- Radial head fracture (17%)
- Management: posterior long arm splint with the elbow in 60-90 degrees of flexion

OLECRANON BURSITIS

- Most common bursitis
- Inflammation and swelling of the bursa overlying the tip of the elbow
- If septic bursitis suspected - perform needle aspirate; Ancef or Vancomycin antibiotic
- Aseptic Bursitis Management
  - Rest, ice, and compression
  - Activity modification and elbow protection
  - Nonsteroidal anti-inflammatory drugs (NSAIDs)

SUPRACONDYLAR FRACTURES

- 75% of pediatric elbow fractures
- Gartland classification system
- Type I - nondisplaced fractures
- Type II - minimally displaced fractures with an intact posterior cortex
- Type III - completely displaced fractures with complete cortical disruption

Management
- Nondisplaced fractures: nonoperatively as an outpatient
- Most displaced fractures require hospital admission for close neurovascular checks and operative stabilization

Complications
- Median nerve = most commonly injured nerve
- Brachial artery injury
- Volkmann ischemic contracture (permanent flexion contracture of the hand at the wrist)
- Compartment syndrome

LATERAL EPICONDYLITIS - TENNIS ELBOW

- Confirmed: reproduce pain with elbow in extension, wrist flexion and forearm pronation against resistance or
- With forearm pronated actively extend fingers or wrist against resistance or
- Pinching with the wrist in extension
- Management: Rest, NSAIDS; steroid injections

MEDIAL EPICONDYLITIS - GOLF ELBOW

- Pain over the medial epicondyle and pain with passive wrist extension and resisted wrist flexion when the elbow is fully extended
- Management: Rest, NSAIDS; steroid injections

LITTLE LEAGUE ELBOW

Medial elbow problems in adolescents from throwing baseballs frequently
a) medial epicondyle avulsion fractures
b) ulnar collateral ligament tears
C) medial epicondyle apophysitis (similar to Osgood-Schlatter disease of the knees)

PROXIMAL FEMUR FRACTURES

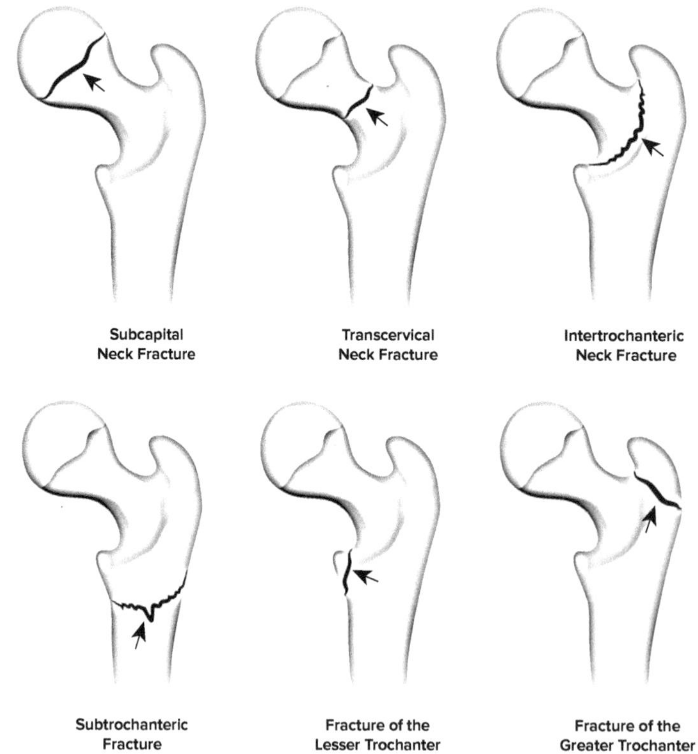

- **PEARL:** Most common complication with **Femoral Neck Fracture** = avascular necrosis
- **PEARL: Femoral shaft fracture** may result in loss of > 1 liter of blood
- **PEARL**: Most hip fractures are intertrochanteric or femoral neck

POSTERIOR HIP DISLOCATION

Most common dislocation of the hip: posterior (80%)
10% of patients with posterior hip dislocations will have associated sciatic nerve injury; femoral head / acetabular fractures commonly occur with hip dislocations

Mnemonic - (DIP)

Patients who take a "DIP" may have a posterior hip dislocation, most common hip dislocation 80%.

D	**AD**Ducted
I	**I**nternally rotated
P	**P**osterior dislocation (most common hip dislocation)

FAT EMBOLISM SYNDROME

- Release of fat globules from long bone fractures —> fat emboli —> lungs
- Diagnosis: clinical; Mortality rate = 20%
- Commonly present within 48 hours: SOB, hypoxia, AMS, agitation, and a petechial rash (most commonly over the chest); Lab: +/- thrombocytopenia
- **Treatment:** Supportive care IVF, O2

PELVIC FRACTURES

- Pelvic fractures include: ring disruptions, sacral fractures, acetabular fractures, and avulsion injuries Significant hemorrhage may accompany any fracture pattern
- Marker for serious concomitant injuries
- Most common cause of mortality from pelvic fracture = hemorrhage
- Pelvic fractures with 2 breaks in the pelvic ring = most unstable
- **Inspection:** search for external bleeding, ecchymosis (flank, perineal, and scrotal), blood at the penile meatus, vaginal bleeding, and the position of the lower extremities and iliac crests
- Rectal and vaginal examination: assess for open fractures; evaluation for palpable bony fragments, integrity of the rectal and vaginal walls, gross blood, and a high riding prostate
- **PEARL**: perform retrograde cystourethrogram: If blood at the urethral meatus, a high riding prostate, or gross hematuria
- Imaging: CT scan remains the preferred method for the evaluation of all hemodynamically stable patients with pelvic trauma
- **Treatment**: Significant pelvis injury + hemodynamically unstable —> pelvis should be "wrapped" with either a sheet or a commercial pelvic binder

KNEE DISLOCATION

- Orthopedic emergency; Popliteal injury is associated 18 to 64% of knee dislocations with 12% of these cases requiring amputation.
- Diagnosis = Emergent arteriography
- Most common nerve injury = Common peroneal (fibular)
- Most common dislocation of **patella** = lateral; Reduction = extend knee, and apply medial pressure on patella

3 WAYS TO INJURE THE EXTENSOR MECHANISM OF THE KNEE

1. **Patellar tendon rupture:** inability to extend the knee, superior patellar displacement, tenderness inferior to the patella; more common in healthy young athletes
2. **Quadriceps tendon rupture:** inability to extend knee, inferior patellar displacement, indentation superior to the patella, and tenderness superior to the patella; More common in individuals > 40 years of age with systemic co-morbidities (obesity, RA, DM, SLE, CKD, steroid therapy local injections or chronic oral, gout, hyperparathyroidsm)
3. **Patellar fracture:** pain, swelling, and ecchymosis over patella; Most commonly a transverse fracture; the quadriceps tendon pulls the superior patella upward and causes a wide displacement of the fracture fragments

KNEE EXTENSORS

- Quadriceps femoris, made up of 4 muscle: rectus femoris, vastus lateralis, vastus medialis, and vastus intermedius

KNEE FLEXORS

- 3 Hamstring muscles: biceps femoris, semitendinosus, and semimembranosus muscles (also, extend the hip)
- Most common ligamentous knee injury = **medical collateral**
- Most common cause of *acute* traumatic knee hemarthrosis = injury to **anterior cruciate ligament (ACL)**
- Accuracy increases from 70 % using **Anterior Drawer test** to 99% using **Lachman's Test** in the diagnosis of ACL injury

LACHMAN'S TEST

- Knee flexed to 20 - 30°, one hand examiner stabilizes thigh the other hand pulls the tibia anterior to identify inappropriate tibial excursion = loss of ACL integrity

POSTERIOR SAG SIGN TEST

- Evaluate the posterior cruciate ligament **(PCL)**
- Patient supine, pillow under the distal thigh and the heel resting on the bed
- The knee is then flexed to the point of maximal relaxation (45 to 90 degrees) and the tibia is observed for posterior sag. If the tibia sags backwards = positive test

MCMURRAY'S TEST

- Evaluate for a **meniscal tear**
- Patient supine, knee hyperflexed
- One hand examiner holds the foot and the other grasps the knee
- At the same time, examiner flexes and extends the knee while internally and externally rotating the tibia on the femur
- Positive test = clicking is heard or the knee locks
- Most common meniscal injury = medical meniscus; less mobile. Knee locks up; get delayed swelling

TERRIBLE TRIAD ("O'DONOGHUE'S TRIAD")

1. Medial collateral ligament injury
2. Medial meniscus injury
3. Anterior cruciate ligament (ACL) rupture

OPEN KNEE JOINT INJURY

- Orthopedic surgical emergency
- Diagnosis: CT scan of knee to look for intra-articular air
- Normal saline and methylene blue injection into the joint space is outdated
- Most frequent site of injury to the common peroneal (common fibular) nerve = just below the knee as the nerve wraps around the lateral aspect of the fibula; foot drop

TIBIAL PLATEAU FRACTURES

- Direct force driving femoral condyles into articulating surface of the tibia or direct trauma; depressed > 5 mm = surgical repair; lateral more common; lipohemarthrosis on x-ray; Check common peroneal nerve (drop foot)
- **Tibial PEARL:** Most common long bone fracture = **tibia**
- **Tibial PEARL:** Most common open bone fracture = **tibia**
- **Tibial shaft fractures** have high incidence of compartment syndrome & poor healing

COMPARTMENT SYNDROME

Most common site for compartment syndrome in **lower extremity = anterior compartment** (anterior tibial artery, deep peroneal nerve also called deep fibular nerve; anterior tibialis muscle, extensor hallucis longus and extensor digitorum longus muscles)

COMPARTMENT DELTA PRESSURE

- Diastolic blood pressure (DBP) - measured intracompartmental pressure
- ≤ 30 mm Hg as indicative of the need for fasciotomy or
- **Absolute compartment pressure** > 30–40 mm Hg
- Needle compartment pressure measurement is performed by inserting a needle at a 90 degree angle to the skin overlying the compartment
- **PEARL:** Delta Pressure = more reliable than direct pressure alone
- Treatment: surgical fasciotomy; then wound is left open
- Delayed closure or skin grafting is performed after edema has resolved
- #2 most common site for compartment syndrome = volar compartment of the forearm
- Most common presenting symptom of compartment syndromes = pain
- Other Ps: paresthesias, paresis/paralysis, pallor and pulselessness
- Pain out of proportion to the injury is the earliest finding

MAISONNEUVE FRACTURE

- Eversion mechanism → proximal fibular fractue + disruption of the deltoid ligament or a medial malleolar fracture + partial or complete disruption of the syndesmosis; ; management: post mold; consult orthopedics for surgery
- **PEARL**: Complication = peroneal nerve palsy

PILON FRACTURE

- Intra-articular comminuted fracture of the distal tibia combined with disruption of the talar dome
- Mechanism: axial force that drives the talus into the distal tibia
- Immobilize with well-padded posterior leg splint + stirrup splint to prevent dorsiflexion, plantar flexion, inversion, and eversion; consult orthopedics for surgery
- **PEARL**: 25% of pilon fractures are open fractures
- **PEARL**: Pilon fractures are frequently associated with polytrauma and other compressive fractures (calcaneus, tibial plateau, acetabular and spinal fractures)

THE OTTAWA ANKLE RULES

Ankle x-ray series are only required if there is pain in the malleolar zone and any one of the following findings:

1. Bone tenderness along the distal 6 cm of the posterior edge of the fibula or tip of lateral malleolus
2. Bone tenderness along the distal 6 cm of the posterior edge of the tibia or tip of medial malleolus
3. Inability to bear weight both immediately and in the ED for 4 steps

Foot x-ray series are only required if there is tenderness in the midfoot zone and any one of the following findings:

1. Bone tenderness at the base of the fifth metatarsal
2. Bone tenderness at the navicular bone
3. Inability to bear weight both immediately and in the ED for 4 steps

- Ottawa Ankle Rules not developed for patients < 18 years old
- Clinical judgment should prevail = if exam is unreliable (ETOH, lack of cooperation, distracting injuries or diminished sensation in the leg) get x-rays

ANKLE SPRAINS

Grade 1: Minimal tenderness & swelling; minimal impairment. Microscopic tearing of collagen fibers.
Treatment: weight bearing as tolerated, PT

Grade 2: Moderate tenderness & swelling, painful/ decrease ROM, possibly mild instability; moderate impairment. Partial tear of a ligament.
Treatment: Air splint, PT

Grade 3: Significant tenderness & swelling and an absence of end points with complete ligament tear or rupture (instability); severe impairment.
Treatment: Immobilization, PT and possible surgical reconstruction

- **Inversion ankle injuries** = typically cause sprains
- **Eversion ankle injuries** = typically cause fractures
- Most commonly injured ankle ligament = **anterior talofibular ligament**
- **Ankle dislocations** have a high incidence of vascular injury and avascular necrosis of the talus

ACHILLES TENDON RUPTURE

- Mechanism: sudden plantar flexion against resistance (taking a jump shot in basketball) or stepping into a hole; Audible "snap" or "pop"; severe pain in the lower calf; **Examination**: palpable defect (gap) in the middle portion of the tendon
- **Ultrasound**: shows separation of torn ends with a contour change of the tendon

- **Thompson test:** patient prone with the distal portion of the leg extending past the stretcher. Provider squeezes mid portion of the calf which should cause plantar flexion of the foot
- Complete rupture: plantar flexion is absent (positive Thompson's test)
- Partial ruptures may have a negative test
- **Treatment: Gravity Equinus Splint:** below-the-knee posterior splint with 20 to 30 degrees of plantar flexion (equinas position)
- Most common tarsal bone fracture = **calcaneus**; 75% intraarticular

CALCANEAL FRACTURES

- Rule of 10's = 10% bilateral, 10% vertebral compression fractures, 10% compartment syndrome; 25% lower extremity injuries (tibial plateau fracture)
- **Bohler's angle:** normal 20 to 40 degrees, if less suspect calcaneal fracture
- 2 bones in the **hindfoot** (calcaneus, talus)
- 5 bones in the **midfoot** (navicular, cuboid, 3 cuneiforms)
- 19 bones in the **forefoot** (5 metatarsals, 14 phalanges)
- Hindfoot connects to the midfoot at the **Chopart** joint
- Forefoot connects to the midfoot at the **Lisfranc** joint
- Most common **midfoot** fracture = Navicular (uncommon)
- Most common **forefoot** fracture = Phalangeal fractures
- Most common **metatarsal** base fracture = 5th metatarsal tuberosity fracture (Pseudo-Jones)
- Most common **metatarsal** fractured = 3rd metatarsal

JONES FRACTURE

- Transverse fracture through the base of 5th metatarsal, 1.5cm distal to the proximal part of the metatarsal; treatment: NWB cast for 6 weeks
- 35-50% patients develop persistent nonunions requiring bone grafting and internal fixation

PSEUDO-JONES (TUBEROSITY FRACTURE)

- Avulsion fracture, more common, peroneus brevis (fibularis brevis) tendon pulls off a portion of the bone where it inserts; treatment: cast shoe
- Most common undisplaced **metatarsal shaft fracture** 2cd-5th
- Treatment: below-knee walking cast 2 to 4 weeks; Non-displaced 1st metatarsal fractures treated with cast 4 to 6 weeks and NWB
- Most common metatarsals involved in stress – "March" – fractures = 2nd and 3rd (fixed)

LISFRANC FRACTURE/DISLOCATION

- Disruption of tarsal-metatarsal joint, fracture at base of 2cd metatarsal
- Xray: separation of the 1st and 2cd metatarsals

RHEUMATOID ARTHRITIS (RA)

- Inflammatory, involves multiple joints at a time
- Pain and swelling: MCP & PIP joints, usually symmetrical
- Bone erosion, cartilage loss = Swan neck, Boutonniere deformity, Bow string sign
- "Morning stiffness" that improves with movement

Treatment of RA

- Mild: NSAIDs or steroids
- Severe: Methotrexate + anti-TNF (tumor necrosis factor) medication - Etanercept (Enbrel) = risk for sepsis, infections including TB

OSTEOARTHRITIS

- Most common presentation: symmetric, polyarticular, mild joint pain, and stiffness; worsens with use; most commonly affects the distal interphalangeal (DIP) joints, the thumb, knees, and hips
- **Heberden nodes** (bony, hard swelling of the DIP joints) = pathognomonic
- **Treatment**: Oral / topical NSAIDs, topical capsaicin, intra-articular corticosteroid injections
- **Xray**
    - RA: periarticular bone
    - OA: loss joint space narrowing and osteophytes

PSORIATIC ARTHRITIS

- Psoriatic extensor surface plaques, nail pitting, asymmetric arthritis, and dactylitis; uveitis

SEPTIC ARTHRITIS

- Most common bacteria causing septic joint = Staph aureus
- Most common septic joint involvement = knee

- **PEARL:** Most common **viruses causing arthritis** = Rubella (German measles) and HBV; others: Parvovirus B19, EBV, mumps, adenovirus and enteroviruses

GOUT / PSEUDOGOUT

- Most common joint involved in **Gout** = Toe
- Crystals: uric acid; needle shaped, blue; negative birefringence

- Most common joint involved in **Pseudogout** = knee
- Crystals: calcium pyrophosphate; rhomboid, yellow; positive birefringence

- **Treatment**: NSAIDs (Indomethacin), oral colchicine (more effective with Gout; side effects strong V/D), cold compresses

- If contraindication to NSAIDs
  a) Oral prednisone 30 -60 mg daily with taper over 10 to 14 days
     If > 5 joints involved → 3 week taper
  b) Intra-acticular steroid injection – triamcinolone 10mg in knees, 8 mg in smaller joints

- Long term Gout/ Pseudogout therapy: allopurinol (↓uric acid production) or probenecid (↑uric acid excretion)

SYNOVIAL FLUID ANALYSIS

Condition	Appearance	WBC's/mm	% PMN's	Glucose; % Serum Level	Crystals Under Polarized Light
Normal	Clear	<200	<25	95-100	None
Non-Inflammatory (i.e. DJD)	Clear	<400	<25	95-100	None
Acute Gout	Turbid	2000-5000	>75	80-100	Negative birefringence; needle-like crystals Blue needle-shaped, uric acid
Pseudogout	Turbid	5000-50,000	>75	80-1000	Positive birefringence; rhomboid crystals Yellow, calcium pyrophosphate
Septic Arthritis	Purulent/ turbid	>50,000	>75	<50	None
Inflammatory (i.e. Rheumatoid arthritis)	Turbid	5000-50,000	50-75	Approx. 75	None

Reference: Clinical Procedures in Emergency Medicine, Roberts et al., 2nd Edition. Harrison's Principles of Internal Medicine, 14th Edition.

KANAVEL'S 4 CARDINAL SIGNS FOR FLEXOR TENDON SHEATH INFECTION

1. Slight flexion of digit
2. Symmetrical swelling ("Sausage Finger")
3. Tenderness over flexor tendon sheath
4. Pain on passive extension

ORTHO ID PEARLS

- Plantar **puncture wounds** while wearing tennis shoes: Pseudomonas aeruginosa (moist inner sole of the shoe provides suitable environment for growth of Pseudomonas; this has recently been challenged-however good boards question)
- Most common cause of **osteomyelitis**: *Staph aureus;* in sickle cell patients, think Salmonella after staph; In young adults think GC after Staph
- Most common **complication associated with leg fractures:** infection
- **Fight bite injury** = *Eikenella corrodens*
- **Cat bite:** *Pasteurella multocida;* 80% get infected. Infection develops within 24 hours
- **Dog bite**: *Pasteurella canis;* only 5% of dog bites get infected; consider prophylaxis or treatment if severe bite or patient has co-morbidity
- **Prophylactic antibiotic after dog or cat bite:** Amoxicillin-Clavulanate 875/125 mg po bid; if beta-lactam allergy: Clindamycin 300mg po tid + Cipro 500mg po bid; Pediatric Clindamycin + TMP-SMX
- Sepsis or gangrenous wound after **dog bite**: *Capnocytophaga canimorsus*
- **Functional or anatomic splenectomy:** *Capnocytophaga canimorsus*
- **Felon:** infection of the deep space of the fingertip: treatment: I&D. MRSA coverage while waiting for culture results.
- **Paronychia**: infection of the dorsal aspect of the nail area; treatment: I&D. MRSA coverage while waiting for culture results

RED FLAGS OF BACK PAIN

- Age < 18 or > 60
- Symptoms or history of cancer
- Pain that gets worse when laying down = spinal cord compression (thoracic vertebrae most common 70%)
- Immunodeficiency (IVDA, prolonged steroid use, HIV = bone or disk infection)
- Recent spinal instrumentation (surgery, lumbar puncture, or epidural anesthesia = spinal epidural abscess or hematoma)
- History of trauma
- Coagulopathy = spinal epidural hematoma
- Cauda equina symptoms = urinary / bowel retention, saddle anesthesia
- Night pain and weight loss = tumor
- Fever / chills = bone or disk infection
- Bondy tenderness = fracture
- Morning stiffness > 30 min in young adult = seronegative spondyloarthropathy (ankylosing spondylitis (AS); reactive arthritis (formerly Reiter syndrome)

LUMBAR RADICULOPATHY

Nerve roots can be injured at any disc level, from the L1-2 level → to the level of they exit into their neural foramina

For Example:

L5 NERVE ROOT COMPRESSION (symptoms upper leg to great toe) can occur as a result of various disc protrusion scenarios:

a) Central disc herniation at the L2-3 level
b) Central disc herniation at the L3-4 level
c) Postero-lateral disc herniation at the L4-5 level
d) Disc herniation into the foramen at the L5-S1 level

L4 NERVE ROOT COMPRESSION

(symptoms on the anteromedial aspect of the leg to below the knee)
a) Far lateral unilateral disc herniation at the L4-L5 level
b) Unilateral disc herniation at the L3-L4 level

L3 NERVE ROOT COMPRESSION

- (symptoms upper leg to knee)
- Unilateral disc herniation at the L3-L4 level

Most common location of disc herniation and cause of lumbar radiculopathies

- L4-L5 and L5-S1 (95%)
- Most commonly caused by herniation of the nucleus pulposus into the lumbar spinal canal

L2/L3/L4 Radiculopathy

- Considerable overlap of the L2, L3, and L4 innervation - so these radiculopathies are generally considered as a group
- Acute back pain = most common presenting complaint
- Pain radiates around the ANTERIOR / MEDIAL aspect of the thigh down into the knee
- **Exam:**
  Weakness of hip flexion, knee extension, and hip adduction
  Sensation reduced over the anterior/medial thigh down to the medial aspect of the lower leg
  Patellar tendon (knee) reflex (L2-4) = reduced

L5 Radiculopathy

- The most common radiculopathy of lumbosacral spine
- Acute back pain
- Rradiates down the LATERAL aspect of the leg into the foot
- **Exam:**
  Weakness of foot dorsiflexion (heel walk), toe extension (toe dorsiflexion), foot inversion, and foot eversion
  Atrophy may be present in the extensor digitorum brevis muscle of the foot and the tibialis anterior muscle of the lower leg
  In severe cases, "tibial ridging" = the normal convexity of the anterior compartment of the leg is lost because of atrophy, leaving a prominent sharp contour of the medial aspect of the tibial bone
  Sensory loss is confined to the lateral aspect of the lower leg and dorsum of the foot
  Sensory loss may be obvious only when testing sharp sensation in the web space between the first and second digits
  Reflexes = generally normal

S1 Radiculopathy

- Pain radiates down the POSTERIOR aspect of the leg into the foot from the back
- **Exam:**
  Weakness of plantar flexion (gastrocnemius muscle) is most specific; toe flexion (toe plantar flexion)
  Sensation reduced on the posterior aspect of the leg and the lateral edge of the foot
  Ankle reflex = reduced
- **Positive straight leg raise test** = tenderness in the sciatic notch, and limited ROM on affected side
- **Crossed straight leg raise test** = is more SPECIFIC for disc herniation than is the straight leg test

  Pearl: Spinal cord terminates at lumbar nerves L1 and L2 (conus medullaris)
  Pearl #2: The spinal nerves continue as a bundle of nerves = the cauda equina

SCLERODERMA (PROGRESSIVE SYSTEMIC SCLEROSIS)

CREST syndrome

C	**C**alcinosis
R	**R**aynaud phenomenon
E	**E**sophageal dysmotility
S	**S**clerodactyly
T	**T**elangiectasias

- Autoimmune; Women > men
- Supportive treatment; +/- some evidence for methotrexate

POLYMYOSITIS

- Idiopathic inflammatory disease causing inflammation and degradation of muscles
- *Proximal* muscle weakness and myalgias
- Most commonly involved muscles = deltoid, neck, and hip flexors
- Symptoms progress over weeks to months
- Sensory system is preserved
- Elevated CPK and LDH (muscle injury)
- **Treatment:** corticosteroids

DERMATOMYOSITIS

- Another inflammatory myopathy; associated with malgnancy
- Similar to polymyositis in presentation but includes skin rashes
- **Gottron papules:** symmetric erythematous papules on the extensor surface of the hands
- Heliotrope rash: erythematous eruption around the eyes and the nasolabial fold
- Diagnosis: EMG, muscle biopsy
- Treatment: corticosteroids or immunosuppressive therapy (DMARDs) IVIG if refractory
- Mild symptoms: discharge home; neurology or rheumatology in one week
- Severe symptoms: severe weakness, respiratory muscle involvement or rhabdomyolysis and admit to the hospital
- **PEARL:** Polymyalgia rheumatica (PMR) associated with temporal (giant cell) arteritis

FELTY'S SYNDROME

Mneomonic - (FAULTS)

F	Felty syndrome
A	Arthritis – chronic Rheumatoid arthritis (affects < 1% patients with RA)
U	Ulcers of leg (pyoderma gangrenosum) may respond to dapsone
L	Leukopenia and neutropenia (low PMN's)
T	Thrombocytopenia
S	Splenomegaly (spleen is often FELT)

PSYCHOBEHAVIORAL

SUICIDE

- Nearly 45,000 people in the United States and > 800,000 worldwide die by suicide each year
- 10th leading cause of death in the US and 14th leading cause of death worldwide
- Among patients who committed suicide, 80% had contact with primary care clinicians within one year of their death
- Females attempt more frequently; males succeed more often
- 20% retry within one year
- 5% of repeaters succeed
- Personality disorders (antisocial, histrionic, narcissistic and paranoid) least likely to commit suicide
- Suicide screening is *not* the same as suicide risk assessment
- Suicide risk assessment: includes review of dynamic, static and protective risk factors

RISK FACTORS FOR SUICIDE

Mnemonic - (SAD PERSONS)

	Mnemonic	Score
S	**S**ex - Male	1
A	**A**ge - 19 or > 45	1
D	**D**epression or hopelessness	2

P	**P**revious attempt = highest risk factor / **P**sychiatric care	1
E	**E**xcess alcohol or substance abuse	1
R	**R**ational thinking loss	2
S	**S**eparated divorced or widowed	1
O	**O**rganized attempt or serious attempt	2
N	**N**o social support	1
S	**S**tated future attempts	2

- Total Score: 0-4 = low risk
- Total Score: 5 to 6 = medium risk; strongly consider hospitalization, depending on confidence in the follow-up arrangement
- Total Score: > 7 = strong risk; psychiatric hospitalization from the ED

DEPRESSION

- Depressed mood or loss of interest or pleasure + 4 or more other symptoms for 2 weeks or longer

Mnemonic - (IN SAD CAGESP)

IN	**In**terest decrease in everything (loss of interest or pleasure)

S	**S**leep disorder (insomnia or hypersomnia)
A	**A**ppetite alteration (weight gain or loss)
D	**D**ysphoric mood (a state of feeling uneasy, unhappy, or unwell; depressed mood)

C	**C**oncentration decreases
A	**A**ffect blunted
G	**G**uilt (feeling inappropriate guilt or feeling worthless)
E	**E**nergy diminishes (fatigue or loss of energy)
S	**S**uicide risk
P	**P**sychomotor - (agitation or retardation)

PEARL: Most common psychiatric disorder is depression

ANXIETY

Generalized Anxiety

- Frequent and prolonged (> 6 months) periods of worry and anxiousness

Panic Disorder

- Sudden, episodic, brief episodes of intense fear with a variety of somatic complaints; +/- agoraphobia

Illness anxiety disorder

- New diagnosis introduced with DSM-5 it replaced reactive hypochondriasis = excessive worry about having or acquiring a serious undiagnosed general medical disease

PERSONALITY DISORDERS

3 Clusters of Personality Disorders

- Cluster A (odd, eccentric)
- Cluster B (dramatic and emotional)
- Cluster C (anxious, fearful)

- 3 Personality disorders in Cluster A = Paranoid, schizoid and schizotypal
- 3 Personality disorders in Cluster C = Dependent, obsessive-compulsive and avoidant

- 4 Personality disorders in Cluster B = Narcissistic, antisocial, borderline and histrionic

CLUSTER A

Mnemonic: (PSS): odd, eccentric

P	**P**aranoid: suspicious, cold, humorless, secretive, hypersensitive
S	**S**chizoid: socially withdrawn, isolated, "loners", aloof and apathetic / lack of concern; indifferent; passive; more common in men > women
S	**S**chizotypal: magical thinking; bizarre fantasy; peculiar language, metaphoric speech

CLUSTER B

Mnemonic: (NAB His): dramatic and emotional

N	**N**arcissistic: can't apologize, grandiose, lacks empathy, exploits others to fulfill own needs
A	**A**ntisocial: breaks laws, no remorse or guilt, appears friendly on the surface, often lie and manipulate situations, blatant disregard of others
B	**B**orderline = unstable interpersonal relationships, impulsivity and a distorted self-image (see section on BPD)
HIS	**His**trionic = Impulsive, false emotions, dramatic, center of attention, inappropriate sexual behavior

CLUSTER C

Mnemonic: (DOA): anxious, fearful

D	**D**ependent (submissive, indecisive)
O	**O**bsessive-Compulsive (perfectionist, passive-aggressive, rigid)
A	**A**voidant (fears criticism, overly serious, withdrawn)

HISTRIONIC PERSONALITY DISORDER

Mnemonic: (PRAISE ME)

P	**P**rovocative behavior (flirtatious, sexually seductive)
R	**R**elationships (considered more intimate than they actually are)
A	**A**ttention (like to be the center of attention)
I	**I**nfluenced easily
S	**S**tyle of speech (impressionistic)
E	**E**motional (rapidly shifting, shallow, excessively emotional, overly dramatic)

M	**M**ade up; manipulative behavior to meet their needs
E	**E**xaggerated emotions (10/10 pain while texting on phone)

- More common in women
- Affects approximately 3% of the general population

BORDERLINE PERSONALITY DISORDER (BPD)

Diagnostic & Statistical Manual (DSM) V Criteria

Unstable interpersonal relationships, impulsivity and a distorted self-image beginning by early adulthood and present in a variety of contexts, as indicated by *five (or more)* of the following:

1. Frantic efforts to avoid real or imagined **abandonment**. Note: Do not include suicidal or self-mutilating behavior covered in Criterion 5.
2. A pattern of **unstable** and **intense interpersonal relationships** characterized by alternating between extremes of idealization and devaluation (**Splitting**)
3. Identity disturbance: markedly & persistently **distorted self-image or sense of self**
4. **Impulsivity** in at least two areas that are potentially self-damaging (e.g., spending, sex, substance abuse, reckless driving, binge eating). Note: Do not include suicidal or self-mutilating behavior covered in Criterion 5.
5. Recurrent **suicidal behavior**, gestures, threats, or self-mutilating behavior
6. Affective **instability due to a marked reactivity of mood** (e.g., intense episodic dysphoria, irritability or anxiety usually lasting a few hours and only rarely more than a few days)
7. Chronic feelings of **emptiness**
8. **Inappropriate, intense anger** or difficulty controlling anger (e.g., frequent displays of temper, constant anger or recurrent physical fights)
9. Transient, stress-related **paranoid ideation** or severe **dissociative symptoms**

- **PEARL:** Enhanced **Emotion-Induced Amnesia** is also seen in patients with BPD

TRIAD BULIMIA NERVOSA

1. Caloric restriction
2. Uncontrolled binge eating followed by
3. Purge (Self-induced vomiting) recurrent cycles

- Patient's have distorted body image, normal or slightly overweight vs anorexia (thin)
- **Compensatory behaviors:** Self-induced vomiting; use diuretics and laxatives; excessive exercise
- Dental erosions, calloused knuckles
- 1 episode/week x 3 months
- Normal / slightly overweight
- Cardiac dysrhythmias secondary to electrolyte abnormalities (hypokalemia)

ANOREXIA NERVOSA

- Patients do not eat; significantly underweight, dancers, gymnasts, model, jockeys
- Amenorrhea > = 3 cycles
- Check for hypochloremic, hypokalemic alkalosis

MALINGERING

- Intentional invention or exaggeration of physical or psychological symptoms for external gain (avoid work or to obtain drugs)

PHOBIC DISORDER

- Clinically significant anxiety provoked by exposure to a specific feared object or situation leading to avoidance behavior

SOMATIC SYMPTOM DISORDER (SSD)

- Formerly somatization or somatoform disorder
- Patients have a variety of complaints and a long, complicated medical history with no apparent medical cause; Nondeliberate; patients strongly convinced they are ill; acquiesce to invasive diagnostic tests

FACTITIOUS DISORDER

- Formerly Munchausen Syndrome
- Most common in men 20–40 y/o
- Patients view themselves as important people and usually have extensive knowledge of medical terminology. Want to assume the "sick role" to gain attention, sympathy or reassurance to themselves; usually well spoken/intelligent/extensive visits

CONVERSION DISORDER

- Disorder involving persistent physical symptoms with no identifiable cause
- Often associated with recent trauma or stressor
- Lack of concern = la belle indifference, has been associated with CD but is NOT specific and should NOT be used to make the diagnosis

PSYCHOSIS

Mnemonic - (DAD HN)

D	**D**elusions
A	**A**bnormal motor behavior (agitation to catatonia)
D	**D**isorganized thinking

H	**H**allucinations (auditory)
N	**N**egative symptoms: decrease motivation (avolition), decreased speech (alogia) and decreased ability to experience pleasure (anhedonia)

- **Psychosis** is a symptom
- **Schizophrenia** is an illness diagnosis
- **PEARL**: Patients diagnosed with schizophrenia may have symptoms of psychosis but not everyone with psychosis will be diagnosed with schizophrenia
- Acute psychotic patients often are not disoriented

DELIRIUM VS DEMENTIA

	DELIRIUM	DEMENTIA
Onset	Abrupt	Gradual
Course	Fluctuating	Slow decline
Duration	Hours to weeks	Months to years
Attention	Impaired	Intact early/impaired late
Sleep-wake	Disrupted	Normal
Alertness	Impaired	Normal
Orientation	Impaired (AMS)	Intact early/impaired late
Behavior	Agitated/depressed	Intact early/impaired late
Speech	Incoherent, rapid/slow	Word finding problem
Thoughts	Disorganized/delusions	Impoverished
Perceptions	Hallucinations (*visual)	Intact early

Most common cause of dementia in elderly patients = **Alzheimer's disease**
* Psychosis = Auditory hallucinations

DEMENTIA - DIAGNOSIS

1. Cognitive deficit
2. Memory impairment (earliest sign!)
3. One of the following: aphasia, apraxia, agnosia or impaired executive function
    - Agitated due to lack of awareness of surroundings or the intent of others
    - No alteration of consciousness

AGITATED PATIENT

PROTECT YOURSELF

- Decrease stimulus: offer food, remove family or police
- Calm voice, reassure expectations of self control
- Stay > 8 feet away Use verbal de-escalation first in the treatment process
- Need very good documentation for restraints
- Your safety is top priority and may need to consider chemical options:
- Ziprasidone (Geodon) 20 mg IM
- B52:Haloperidol (Haldol) 5mg + Lorazepam (Ativan) 2mg + Benadryl (diphenhydramine) 50mg IM
- Haldol and ativan are "compatible" and can be mixed and administered through same syringe
- Olanzapine (Zyprexa) 10mg IM
- In the combative excited delirium patient consider Ketamine 1 mg/kg IV or 5 mg/kg IM
- Consider your medical-legal environment, consider the BPD PEARL below, consider the number of narcotic seeking behavior patients you will encounter and other patients who have their own agendas and this will lead to an important point to remember: **you don't have to do anything to be accused of doing something**. So, protect yourself by including other team members during your patient encounters and develop safeguards to protect you and your team.
- **PEARL:** If you have a "difficult patient" with insolvable problems, multiple visits, hostility, name dropping excessive need for attention and threats consider Borderline Personality Disorder (BPD)

PSYCHOBEHAVIORAL PEARLS

- Psychiatric illness ("functional") vs medical illness ("organic")
- Assume medical etiology until proven otherwise; 20% of all psychiatric referrals have organic etiologies
- **Medical features:** abrupt onset, age > 40, visual or tactile hallucinations, abnormal vital signs
- **Auditory hallucinations** suggest psychiatric disease = schizophrenia
- Psychiatric presentation: normal cognitive, normal vital signs and normal physical exam
- **Disorientation** is more common with medical illness (delirium); psychiatric illnesses generally regain orientation
- The most common DSM-V diagnostic group for pediatric patients in the ED = substance disorders
- Mania (Biploar) patients - have flight of ideas
- Mania
  - Drug causes: steroids, antidepressants, psychostimulants, PCP
  - Medical conditions: hyperthyroidism. Cushing's syndrome and CNS tumors
- Classic "fakers" of Psychiatric Illness
  - Acute intermittent porphyria (AIP): psychosis + abdominal pain
  - Pheochromocytosis
  - MS
  - Cushing's disease
  - Syphilis, AIDS
  - SLE

MEDICAL LEGAL / LEADERSHIP

Success in Medical School and Beyond / Mnemonics and Pearls

FOUR ELEMENTS OF NEGLIGENCE

Mnemonic: (B,C,D_2)

B	**B**reach of Duty - failed to act in accordance with "standard of care" = exercising the skill, care and knowledge that a reasonably well qualified practitioner in the same specialty would apply under the same or similar circumstances
C	**C**ausation a) Actual Cause - direct causal relationship between negligent act and the injury b) Proximate Cause - direct temporal relationship between the negligent act and the injury
D	**D**amages
D	**D**uty - created by the physician-patient relationship

PEARL: Defenses to Negligence = Statutes of Limitation and Good Samaritan Laws

THREE BASIC REQUIREMENTS EMTALA

Emergency Medical Treatment and Active Labor Act (EMTALA)
Patient is anywhere within 250 yards of main hospital

1. Medical Screening Exam (MSE): by qualified medical personnel; must include H&P
2. Stabilization
3. Transfer (patient request after stabilized, or benefits of transfer to a center with more resources outweigh the risks of transfer)

EMTALA ends when: patient is stabilized, arrives at receiving hospital or patient refuses care; does not apply to admitted patients

CONSENT

1. Express Consent = oral or written agreement between parties with full disclosure of information
2. Implied Consent = consent is implied by patient's actions (example: rolling up one's sleeve for injection)
3. Emergent Consent
4. Informed Consent = patient must understand all the reasonable risks and benefits inherent to a treatment or procedure; patient must be competent to make decision

EMANCIPATED MINORS

May not require parental consent

1. Marriage
2. Pregnancy
3. Parent
4. "Mature Minors" - capable of understanding risks/benefits of treatment and making rational decision yet < 18 years old
5. Military service
6. High School graduate

- Other exceptions: public policy concern: drug/alcohol addiction or abuse, STD, birth control and physical/sexual abuse - varies state by state.

HEALTH INSURANCE PORTABILITY AND ACCOUNTABILITY ACT (HIPAA)

- Protected health information - individually identifiable demographic data relating to provision of health care to individual
- (name, address, DOB or SS#). Data which could be reasonably used to identify patient

Permissible disclosures: disclosures for treatment, payment, court orders, some law enforcement requests, public interest / public health activities. Patient request is not required

AGAINST MEDICAL ADVICE (AMA)

properly completed AMA forms should show the process of determining patient's decision-making capacity and that the patient has been fully informed of the risks, benefits, and alternatives to treatment. AMA forms do not provide immunity to malpractice suits

LIVING WILL

Legal document directing healthcare staff on treatment preferences of patient when patient is unable to make this decision. Living wills may be revoked at any time. DNR does not "mean do not treat"

DURABLE POWER OF ATTORNEY

Legal document used in some states to specify an agent to help patients make healthcare decisions when patients are no longer capable of making decisions by themselves. Patient may limit agent's powers
Assault: Reasonable fear of harmful touching without consent

BATTERY

Harmful touching / blood draw without consent

FALSE IMPRISONMENT

Intentionally detaining in an unlawful manner or otherwise restricted in movement without consent

Agency, vicarious lability, respondeat superior (Latin:"let the master answer"), captain of the ship = all involved liability for one person acting on behalf of another person (In a workplace context, an employer can be liable for the acts or omissions of its employees)

Res Ipsa Loquitur = "the thing speaks for itself"

MALPRACTICE INSURANCE

- Occurrence-based = protects physicians against negligent acts that occurred while the insurance was in effect
- Claims–made coverage = must be in effect when negligent act occurred and when "claim was made"
- Tail insurance = additional insurance that provides protection when "Claims-made" policy lapses
- Claims made policy + Tail insurance = Occurrence-based insurance

CORE: Communicate Openly; Resolve Early

DISCLOSURE OF UNANTICIPATED OUTCOMES

Begin with AID discussion

A	**A**cknowledge (acknowledge the outcome)
I	**I**nvestigate (promise to investigate; complete within 45 days)
D	**D**isclose (commit to disclose findings)

After Investigation determine if *Reasonable Care* **vs** *Unreasonable Care*

REASONABLE CARE – harm not preventable

Mnemonic (ALEE)

A	**A**nticipate and Adjust
L	**L**isten
E	**E**mpathize
E	**E**xplain

UNREASONABLE CARE – harm preventable

STOP – contact Risk Manager prior to any contact with patient / family

Next step: **ALEE + TEAM**

T	**T**ruth, Transparency, Teamwork
E	**E**mpathy
A	**A**pology & **A**ccountability
M	**M**anagement

LEADERSHIP PEARLS

CHARACTER + COMPETENCE = LEADERSHIP

Watch your thoughts, they become your words.
Watch your words, they become your *actions.
Watch your actions they become your **habits.
Watch your habits, they become your CHARACTER
Mahatma Gandhi

When I think of various *actions ... I think of "The Tao of Pooh", Benjamin Hoff
While Eeyore frets ....
... and Piglet hesitates
... and Rabbit calculates
... and Owl pontificates
Pooh just is

When I think of **habits .... *I think of 6 Habits That Make or Break a Leader at Work and Home,* Dave Anderson

6 HABITS OF CHARACTER

Mnemonic: (D – CHIPS)

D	**D**uty

C	**C**ourage
H	**H**umility
I	**I**ntegrity
P	**P**ositivity
S	**S**elflessness

Leaders → **influence** (moral/ethical vs. bad) → GOALS

VAGINAL BLEEDING

DEFINITIONS

- Menorrhagia: menstruation at regular cycle intervals but with excessive flow and duration
- Metrorrhagia: irregular vaginal bleeding outside normal cycle
- Menometrorrhagia: irregular vaginal bleeding, excessive bleeding, outside normal cycle
- Polymenorrhea: frequent, light, bleeding at intervals < 21 days
- Dysfunctional uterine bleeding: abnormal vaginal bleeding due to anovulataion
- Hypomenorreah: scanty menstruation; causes: emotional stress, excessive exercise and dieting, Asherman's syndrome, and post- myomectomy
- Oligomenorrhea: infrequent menstruation with cycles of greater than 35 days; associated with prolactinomas, thyrotoxicosis, perimenopause, Prader-Willi syndrome, Graves disease, athletes, excessive exercise, breastfeeding, polycystic ovarian syndrome, and eating disorders

MISCARRIAGE

- 80% of miscarriages occur during the first trimester
- 50% of women who bleed during early pregnancy miscarry

TYPES OF SPONTANEOUS ABORTIONS

- **Threatened abortion:** vaginal bleeding < 20 weeks of gestation and a *closed* internal cervical os; risk of miscarriage in this population is up to 50%
- **Inevitable abortion:** vaginal bleeding < 20 weeks of gestation, with an *open* internal os, and no passage of placental or fetal parts
- **Incomplete abortion:** vaginal bleeding < 20 weeks of gestation, with an *open* internal os, with products of conception (POC) present at the cervical os or in the vaginal canal
- **Complete abortion:** vaginal bleeding < 20 weeks of gestation, with a *closed* internal os, with complete passage of POC; uterus contracted
- **Missed abortion:** fetal death < 20 weeks without POC passage
- **Septic abortion:** any type of abortion accompanied by a uterine infection

ECTOPIC PREGNANCY (EP) PEARLS

- 15% of clinically recognized pregnancies terminate in miscarriage
- Mean gestational age for ectopic rupture = 8.0 to 10 weeks
- Isthmic ectopic pregnancies rupture *earlier* = 6 to 8 weeks
- Cornual ectopic pregnancies rupture *later* = 14 to 16 weeks
- Recent estimate of heterotopic pregnancy = 1 in 4,000 pregnancies
- If women have undergone embryo transfer or use of ovulation-inducing drugs incidence or heterotopic pregnancy = 1 in 100 pregnancies

- Most common site of EP implantation = ampullary (80%) portion of the fallopian tube
- ↑maternal mortality rate if EP implantation = cornual location
- Monoclonal antibody assays detect presence of β-hCG as soon as 2-3 d post-implantation
- The earliest a serum beta-hCG test can detect pregnancy = shortly before missed period; usually reaches 200 IU/ml at time of menses
- In a normal pregnancy, β-hCG doubles every 2 days or increase by 66% every 3 days for the first 6-7 weeks beginning 8-9 days after ovulation
- After 9-10 weeks gestation, beta-hCG levels decline
- 10% of normal pregnancies can manifest abnormal doubling times
- 15% of EP's can have normal doubling times
- Evidence of IUP should be seen by transabdominal ultrasound with beta-hCG levels of 6,500 mIU/mL, or at least 1,500 mIU/mL using TVUS (discriminatory threshold)
- Rupture can occur in patients with beta-hCG levels as low as 100 mIU/mL
- The most common clinical presentation of patients with EP = abdominal pain (80%); vaginal Bleeding (50-80%)

RISK FACTORS FOR ECTOPIC PREGNANCY

LESSER RISK	GREATER RISK	GREATEST RISK
Previous pelvic or abdominal surgery	Previous PID	Pervious ectopic pregnancy
Cigarette smoking	Infertility (IVF)	Pervious tubal surgery or sterilization
Vaginal douching	Multiple sexual partners	Diethylstilbestrol exposure to utero
Age of 1st intercourse < 18 yrs		Documented tubal pathology (scarring)
		Use of IUD

ECTOPIC PEARLS

TV Ultrasound findings	beta-hCG (mIU/mL)	Gestational Age
Gestational sac (GS) First sonographic finding	1,000	4-5 weeks
Yolk sac = earliest sonographic finding of an IUP Small hyperechoic ring in GS with anechoic center (looks like a "cheerio" sitting in gestational sac)	1,000 to 7,000	5 weeks
Fetal pole (embryo) Seen adjacent to yolk sac	1,000 to 7,000	5-6 weeks
Fetal cardiac activity Normal heart rate in early pregnancy = 112 to 136. Slower heart rates in 2nd and 3rd trimester	10,000 to 23,000	6 weeks

Menstrual age = 2 weeks older than embryonic age (ovulation typically takes place at midpoint of a typical 28-day menstrual cycle)

- **Double-decidual sac sign (DDSS) ("double ring sign"): 2 distinct echogenic rings surrounding the hypoehoic gestational sac**
  Inner ring: decidua capsularis; outer ring: decidua parietalis (also called decidua vera)
  The earliest reliable US finding seen in normal intrauterine pregnancies
  Should be visualized by 5 weeks after last menstrual period
- Earliest definitive sign in the initial diagnosis of an IUP = **yolk sac** in the uterus. Should be visualized by 5.5 weeks after last menstrual period
- Most common cause of misdiagnosis of ectopic pregnancy by TVUS = misinterpretation of the **pseudogestational sac** as an IUP
- **Pseudogestational sac:** anechoic fluid collection without a clear double decidual reaction
  Seen in 10 to 20% of ectopics
- Double-decidual sac sign can be used to differentiate true GS from pseudo-GS
- Other US findings in Ectopic = free fluid, adnexal mass, or tubal ring
- Ectopic pregnancies are due to anatomic abnormalities of the salpinx (tube), prior tubal infection or an abnormal endometrium

3RD TRIMESTER VAGINGAL BLEEDING

PLACENTAL ABRUPTION

- Placental abruption: premature separation of a normally implanted placenta
- Usually occurs spontaneously (though trauma can cause abruption)
  - HTN is the most common risk factor
  - Other risk factors: trauma, cocaine, multiparity, smoking, advanced maternal age, chronic ETOH, previous abruption
- Manifests clinically as painful third trimester vaginal bleeding
- Clinical diagnosis:
  - Dark VB, uterine pain or tenderness is seen in 2/3
  - Uterine irritability or contractions are seen in 1/3
  - US only 50% accurate in the diagnosis
  - Cardiotocographic monitoring most reliable for the diagnosis
- Complications of placental abruption: fetal/maternal death, DIC, amniotic fluid embolism, and fetal/maternal hemorrhage
- Treatment: delivery

PLACENTA PREVIA

- Most common cause of third trimester vaginal bleeding
- Painless vaginal bleeding occurs
- Do not perform vaginal exam if suspected previa/abruption ... it may lead to worsened bleeding
- Risk factors for placental previa
  - Advancing age
  - Multiparity

ANTI-D IMMUNE GLOBULIN (RHO-GAM®)

- Rh-isoimmunization occurs when an Rh-negative woman is exposed to Rh+ fetal blood
- Anti-D immune globulin (Rho-GAM®) is indicated for Rh-negative mothers who are exposed to a clinical sensitizing event including: termination of pregnancy, amniocentesis, threatened miscarriage, spontaneous miscarriage, ectopic, placenta previa, abruptio placenta, during term pregnancy delivery, abdominal trauma)
- These events put patients at risk for Rh isoimmunization which can negatively impact both current and subsequent pregnancies (fetal anemia, hydrops fetalis and death)
- RhoGAM must be administered within 72 hours of the event to be effective in preventing anti-Rh antibody formation secondary to Rh-isoimmunization
  - 50 mcg IM < 12 weeks gestational age
  - 300 mcg IM > 12 weeks gestational age

POSTPARTUM HEMORRHAGE

- Cumulative blood loss of > 500 mL after vaginal delivery or > 1,000 mL after cesarean delivery within 24 hours of birth process. All blood loss should be weighed (1mg = 1mL)
- American College of Obstetricians and Gynecologists defines postpartum hemorrhage as either:
  - Cumulative blood loss ≥ 1,000 mL (regardless of mode of delivery)
  - Blood loss accompanied by signs or symptoms of hypovolemia within 24 hours after birth
- Tachycardia and hypotension do not present until a woman has lost 25% of blood volume ~ 1500mL
- Most common early (< 24 hours after delivery) cause = **uterine atony** (uterus will feel boggy)
- Most common late / delayed postpartum hemorrhage (> 24 hours and up to 6 weeks): r**etained uterine products of conception**
- Risk Factors for retained uterine products of conception = c-section, previous curettage, multiple births, endometrial infection and injury
- **Treatment:** initiate massive transfusion protocol; see uterotonic medications below; consider TXA

POST PARTUM HEMORRHAGE
MNEMONIC - 5T'S

T	Tone	Uterine atony Occurs immediately post-partum Most common cause < 24 hours and most common cause overall of postpartum hemorrhage **PEARL**: Vigorous bimanual uterine massage of "boggy" uterus while waiting for utertonic agents
T	Tissue	Retained products of conception: most common cause > 24 hours and up to 6 weeks after delivery
T	Traction	Uterine inversion
T	Trauma	Lacerations
T	Thrombosis	Coagulation disorders

DRUGS THAT STIMULATE UTERINE CONTRACTION

USED TO INDUCE LABOR AND CONTROL POST-PARTUM HEMORRHAGE (UTEROTONIC AGENTS)

- Oxytocin (Pitocin): 10 to 40 units in 500 – 1,000 mL normal saline as continues infusion or 10 units IM
- Methylergonovine (Methergine): 0.2 mg IM every 2-4 hours
- Carboprost (Hemabate); chemical name: 15-methyl PGF2α: 0.25 mg IM every 15-90 minures to a maximum 8 doses
- Misoprostol (Cytotec): 600-1,000 micrograms oral, SL or rectal

- **PEARL:** Most common cause of vaginal bleeding related to primary coagulation disorder: Von Willebrand's disease
- **PEARL:** Most common causes of vaginal bleeding in prepubertal girls (without precocious puberty): vulvovaginal abnormalities (vaginitis, vaginal FBs, trauma, and tumors)

TOCOLYTIC AGENTS

- Used to stop premature labor (labor that starts before 32), by causing myometrial relaxation
- Based on "viability" and corticosteroid effectiveness the The American College of Obstetricians and Gynecologists (ACOG) does not recommend treatment before 24 weeks
- Delay delivery by at least 48 hours; antenatal corticosteroids given to the mother will have time to achieve their maximum fetal/neonatal effects
- Predelivery betamethasone reduces the risk of neonatal death, respiratory distress syndrome, intraventricular hemorrhage, and necrotizing enterocolitis in premature neonates

24 to 32 weeks gestation
1) Indomethacin - first-line
2) Nifedipine

32 to 34 weeks gestation
1) Nifedipine - first-line
2) Terbutaline (beta 2 agonist)

- In women with an acute episode of preterm labor, bedrest, hydration, sedatives, antibiotics, and progesterone supplementation are NOT effective for preventing preterm birth
- Discontinue tocolytics 48 hours after administration of first corticosteroid dose
- Magnesium, Nitrous Oxide and oxytocin receptor anatgonists are LESS effective tocolytic drugs

CONFIRMING RUPTURE OF MEMBRANES

1. Pooling of amniotic fluid in vaginal vault (not specific; could be: amniotic, vaginal or urinary fluid)
2. Nitrazine test + (non-specific, a lot of false +, could be: lubicrants, semen, blood, cervical mucus)
3. Ferning (NaCl crystal precipitation) on microscopic analysis of amniotic fluid is the most specific test to confirm rupture of membranes)

When exposed to a Flame:

- Vaginal secretions turn brown
- Amniotic fluid turns WHITE, displays crystallized FERNING pattern

Nitrazine strips (pH indicator):

- Vaginal fluid: Mildly acidic pH 4 to 5
- Amniotic fluid = Basic pH of 7 to 7.5
- Vaginal fluid: Nitrazine strip remains yellow or turns slightly red
- Amniotic fluid: Nitrazine strip turns BLUE

EMERGENCY CONTRACEPTION

- Progestin only (levonogestrel) (Plan B, Plan B One Step, Fallback Solo, among others) = most commonly used in ED; does not require prescription
- Anti-progestin as equally effective as Progestin only (if given early)
- Anti-progestin more effective than Progestin only, if taken later and has less caustic side effect profile
- Combined estrogen-progestin emergency contraception pill more likely to cause N & V; less effective than 2 options above
- If > 5 days (120 hours) since unprotected intercourse: the Copper IUD (brand name = Paragard) is the BEST contraception

RISK FACTORS FOR ENDOMETRIAL CANCER

- Obesity
- Nulliparity
- Early Menarche
- Late menopause
- Anovulatory cycles

RISK FACTOR FOR CERVICAL CANCER

- Multiple sex partners (HPV)

PREECLAMPSIA AND ECLAMPSIA

- Preeclampsia = gestational HTN & proteinuria
- Blood pressure ≥ 140/90 mm Hg on 2 occasions ≥ 4 hours apart
- Proteinuria defined as either:
  - ≥ 300 mg per 24 hour urine collection
  - Protein/creatinine ratio ≥ 0.3 mg/dL or
  - Dipstick reading of 2+ (should be used only if other quantitative methods are not available)
- Preeclampsia and eclampsia occur at > 20 weeks gestation
- Can also occur several weeks POST-partum
- 7% of all pregnancies
- More common in primigravida patient
- Most common cause of death in toxemia = cerebral hemorrhage
- Treatment of ecclamptic seizures or prophylactic treatment of patients with severe preeclampsia: **magnesium sulfate** first-line agent
  Loading dose 4 to 6 grams over 15 minutes, followed by IV infusion of 1 to 2 gm/hour maintained for 24 hours after the last seizure
- Observe for nausea, somnolence and loss of deep tendon reflexes
- First sign of **magnesium sulfate toxicity** = hyporeflexia (loss of deep tendon reflexes) and occurs at serum concentrations > 8 mEq/L
- At serum concentrations > 10 mEq/L, patients can develop respiratory depression/apnea

- **Antidote for magnesium sulfate toxicity** = calcium gluconate 1.5-3 grams IV over 5 minutes
- Side effects of rapid intravenous calcium gluconate injection = vomiting, vasodilation, dysrhythmia, hypotension and bradycardia
- **HTN Management:**
  - **Labetalol algorithm**: Labetalol 20 mg, if needed repeat 40 mg in 10 minutes, if needed repeat 80 mg in 10 minutes, if needed switch to Hydralazine 10 mg IV
  - **Hydralazine algorithm**: Hydralazine 5-10 mg, Hydralazine 10mg then switch to Labetalol 20mg then Labetalol 40mg IV
- **Anticonvulsants** (for recurrent seizures or when magnesium is contraindicated:
  - Lorazepam: 2-4 mg IVx1, may repeat x1 after 10 minutes
  - Diazepam: 5-10 mg IV every 5-10 minutes to max of 30 mg
  - Keppra: 500 mg IV
  - Phenytoin: 15-20 mg/kg IV x1, may repeat 10 mg/kg IV after 20 minutes if no response

7 CARDINAL MOVEMENTS OF FETAL DESCENT DURING LABOR

1. Engagement: Delivery is imminent if pelvic examination shows a completely effaced cervix and the fetal head is visible at the introitus
2. Descent
3. Flexion
4. Internal rotation of the fetus: the occiput moves anteriorly
5. Extension of the head as it exits the introitus. Clinician support sthe face with the inferior hand
6. External rotation of the fetus bringing the thorax into the anteroposterior diameter of the pelvis
7. Expulsion

GESTATIONAL TROPHOBLASTIC DISEASE

- Molar pregnancy = 1 in 1,700 pregnancies
- Present 1st or 2nd trimester
- Spectrum of conditions caused by neoplastic mutation of the trophoblastic cells of the placenta:
  a) Complete hydatidiform mole (most common); 80 % present as hydatidiform mole and follow benign course
  b) Partial hydatidiform mole
  c) Malignant forms = invasive mole (12-15%) and choriocarcinoma (5-8%)
  Choriocarcinoma may metastasize to vagina/lung/liver/brain and is sensitive to chemotherapy
- **Risk factors**
  - Advanced maternal age and prior gestational trophoblastic disease
- **Signs / Symptoms**
  - Hyperemesis gravidarum, VB, pelvic pressure / pain, and uterine size greater than > dates; βhCG is structural similar to TSH → thyroid overstimulation → **hyperthyroidism**
- **Gestational HTN** < 20 weeks gestation (preeclampsia) is highly suggestive of gestational trophoblastic disease
- **Lab**: ↑ β-hCG levels are markedly elevated (>100,000 mIU/mL) and significantly above expected levels for gestational age
- **US findings:** intrauterine echogenic mass with multiple small hypoechoic vesicles interspersed ("grape-like" appearance or "snowstorm appearance")

HYPEREMESIS GRAVIDARUM

- Etiology
  - Hormonal hCG stimulation of estrogen production
  - Abnormal gastric motility
- First trimester, usually starts at 5 to 6 weeks gestation and peaks at 9 weeks

HYPEREMESIS GRAVIDARUM – TREATMENT OPTIONS

- IV Hydration
- Glucose with thiamine (B1) IV
- Must have glucose to break ketosis
- Antiemetics
- Pyridoxine (Vitamin B6) 50mg po + Doxylamine (Unisom) 50mg po
- Ginger

CERVICITIS, URETHRITIS, PID

- Two most common causes of STDs: Neisseria gonorrhoeae and Chlamydia; Chlamydia: most common overall
- **Acute complications of cervicitis:** PID, Bartholin abscess, tubo-ovarian abscess (TOA), peritonitis, peri-hepatitis (Fitz-Hugh-Curtis syndrome), prostatitis, epididymitis and reactive arthritis (formerly known as Reiter's syndrome)
- **Chronic PID complications:** chronic pelvic pain, infertility, ectopic pregnancy (risk for ectopic pregnancy is 7 to 10x greater in women with a history of PID)
- Nucleic acid amplification techniques (NAATs): diagnostic test of choice NAATs
- Sn better than culture (>90% versus 60-80%); Sp 99%
- Performed on endocervical swabs and urine
- 70% of women infected with C. trachomatis are asymptomatic
- Chlamydia urethritis: 20% of women will present with dysuria (sterile pyuria)
- **Treatment Simple Cervicitis / Urethritis / Proctitis**
- Gonorrhea: Ceftriaxone 500 mg IM x1 dose (or if >/= 300 lbs treat with 1gm IM)
- Chlamydia: Doxycycline: 100 mg po bid x 7 days (alternative regimen Azithromycin 1gm po is effective for chlamydia)
- Dual therapy for GC is no longer recommended; if concomitant Chlamydia infection is not excluded treat with Ceftriaxone + Doxy
- **Outpatient PID Treatment**
  - CDC recommends ceftriaxone 250 mg IM + doxycycline 100mg pd bid for 14 days with or without metronidazole 500 mg orally twice daily for 14 days
- **Inpatient PID Treatment**
  - Cefoxitin 2 g IV every 6 hours or cefotetan 2 g IV every 12 hours, PLUS doxycycline 100 mg orally every 12 hours

CDC Hospital Admission Criteria for Patients With PID

- Pregnancy, severe illness, persistent N/V, high fever, TOA, cannot exclude surgical emergencies (appy), unable to tolerate outpatient antimicrobial therapy, no clinical response to oral antimicrobial therapy
- **PEARL:** cervical motion tenderness: "Chandelier sign"
- **PEARL:** Gestational age pregnant women with **HSV** should begin suppressive therapy to reduce the likelihood of lesions during labor = 34-36 weeks of gestation

RISK FACTORS FOR ENDOMETRITIS

- Cesarean delivery (*most frequent*), retained products of conception (POC) or placenta, young maternal age, PROM, frequent vaginal examinations and use of intrauterine monitoring devices
- Begins 3 to 5 days post delivery; foul smelling lochia, fever, pelvic pain & uterine tenderness
- **Complications:** parametrial or pelvic abscesses, septic thrombophlebitis of pelvic veins
- **Treatment**: Clindamycin OR Ampicillin + Gentamycin OR Unasyn OR Zosyn
- Gestational age pregnant women with HSV should begin suppressive therapy to reduce the likelihood of lesions during labor = 34-36 weeks of gestation
- **PEARL:** Chorioamnionitis: infection of fetal membranes; associated with PROM; Maternal tachycardia, fever and abdominal pain; fetal tachycardia

ENDOMETRIOSIS

Disease of ectopic endometrial tissue

Mnemonic: 3 - D's

D	**D**ysmenorrhea (painful menstruation)
D	**D**yspareunia (painful sexual intercourse)
D	**D**yschezia (painful bowel movement)

ENDOMETRIOSIS TREATMENT

- NSAIDs
- Hormonal contraceptives
- Gonadotropin-releasing hormone (GnRH) agonists
- Aromatase inhibitors
- **PEARL**: catamenial hemoptysis: hemoptysis due to ectopic endometrial tissue in the pulmonary system

UTERINE RUPTURE

- Most common cause = previous cesarean section; other causes = trauma, congenital uterine anomalies, use of medications for labor induction
- Maternal shock, severe abdominal, pelvic pain and VB or minimal pain and VB
- Loss of fetal station, abnormal fetal lie, palpable uterine defect, and ability to palpate fetal anatomy = suspicion of a uterine rupture
- Termination of uterine contractions, decreased amplitude of contractions on tocodynamometry can be seen, however fetal heart rate is more reliable sign
- Non-reassuring FHT = most reliable sign of uterine rupture
- Time for intervention to prevent fetal mortality = < 30 minutes

PERIMORTEM C-SECTION

- Midline vertical incision from pubic symphysis to → 4-5cm below the xyphoid process
- #10 scalpel
- Incise down to peritoneal cavity
- After bladder is reflected inferiorly
- Vertical incision in the uterus

Remember 24 and 4

- > 24 wks gestation (FHTs present)
- Start within 4 min of arrest (70% children who survived were delivered < 5 min)

Prolonged CPR > 25 minutes = near certain non-viability of the fetus

COMPLICATIONS OF INTRAUTERINE DEVICES (IUDS)

- Device migration and malposition (10%)
- IUDs can be partially expelled into the cervix, rotate on their axes, can migrate and embed in the myometrium and even translocate through the uterus into the
- abdominal cavity; migration to adjacent organs can lead to bowel obstruction, peritonitis, fistula formation, obstructive uropathy, and intraperitoneal adhesions
- Malpositioned IUDs can cause significant pain; Order ultrasound (US) and/ or CT scan to evaluate its specific position
- Malpositioned IUDs should be removed
- IUDs positioned in the cervix have a 14-fold increased risk of pregnancy, so patients should be instructed to use alternative means of contraception
- IUD removal is recommended in women who get pregnant with an IUD desiring pregnancy continuation; Retained IUDs have increased risk of spontaneous abortion, septic abortion, chorioamnionitis, placental abruption, placenta previa, low-birth-weight infants, and preterm delivery; if strings are visible the IUD should be removed from the cervical canal; if the strings retract into the uterus, US-guided IUD removal should be performed but may disrupt a wanted pregnancy

SHOULDER DYSTOCIA = OBSTETRICAL EMERGENCY

- Obstructed labor = the shoulders become trapped at the pelvic outlet after delivery of the head
- The fetal head retracts tightly against the perineum = "turtle sign"
- This can lead to fetal hypoxia and fetal demise if delivery is not prompt (compression of the umbilical cord in the birth canal)
- Additional complications include: fetal brachial plexus injury, clavicular fracture, and postpartum hemorrhage

SHOULDER DYSTOCIA RISK FACTORS

Mneumonic - DOPE

D	**D**iabetes (maternal diabetes)
O	**O**besity fetal (maternal obesity)
P	**P**ost-date delivery
E	**E**xcessive growth (fetal macrosomia)

Shoulder Dystocia Management

a) Episiotomy incision location = mediolateral
b) Empty bladder
c) Hyperflex mother's legs and pull them up towards the abdomen (**McRobert's maneuver)**
d) Firm suprapubic pressure applied
This rotates the pelvis and facilitates release of the trapped shoulder

If McRobert's maneuver fails to deliver the infant → attempt **Gaskin maneuver**

a) Mother should be placed in the all-fours position (this increases pelvic dimensions and may allow fetal position to shift)
b) Gentle downward traction applied to fetal head

If Gaskin maneuver fails → go to last resort option or try **clavicle fracture** before last resort
Clavicular fracture — The clavicle can be intentionally fractured to shorten the bisacromial diameter

If all fails → "last resort" option → **Zavenelli maneuver**

a) Reinsert fetal head
b) Followed by C-section

UMBILICAL CORD PROLAPSE

- < 1 % of deliveries
- More likely in compound, shoulder, or breech presentations as the presenting fetal part does not completely fill the birth canal
- Cord is visualized at the perineum or protruding from the cervix Emergency cesarean section is the delivery method of choice

Maneuvers to decrease compression of the cord

a) Trendelenburg position
b) Knee-chest position (the patient prone with knees at right angles to the bed and her chest flat; on knees and elbows with chest flat to ground)
   - Presenting part should be manually lifted off the cord;
   - Mother should refrain from pushing
   - Perinatal mortality rates correlate with time from diagnosis to delivery
   - If obstetric backup is not available or surgical delivery will be delayed, careful manual replacement of the cord into the uterus and vaginal delivery may be the only option
   - Prepare for resuscitation of the likely distressed infant

NUCHAL CORD (UMBILICAL CORD LOOPS AROUND FETUS'S NECK)

- Common = 1/3 of deliveries
- Manual reduction of the cord by slipping the cord over the fetal head = Type A (cord in an unlocked pattern)
- If the cord cannot be reduced (Type B, "locked" pattern)

a) **"Somersault maneuver:** place your palm on the fetal occiput and push the face into the mother's thigh (or pubic bone), which allows the shoulders, then body, then legs to deliver - in "somersault" motion
b) **Clamp and cut the cord**
   - Two clamps are applied at the area of best access, and the cord is cut between the 2 clamps
   - Fetus must be rapidly delivered after cutting the cord (cord without blood supply at this point)
   - Some studies have shown a mild increase in cerebral palsy in patients with prolonged or tight nuchal cords

OB /GYN PEARLS

- Blighted ovum = inability to visualize yolk sac or fetal pole (embryo) in a large gestational sac on TV ultrasound → major criteria for fetal demise

- Subchorionic hematoma = more than ↑double the chance pregnancy loss in threatened abortion
- HELLP Syndrome = **H**emolysis, **E**levated **L**iver Enzymes, **L**ow Platelets
  More common in *multigravid* patient
  Can also occur postpartum
- Leading non-OB cause of maternal death: blunt trauma; the most common cause (50%) of blunt trauma = MVC; #2 domestic violence (abdomen most common site of trauma) and #3 falls
- Cardiotocographic monitoring: Most SENSITIVE modality for identifying occult trauma to the uterus or to the fetus
- 45% of women report assault or abuse during pregnancy
- Intimate partner violence (IPV) > if separated vs married or even divorced and increased if weapons in home
- Nearly 50% of intimate partner homicide victims visited a health care provider within 1 year of their death
- Most common cause of death in toxemia: cerebral hemorrhage
- Most common medical cause of death in pregnant patient = PE
- Most common cause of death in pregnant patient overall = injury (homicide most common injury)
- The leading cause of death in first trimester is ectopic pregnancy
- Most common organism in lactational mastitis: *S. aureus;* Treatment = penicillinase-resistant antibiotic and continued emptying of the breast milk (continued nursing or manual extraction). The breast milk will not harm the nursing infant. Women are encouraged to continue to nurse if able.
- Threshold for human teratogenesis = 5-10 rad; fetus most vulnerable 8 to 15 weeks gestation, 1mGy = 0.1 rad
- V/Q = Total fetal exposure to xenon-133 and technetium-99m = 0.5 rad
  CXR = 0.00005 rad; CT head < 0.1 rad, CT chest = < 1 rad; CT abdomen = 3.5 rad
- British Journal of Radiology (2006) [79, 441-444] recommends: D-dimer → + → bilateral lower extremity venous doppler → non-diagnostic → CT chest over V/Q to diagnose PE
- Expected physiological changes in pregnancy
  - ↑ HR
  - ↓ SVR
  - ↑ Cardiac Output (HR x SVR)
  - ↑ Blood volume
  - ↓ CVP
  - ↓ SBP which normalizes near term
  - ↑ Minute Ventilation
  - ↑ WBC – mild
  - ↓ BUN / Cr
- 10% of insulin-dependent patients will develop DKA during pregnancy; occurs more rapidly and lower levels of glucose in pregnant patients; hyperemesis and non-compliance most common causes
- pH may be normal in DKA, because the initial pH is ↑ in pregnancy due to physiologic hyperventilation
- **Mondor's Syndrome** = superficial phlebitis of the veins in the SQ tissue of the breast; may occur post-op or minor trauma. (Mondor's disease of penis also described)

ACUTE VISUAL LOSS

Mnemonic - (CAN U GO STARE AT HIM) [http://canadiem.org/2016/01/12/tiny-tip-can-u-go-stare-at-him/ and Dr. Postel]

C	CRVO/CRAO	**S**	Scleritis	**H**	Hemorrhage (Hyphema / Vitreous)
A	Abrasion (Corneal)	**Ta**	Temporal Arteritis	**I**	Iritis
N	Neuritis (optic)	**R**	Retinal Detachment	**M**	Migrane / Meds / Drugs
U	Ulcer (Corneal)	**E**	Epscleritis		
G	Glaucoma (Acute)	**At**			
O	Object (Foreign)				

PEARL: most common cause of vision loss from retinal vascular disease = diabetic retinopathy

ACUTE ANGLE-CLOSURE GLAUCOMA (AACG)

Classic history: patient walks into dark room from daylight or by administering a mydriatic → pupil dilation → occlusion of the chamber angle (the canal of schlemm) → aqueous humor build up → ↑IOP → AACG → periorbital pain, ipsilateral HA, blurry vision / vision loss / halos, abdominal pain

TREATMENT ACUTE ANGLE-CLOSURE GLAUCOMA (AACG)

1) **Block aqueous humor production**
   a. Topical beta-blocker (Timoptic 0.5% one drop) ↓ IOP in 30 to 60 minutes
   b. Topial alpha-2 agonist – Apraclonidine (Iopidine) one drop
   c. Oral /IV Acetazolamide (Diamox) 500mg

Mneumonic (DATE)

D	**Diamox**
A	**A**praclonidine
T	**Timolol**
E	**E**ye will make less aqueous humor

2) **Reduce vitreous humor volume**
   a. Systemic hyperosmotic agent = Mannitol 1 – 2 gm/kg IV

3) **Facilitate aqueous outflow**
   a.Pilocarpine 1 or 2% one drop 4x daily → after pressure reduced < 40 mm Hg → makes pupil miotic → pulling the peripheral iris away from the angle (will not work if given early because pressure induced ischemic paralysis of iris); *this is the only emergent use of a miotic agent (green caps)*

4) **Decrease the inflammatory reaction and reduce optic nerve damage**
a.Topical steroid: Pred Forte 1% one drop every 15 min for four doses then hourly
Other: analgesics, antiemetics and supine position (the lens falls away from the iris decreasing pupillary block)

PEARL: Differentiate AACG vs Iritis
Iritis has normal cornea, constricted to mid-range pupil, normal IOP, ciliary flush (perilimbal injection: dilation of the blood vessels adjacent to cornea), debris in anterior chamber (cell and flare)

HYPHEMA

Collection of RBC's in the anterior chamber. Most often due to trauma (traumatic forces cause mechanical tearing of iris or ciliary body vasculature) and promotes bleeding

Grading hyphema on amount of blood layering in Anterior Chamber (AC)

Grade 0	Microhyphema (RBCs in AC)
Grade I	< 1/3 of AC
Grade II	1/3 to 1/2 of AC
Grade III	Slightly less than total AC
Grade IV	"Eight Ball" hyphema (blood fills entire AC)

- If hyphema < 1/3 the anterior chamber (Grade I) - manage outpatient: bedrest, elevate HOB 30 to 45 degrees, limit eye movement (reading). Ophthalmology should be consulted for all hyphemas of Grade > 2
- **PEARL:** AACG patient should be supine
- Symptoms: blurry vision, ocular pain, photophobia and tearing
- Exam: unequal pupils, injected conjunctiva/sclera, blood in anterior chamber, absence of red reflex
- Treatment of ↑ IOP: use approach above for **AACG** except the pupil needs to be dilated with Atropine 1% one drop three times daily. Atropine will help avoid **pupillary play** (pupillary play = constant constriction and dilation of pupil stretching the previously injured vessels and leading to re-bleeding)
- **PEARL:** AACG treatment: miotic agent (pilocarpine)
- Avoid aspirin, NSAIDs, and anticoagulants
- Antifibrinolytic: aminocaproic acid (AMICAR) per ophthalmologist
- **PEARL:** Avoid Acetazolamide (Diamox) if etiology of hyphema is due to sickle cell disease or if patient is allergic to sulfa
- **PEARL:** Major complication: **rebleeding** after 3 to 5 days; other complications: corneal blood staining, acute/chronic glaucoma, and anterior or posterior synechia formation
- **PEARL:** Hyphema >25% of the anterior chamber = risk for **traumatic glaucoma**

CENTRAL RETINAL ARTERY OCCLUSION (CRAO)

- CRAO is a true ophthalmologic emergency
- Acute, painless vision loss
- Episodes of **amaurosis fugax**
- Pale/gray retina with macular **"cherry red spot"** (macula is thinnest portion of retina; intact choroidal circulation remains visible through this section of retina)
- Optic disc: **boxcar segmentation**
- Afferent pupillary defect (APD) (usually not seen with CRVO)
- **Causes**: embolus (carotid, heart), thrombosis, giant cell arteritis, vasculitis (Lupus), sickle cell disease, hyperviscosity syndromes and trauma

CRAO TREATMENT

1. Emergent ophthalmology consultation
2. Massage 15 seconds with sudden release (attempt to dislodge clot)
3. Topical beta-blocker (Timoptic 0.5% one drop) ↓ IOP
4. Oral /IV Acetazolamide (Diamox) 500mg ↓ IOP
5. Vasodilators: Pentoxifylline (Trental), Isosorbide (Imdur)
6. Anterior chamber (AC) paracentesis will immediately decrease IOP; problem = increase retinal perfusion may propagate the clot more distally limiting the visual deficit. Reserved for cases refractory to medical management

PEARL: Treatment futile if > 90 minutes

CENTRAL RETINAL VEIN OCCLUSION (CRVO)

Acute painless vision loss, NOT an ophthalmologic emergency
Venous stasis → increased vascular back pressure → results in decreased arterial flow to retina → ischemia

Ischemic CRVO

- Severe visual loss, extensive retinal hemorrhages and cotton-wool spots, dilated tortuous retinal veins, macular edema, and optic disc edema.
- Retinal hemorrhages may be mild, moderate or large giving a "blood and thunder appearance".
- Relative APD (however, usually not seen with CRVO); V/A < 20/100

Complication: neovascular glaucoma

Nonischemic CRVO

- Milder form of the disease, less vision loss, no APD
- Good retinal perfusion; can progress to ischemic type
- Causes: HTN, DM, CVdisease, Polycythemia vera, Lymphoma, Leukemia, Clotting disorders, Multiple myeloma, Syphilis, Sarcoidosis, Autoimmune disease – SLE; Oral contraceptive use

Treatment: Identifying and treating any systemic medical problems to reduce further complications is important; Ophthalmology follow-up → dexamethasone implant; triamcinolone (intravitreal)

RETINAL DETACHMENT

- **History**: Painless visual field deficits, flashing lights, "spider webs" and "floaters" or "curtain lowering"
- **Fundoscopic exam:** pale, grey area of detached retina
- **Risk factors:** advanced age, DM, previous cataract surgery, severe myopia, uveitis, connective tissue disorders, trauma, family history of retinal detachment
- **Ultrasound:** detachment is seen as an echogenic membrane in the posterior and lateral aspect of the globe that moves with eye movements

Treatment: Emergent ophthalmology consultation for possible repair

OPTIC NEURITIS

- Acute demyelinating inflammation of the optic nerve (CN II)
- **Etiologies:** Most common = Multiple Sclerosis (MS); other causes: infectious (Lyme, Herpes, Syphilis); autoimmune (SLE, Neurosarcoidosis); methanol toxicity; B12 deficiency
- **Presentation / exam:** gradual decreased visual loss (monocular partial or complete) over the course of days to weeks; pain with eye movements, severe unilateral central vision loss (with mild to NO peripheral vision loss), fever, headache, and nausea; color perception is decreased (dyschromatopsia) Afferent Pupillary Defect (APD) **(Marcus Gunn pupil); Fundoscopic examination:** normal as the inflammation is often retrobulbar
- Painless visual field deficits, flashing lights, "spider webs" and "floaters" or "curtain lowering"; fundoscopic examintion = pale, grey area of detached retina
- **PEARL: Uhthoff's phenomenon:** transient worsening of vision with increased body temperature
- **Treatment:** admission for intravenous steroids; consults ophthalmology and neurology

IRITIS

Eye terminology:

- **Uvea** = middle portion of the eye; divided into anterior and posterior
- The ***anterior*** portion of uvea includes the iris (the colored part of the eye) and ciliary body (synthesizes aqueous humor)
- The ***posterior*** portion of the uvea is known as the choroid
- **Anterior uveitis** is synchronous with iritis
- **Posterior uveitis** or **chorioretinitis**: inflammation of the choroid and retina
- **Causes**: often idiopathic; may be traumatic, infectious or systemic (Behcet's, Kawasaki, MS, sarcoid, relapsing polychondritis, Sjogren syndrome, SLE and vitiligo)
- Most common **viral causes of uveitis:** CMV (rarely in immunocompetent patients), HZ and HSV
- Most common **illness associated anterior uveitis:** HLA-B27 diseases (ankylosing spondylitis, reactive arthritis (formerly Reiter), psoriatic arthritis, IBD)
- **Exam**: eye pain, redness, consensual photophobia (hallmark symptom), constricted pupils
  Floaters / leukocytes in the anterior chamber (AC): **"cell & flare"**
  The cardinal sign of iritis: **ciliary flush** (marked injection at the limbus, or a red ring around the iris)

- **Treatment for Anterior Uveitis**
  - If infection: treat infection
  - If not infection: topical glucocorticoids (prednisolone acetate 1%)
  - Dilate eye to relieve ciliary spasm or if there is a risk for posterior synechiae (cyclopentolate 1%)

CMV RETINITIS

- Most common cause of retinitis and blindness in AIDS patients
- CMV retinitis leads to blindness in 10% despite therapy. Exam: Cotton wool spots; white/yellow patches with or without hemorrhage ("cottage cheese & ketchup appearance)
- Treatment: Zigran (Ganciclovir) or Foscarnet (Foscavir)

ENDOPHTHALMITIS

- Ophthalmologic emergency
- Purulent inflammation of intraocular fluids usually due to infection
- Causes: ocular procedures, trauma and hematogenous spread of systemic infection
- Most common surgical procedure complicated by endophthalmitis = cataract surgery

NEONATAL CONJUNCTIVITIS

(ophthalmia neonatorum) - First month of life:
  - Day 1-2: chemical
  - Day 3: Gonorrhea
  - Day 6 to first month of life: Chlamydia trachomatis

- GC ophthalmic infections: ocular emergency; loss of vision, corneal perforation
- **Treatment**: admit, IV Ceftriaxone (Rocephin)
- Most common viral cause of conjunctivitis: Adenovirus

CHALAZION

- Lipogranuloma of meibomian gland or a Zeis gland; firm, painless, above eyelashes on the upper lid
- **Treatment:** warm compresses

HORDEOLUM (STYE)

- Acute pyogenic *(Staph aureus)* inflammation of gland of Moll (ciliary gland)
- Teneder, at or near an eyelash follicle
- **Treatment:** warm compresses; topical antibiotics if progression to blepharitis / cellulitis

DACRYOCYSTITIS

- Acute, rapid onset, infectious obstruction of the nasolacrimal duct, most commonly **caused** by *Staph aureus:* Other bugs: *Strep pneumoniae* and viridans, *Staph epidermidis*
- **Symptoms:** unilateral, painful, erythematous swelling inferior and medial to the eye near the nasolacrimal duct, epiphora (overflow of tears)
- **Exam**: Digital massage of the duct = purulent drainage from the puncta
- **Treatment**: Topical and oral antibiotics, warm compresses analgesics; ophthalmologic referral
- Do NOT I&D (could permanently damage the anatomy of the tear duct)

ULTRAVIOLET KERATITIS

- Skier or welder; bilateral decreased visual acuity, pain, and redness; **fluorescein staining:** multiple punctate lesions
- **Treatment**: topical / oral NSAIDs; +/- antibiotics; +/- cycloplegics

CORNEAL ABRASIONS

- Most are self-limiting (most completely resolving within 24–72 hours); perform fluorescein staining and don't forget eversion of eyelid to evaluate for retained foreign body; topical antibiotics, tetanus update and follow-up with ophthalmology
- **PEARL**: Corneal abrasion resulting from prolonged contact lens wear → secondary infection: *Pseudomonas aeruginosa*

CORNEAL ULCER

- **Causes**: bacterial infection: *Staphylococcus, Pseudomonas* (contact lens wearers), *Streptococcus pneumoniae*.
- **Risk factors:** Bell's Palsy (incomplete lid closure); soft contact lens use; trauma
- **Exam**: White hazy irregularity of the cornea; redness & swelling of eyelids; FB sensation; photophobia; secondary iritis.
- **Treatment**: Topical antibiotic(fluoroquinolone); emergent ophthalmologic consultation

OPHTHALMOLOGY PEARLS

- Right eye = OD, left eye = OS. OD acuity appears above the OS acuity when written on the chart
- 20/200 vision OD = right eye sees at 20 feet what a normal eye sees at 200 feet
- Normal intraocular pressure (IOP): 10 to 20 mm Hg
- Most common cause of ***painless*** **red eye**: viral conjunctivitis
- Most common cause of viral conjunctivitis: Adenovirus
- Most common cause of ***painful*** **red eye**: iritis (aka uveitis / iridocyclitis)
- Subconjunctival hemorrhage is very common, asymptomatic and resolves without sequelae
- Afferent pupillary defect (APD) **(Marcus-Gunn pupil)**: affected pupil dilates in response to light. Conditions with APD: CRAO, optic neuritis and retrobulbar hematoma
- **Amaurosis fugax:** Greek amaurosis = darkening, Latin fugax = fleeting, is a transient monocular visual loss
- **Preseptal cellulitis (also called periorbital cellulitis)**
Superficial mild skin infection around the eye
Most common causes: Staphylococcus aureus and group A Streptococcus
Your main goal = distinguish preseptal cellulitis from orbital cellulitis
Treatment: Cephalexin 500 mg po qid; children, 25-50 mg/kg/day po in 4 divided doses
- **Orbital Cellulitis**: proptosis, ophthalmoplegia (paralysis or weakness of one or more of the eye muscles), edema & erythema of the eyelids, pain on eye movement, fever, headache, and malaise;
Diagnostics: CT orbits;
Management: IV antibiotics (Piperacillin-tazobactam), ENT consult; up to 11% of cases result in visual loss
Most common cause of orbital cellulitis: **ethmoid sinusitis** (90%)

PEARL: Dacryocystitis can also cause preseptal or orbital cellulitis

- Orbital Cellulitis complication: **cavernous sinus thrombosis**
    - Cranial nerve III - VI palsies (most commonly VI, impairment of lateral gaze)
    - Rare but life-threatening with mortality of about 30%-50%
    - **Diagnosis** of cavernous sinus thrombosis: MRI/MRV = 1st line; CT venography = 2nd line; "delta" sign on CT without contrast, empty "delta" sign on CT head with IV contrast
    - **Treatment** of cavernous sinus thrombosis: anticoagulation

- **Hutchinson's sign**: Herpes Zoster lesions on tip nose – prognostic of corneal involvement; herpes zoster ophthalmicus → HZ travels down V1 → nasociliary nerve (branches innervate cornea and skin)
- **Ramsey-Hunt Syndrome:** HZ of the geniculate ganglion; painful rash, hearing loss, vesicles on TM CN VII paralysis
- **Synechia**: iris adheres to either the cornea (anterior synechia) or lens (posterior synechia)
- **Anterior synechia** → prevent drainage of aqueous humor → closed angle glaucoma
- **Posterior synechia** → block aqueous from posterior chamber to anterior chamber → increased IOP
- **Causes**: trauma, iritis or iridocyclitis

- Hallmark physical finding in **Behcet's Disease**: **hypopyon uveitis** is seen rarely; recurrent painful aphtous ulcers of oral mucosa and genitals are more common finding
- Amiodarone can cause chemical epididymitis, hypothyroidism/hyperthyroidism, interstitial lung disease (pulmonary fibrosis), blue-grey skin discoloration, **corneal microdeposits**; bradycardia, heart blocks, dysrhythmias, prolonged QT, hypotension
- Blood in the anterior chamber is the characteristic physical exam finding associated with a **hyphema**
- Consensual photophobia ss a classic physical exam finding associated with **iritis**
- A teardrop-shaped pupil is a highly specific physical exam finding associated with a **ruptured globe**
- Treat super glue/crazy glue (cyanoacrylate): erythromycin ointment
- Alkali burns (liquefactive necrosis) more destructive than acid burns → irrigate copiously, check pH (Normal eye pH = 7.0 to 7.4)

EAR / NOSE / THROAT

EPISTAXIS

- Most common site of nosebleeds = anterior nosebleed
- Most common site of anterior nosebleeds = Kiesselbach's plexus (or Little's area)
- Most common site of posterior nosebleeds = sphenopalatine artery

EPISTAXIS MANAGEMENT

ANTERIOR BLEEDING

- Patient releases pressure from nostrils, blows their nose to remove clots
- Instruct patient to pinch nostrils & apply direct pressure to septal area for 10-15 minutes
- Sit and lean forward so blood does not run down posterior pharynx
- Patient holds emesis basin to catch any bleeding
- 0.05% oxymetazoline (Afrin) nasal spray x 2
- Next, insert cotton ball soaked in viscous xylocaine 5% + oxymetazoline x 10 minutes
- Remove cotton ball
- Consider chemical cautery with silver nitrate silver sticks (begin at the periphery and move into center)
- Insert anterior nasal pack to remain in place 24-48 hours
- Discharge with prophylactic antibiotic to cover Staph (controversial) and ENT follow up
- Tranexamic acid (TXA) - soaked pledgets may reduce epistaxis bleeding better in patients taking antiplatelet drugs

POSTERIOR BLEEDING

- Monitor, IV, pulse oximetry; balloon catheter – Epistat
- Inflate the posterior balloon with 10 mL of sterile water
- Retract the catheter gently until it lodges against the posterior choana in the nasopharynx
- Next, inflate the anterior balloon with 30 mL of sterile water
- If the patient experiences severe pain or deviation of the nasal septum or soft palate, gradually deflate the anterior balloon until the pain or deviation resolve

- **PEARL:** Patients with posterior nasal packings are at risk for hypoxemia and dysrhythmias; admit to monitor setting
- **PEARL :** Epistaxis is the most common presenting symptom among patients with hereditary hemorrhagic telangiectasia (Osler-Weber-Rendu disease)
- **PEARL:** Oxymetazoline is unlikely to cause an elevation in blood pressure

OTITIS MEDIA

- Most common bacterial cause of otitis media: *Strep pneumoniae 40%; H. influenzae, M. catarrhalis,* and *S. aureus*
- **Treatment:** High Dose Amoxicillin 90 mg/kg/day div q 12 or q 8 hours
- OM best confirmed: decreased mobility of TM and loss of normal landmarks
- Most common complication of otitis media: hearing (conductive) loss
- Other complications: perforation, which usually heals within 7 days; mastoiditis
- Most common intracranial complication of otitis media = meningitis

OTITIS EXTERNA

- Most common organism = *Pseudomonas aeruginosa*; *#2 Staphylococcus aureus*
- **Treatment:** ciprofloxacin 0.3% plus dexamethasone 0.1%

NECROTIZING OTITIS EXTERNA

(formerly known as "Malignant"Otitis Externa)

- Most common finding: granulation tissue on the floor of the auditory canal at the bone-cartilage junction
- An invasive infection of the external auditory canal that can extend into the base of the skull. Most common cause: *Pseudomonas aeruginosa*; 10% fungal (Aspergillosis)
- Necrotizing OE = an osteomyelitis
- Risk factors include: advanced age, immunocompromised patients, especially uncontrolled DM and those with HIV-AIDS
- As the infection extends into the skull base cranial nerve palsies are common
- CN VII paralysis most common
- **Other Complications:** meningitis, brain abscess and dural sinus thrombosis
- **Labs**: ESR, CRP. suspect NOE in patient who had cultures prior to antimicrobial therapy which were negative and are unresponsive to appropriate antimicrobial therapy
- **Imaging:** CT scan of the temporal bones and skull base (spread of infection to bony external auditory canal, skull base, and adjacent soft tissues (with or without bone erosion)
- **Treatment:** Ciprofloxacin 750 mg orally every 12 hours for 6-8 weeks; Debridement + Ciprofloxacin 400 mg IV every 12 hours if patient is unresponsive to oral meds; in severe cases consider dual therapy against *Pseudomonas aeruginosa* (ciprofloxacin plus ceftazidime) + debridementTreatment for fungal (Aspergillosis) necrotizing otitis externa: prolonged systemic voriconazole 6-12 weeks, in conjunction with surgery

MASTOIDITIS

- Inflammation of the mastoid air cells of temporal bone inside the mastoid process, usually as a complication of acute otitis media
- **Causes**: *Streptococcus pneumoniae* (most common), *Streptococcus pyogenes, Haemophilus influenzae*, and *Moraxella catarrhalis*
- **Exam**: protruding ear, retroauricular erythema, swelling or pain, and fever; hearing loss, ear discharge, and vertigo
- **Diagnosis**: contrast-enhanced computed tomography (CT) imaging of temporal bone or MRI
- **Management**: usually too ill for outpatient management; ENT consult; Piperacillin-tazobactam + Vancomycin
- **Complications include:** cavernous sinus thrombosis, meningitis, epidural /subdural abscess, CN VII palsy, hearing loss, labryinthitis, osteomyelitis

AURICULAR HEMATOMA

- Occur after blunt trauma to the ear (wrestlers)
- Without proper treatment, the cartilaginous structures of the ear can become permanently deformed (cauliflower ear)

- **Treatment:** Regional auricular nerve block followed by incision & drainage of the hematoma by making a small incision in the helix or antihelix, followed by application of a pressure dressing to maintain the contours of the ear
- If acute (< 48 hours) and small (<2cm) = needle aspiration
- Next-day follow-up to ensure hematoma re-accumulation has not occurred

EAR LACERATIONS

Need rapid repair to:

1) Cover the auricular cartilage to limit infection
2) Prevention of auricular hematoma

RELAPSING POLYCHONDRITIS

- Autoimmune disease characterized by episodic inflammation of cartilaginous tissues (external ears, nose, joints, and the upper and lower respiratory tracts)
- When the auricle is affected the ear lobe is spared since it does not have cartilage
- Systemic immune-mediated cause of Uveitis
- 30% of patients present with coexisting autoimmune or inflammatory disease

Ear Piecing Pearl: *Pseudomonas aeruginosa:* the most common organism associated with infections following piercing through ear cartilage; Treatment: Ciprofloxocin

PERICHONDRITIS PEARL: *Pseudomonas aeruginosa*: the most common organism associated with perichondritis; Treatment: Ciprofloxocin

HEARING LOSS

Alport syndrome

- X-linked hereditary disorder; sensorineural hearing loss; glomerulonephritis with progression to chronic kidney disease
- Eye findings: anterior lenticonus (lens becomes cone-shaped); abnormal coloration of the retina (dot-and-fleck retinopathy), possible vision loss

Ruptured tympanic membrane

- Sudden sensorineural hearing loss
- Develops acutely over 3 days or less

PEARL: Conductive hearing loss = impaired conduction
PEARL: Sensorineural hearing loss = dysfunction of the inner ear

Conductive causes are reversible and include otitis media, middle ear effusion, or cerumen impaction

Sudden sensorineural hearing causes

- Idiopathic, infectious, autoimmune disease, neoplasms, CVA, and ototoxic medications
- Viral infections, particularly mumps
- Bacterial meningitis (incidence has decreased in post-immunization era)
- Thromboembolism and hemorrhage
- Neoplastic conditions (vestibular schwannomas or cerebellar angiomas)

Weber and Rinne tests use a vibrating tuning fork to distinguish conductive from sensorineural hearing loss

PEARL: Treatment for idiopathic sudden sensorineural hearing loss: prednisone 60 mg daily for 7-14 days

SINUSITIS

- Most common cause of acute bacterial sinusitis: Strep pneumoniae, H. influenzae
- Most common cause of sinusitis overall: Viral; symptoms usually resolve by 10 days, so management should focus on symptomatic relief (pain management and decongestant therapy (topically = oxymetazoline; systemic therapy: pseudoephedrine), +/- antihistamine is suspect allergic etiology); not antibiotics
- Saline nasal irrigation is beneficial for all forms of acute rhinosinusitis
- **Complications of sinusitis:** orbital cellulitis, meningitis, subdural abscess, cavernous sinus thrombosis (CST)
- **PEARL:** Most common cause of **chronic sinusitis**: allergic, then infectious (mixed flora, anaerobes and fungi)
- **Mucormycosis:** rapidly progressive fungal infection of the sinuses seen in DM and immunocompromised patients; ENT consult for extensive debridement

CAVERNOUS SINUS THROMBOSIS (CST)

- Thrombosis of the dural sinus and/or cerebral veins
- **Causes**: Most common = contiguous spread from nasal furuncle; other causes: sinusitis (most common sphenoid and ethmoid), dental infection; less common: OM and orbital cellulitis
- **PEARL**: most common infectious microbe = *Staphylococcus aureus* (70%); *Streptococcus sp.* #2; *H. influenzae;* Aspergillus sp. less common; rarely anaerobic bacteria or gram-negative bacteria
- **Symptoms:** acute onset headache, decrease or loss of vision, exophthalmos, photophobia, cranial nerve palsies (CN III-VI); life threatening
- **PEARL**: Most common CN palsy with CST = CN VI
- **Diagnosis**: MRI with MR venogram = 1st line diagnostic imaging. CT venography 2cd line
- **PEARL: Delta (Δ)** (non-contrast study) and "empty delta" (contrast study) are signs of dural venous sinus thrombosis of the superior sagittal sinus. Empty delta sign: contrast outlines a triangular filling defect (which represents thrombus)
- **Management:** Heparin used but no definitive evidence of efficacy; Vancomycin + Ceftriaxone 2gm IV q12 hours. If dental source add Flagyl. ENT consult (surgical drainage of sinus infection)

ANGIOTENSIN CONVERTING ENZYME (ACE) INHIBITOR ANGIOEDEMA

- Incidence < 1% in users
- 40% of all emergency department visits for angioedema
- ACE inhibitors result in elevated bradykinin levels → vasodilation and increased vascular permeability → cutaneous and subcutaneous edema
- Majority of cases occur in the first few months of use (however can occur any time)
- **Presentation:** edema of the face, lips, or tongue; pruritus and rash absent
- **Management:** airway priority, discontinue ACE inhibitor
  - Treat with epinephrine, diphenhydramine, and corticosteroids however these treatment options do NOT affect bradykinin levels and are unlikely to be effective
  - Supportive care
- Angioedema usually lasts 24-72 hours

HEREDITARY AND ACQUIRED ANGIOEDEMA

- Problem: Deficiency or dysfunction of C-1 esterase inhibitor
- **Treatment:** Replace C1-esterase inhibitor (FFP)

SIALOLITHIASIS

- Development of stones within the salivary glands or duct system (result of stagnant flow of saliva and increased salivary calcium concentrations)
- **Physical exam:** stone within the salivary duct may be palpated, tenderness, and swelling
- **Risk factors:** dehydration, smoking, severe periodontal disease, prior history of gout or nephrolithiasis, anticholinergics and diuretics
  90% of stones = submandibular gland and duct
- **Diagnosis:** clinical; CT imaging if diagnostic uncertainty, concern for concomitant abscess development, or suspicion of underlying neoplastic etiologies
- **Treatment:** sialogogues (e.g., tart candies, lemon drops), gland massage with warm compresses, and milking of the affected duct
  If these measures fail, outpatient otolaryngology referral is appropriate for potential procedural or surgical intervention
  If infection: bacterial sialadenitis = add amoxicillin-clavulanic acid (Augmentin)

ACUTE NECROTIZING ULCERATIVE GINGIVITIS (ANUG)

- Acute pain in the gingiva, gray pseudomembranes, foul breath metallic taste
- Seen in immunocompromised patients and smokers.
- Antibiotic to cover: anaerobic gram-negative bacilli, *Prevotella intermedia*, Spirochetes, Fusobacteria and Bacteroides = Clindamycin, Pen VK, oral hygiene and chlorhexadine

LUDWIG'S ANGINA

- Most common precipitant = recent extraction or infection of a mandibular molar tooth
- Deep space infection of the floor of the mouth and neck, which can lead to edema and displacement of the soft tissues resulting in upper airway obstruction that can be rapidly fatal
- **Symptoms:** sore throat, fever, dysphagia, odynophagia, tongue swelling, pain and swelling in the floor of the mouth and neck swelling, and a change in voice (dysphonia)
- **Physical examination findings:** swelling of the floor of the mouth, elevation and protrusion of the tongue, a "woody" consistency of the floor of the mouth, bilateral submandiular swelling, and a "bull neck" (edema and induration of the neck above the level of the hyoid bone)
- **Management:** emergent ENT consult, airway management, CT with contrast of neck, broad spectrum antibiotics to cover staph, strep and anaerobes

PERITONSILLAR ABSCESS (PTA)

- Most common deep infection of the head and neck; develops primarily in adolescents and young adults; sore throat, fever, odynophagia, dysphagia, and referred otalgia; inferior and medial displacement of the affected tonsil with deviation of the uvula to the contralateral side; muffled, "hot potato" voice and trismus which can limit the examination. Most common: unilateral (peritonsillar cellulitis: bilateral).

- **Treatment**: Needle aspiration which is easier to perform, less painful for patients than I&D and is effective in 90% of patients + antibiotics to cover both Streptococci and oral anaerobe. Needle aspiration risk: injury to carotid artery
- **Potential serious complications include:** jugular vein suppurative phlebitis (Lemierre's syndrome) and/or erosion into the carotid artery with subsequent hemorrhage

LEMIERRE'S SYNDROME

- Jugular vein suppurative thrombophlebitis; preceded by pharyngitis, usually in association with tonsil or peritonsillar involvement
- Other antecedent conditions include primary dental infection or infectious mononucleosis

EPIGLOTTITIS

Inflammation of the epiglottis and adjacent supraglottic structures
Haemophilus influenzae type B (Hib); *H. influenzae* types A and F, and nontypeable strains; *Haemophilus parinfluenzae, Streptococcus pneumoniae, MSSA* and *MRSA*, Beta-hemolytic streptococci, Herpes simplex virus type 1, Varicella zoster virus, Influenza B, EBV, Parainfluenza. Epiglottitis also may be caused by trauma (foreign body ingestion, thermal injury, or caustic ingestion)

Clinical triad with acute onset high fever - **3D's**

1. **D**rooling (80% of cases)
2. **D**ysphagia
3. **D**istress – Respiratory or air hunger in "sniffing" posture

As the airway diameter decreases due to inflammation, stridor may develop as obstruction worsens; in a worst-case scenario, total airway obstruction can occur.

TRACHEOSTOMY COMPLICATIONS

Accidental decannulation: obstruction (mucous plug = suction); infection; bleeding

Tracheo-innominate artery fistula: usually within first 3 weeks

- Sentinel bleed followed by massive bleeding
- Digital pressure/hyperinflate cuff
- Emergency consultation
- **PEARL:** tracheostomy tract matures around 15-30 days

TEMPOROMANDIBULAR JOINT DISEASE (TMJ)

- Triad: 1) muscle dysfunction 2) problem at TMJ joint 3) cervical spine dysfunction
- Involves the structures of the jaw (masticatory system) and can present with pain in the jaw or jaw malfunction; exact cause is unknown; symptoms acute or chronic including unilateral, dull, constant pain in the muscles or joints of the jaw; dysfunctional chewing, neck stiffness/pain, and headache; ear pain, tinnitus
- **Physical exam:** TMJ tenderness, bruxism, and limited mouth opening; check for crepitus, abscess of teeth, or bony tumors
- **Treatment**: NSAIDs, tricyclic antidepressants, or muscle relaxants
- Referral to a dentist for bite (occlusal) splints

CAUSES OF HYPERKALEMIA

Mnemonic - (RAD MY LAD)

R	**R**enal Insufficiency; RTA type 4
A	**A**drenal Insufficiency
D	**D**rugs K+ sparing = Triamterene and Spironolactone Transcellular shifts = Succinylcholine, β-blockers and digoxin Drug induced hypoaldosteronism = ACE inhibitors, NSAIDs, Heparin, Cyclosporin and Bactrim

MY	**MY**onecrosis / Cell injury (rhabdomyolysis, burns, crush / acute tumor lysis syndrome

L	**L**ack of Insulin → DKA (transcellular shift)
A	**A**cidosis (transcellular shift)
D	**D**igitalis Toxicity (↓K+, ↓Mg2+ and ↑Ca2+→ ↑dig toxicity)

- **PEARL:** Most common cause of markedly ↑ K+ = lab hemolysis
- **Non-Arrest, ECG Findings in Hyperkalemia:**
  Peaked T waves, prolonged PR, dropped P wave, widened QRS, sine wave
- **PEARL:** Normal ECG *does not* rule out hyperkalemia; case studies where normal ECGs were seen in patients with potassium levels > 8 mEq/L

TREATMENT OF HYPERKALEMIA

Mnemonic - (C BIG Potassium DROP)

C	**C**alcium chloride or gluconate Calcium gluconate 10cc of a 10% solution slowly over 2 min (stop if bradycardic) **Calcium Indications:** Moderate to severe hyperkalemia (> 6.5 mEq/L); ECG changes are present or risk of dysrhythmia Pediatric patient: 1.0 mL/kg, not to exceed 10ml, of 10% calcium gluconate solution over 3-5 minutes If CaCl use central line (CaCl hs 3x more Ca2+ than Ca gluconate) Most rapid and effective treatment, stabilizes cardiac membrane without changing serum K+ level; Avoid in Digitals toxicity; can use 2gm of Magnesium sulfate over 5 min if dig-toxic arrhythmia **Onset of action** = < 5 minutes **Duration of action** = 30 to 60 minutes Consider repeat dose if ECG changes do not normalize in 3-5 min

B_2	Shifts potassium into cells **B**icarb Infants: 0.5 mEq/kg IV over 5-10 min Children: 1 mEq/kg IV over 5-10 min In infants use the 4.2% solution and the 8.4% solution in children and adults **Onset of action** = within minutes **Duration of action** = 1 to 2 hours Sodium bicarbonate infusion may be helpful in patients with metabolic acidosis; if blood pH is neutral, bicarb will be inneffective Bolus dosing of sodium bicarbonate is less effective Sodium bicarbonate can potentially increase fluid load, causing hypernatremia and metabolic alkalosis, and should therefore be used with caution in patients with heart failure and CKD because of sodium load Bicarb drip (3 Amps of Bicarb in 1 liter D5W); Infusion preferred over bolus **PEARL:** Bicarb is rarely indicated in DKA, unless pH <7.0 or cardiac arrhythmias **B**eta-2-adrenergic agonist (Albuterol); 10 mg/hr Neb → ↑ activity of Na-K-ATPase pump in skeletal muscle → shifts K+ into cells

I	**Insulin** enhances activity of the Na-K-ATPase pump in skeletal muscle → shifts K+ into cells 5-10 units regular insulin IVP (with the dextrose solution) Pediatric patient: 0.1 U/kg regular insulin (1 unit regular insulin/ per 5 gram of glucose infused) **Onset of action** = 20-30minutes, peaks at 30-60 minutes and **duration of action** = 4-6 hours

G	**Glucose** (prevent hypoglycemia after insulin administration; frequent Accu-cheks given the risk of hypoglycemia) 1-2 amps of D50 Pediatric patient: 0.5 gm/kg (2mL/kg) 25% dextrose solution (with insulin over 30 min) Bicarb/insulin/glucose combo "shifts" K+ into cells

Potassium	**Potassium** Binders Patiromer, brand name Veltassa; gastrointestinal cation exchanger, binds potassium in colon in exchange for calcium; 8.4 gram once Other option: sodium zirconium cyclosilicate (LOKELMA) packet 10 g

Drop$_2$	**D**iuretic - Loop Diuretic - Furosemide (Lasix) **D**ialysis

PEARL: Kayexalate (sodium polystyrene sulfonate (SPS) – has fallen out of favor and should be avoided due to reports of bowel necrosis

CAUSES OF HYPERCALCEMIA

Mnemonic - (VITAMINS TRAP)

V	**V**itamin D intoxication **V**itamin A intoxication (transcription factor in osteoclast stimulation)
I	**I**mmobilization
T	**T**hyrotoxicosis → direct stimulation of osteoclastic bone resorption
A	**A**drenal insufficiency (Addison's) Lack of hypocalcemic effect of corticosteroid → ↑active Vitamin D → ↑bone resorption & ↑GI Ca absorption; also decrease renal clearance of calcium
M	**M**yeloma / Milk-alkali syndrome → excessive consumption of Ca and absorbable antacids
I	Insufficiency → acute renal failure → ↓Ca2+ ↑Phos → ↑PTH → ↑ Ca2+ from bone and GI and ↓ phosphate reabsorption from kidneys → ↑ phos urine excretion In chronic renal failure the calcium will remain ↓low and ↑phos because kidney cannot excrete
N	***N**eoplasm (squamous cell lung, head and neck, breast, renal, multiple myeloma, leukemia)
S	**S**arcoid (other disorders: TB & Granulomatosis with polyangitis (GPA); Fungal: Histoplasmosis, Coccidiomycosis) Overproduction of vitamin D by macrophages and ↑extrarenal alpha1-hydroxylase activity (enzyme, which converts Vit D to active form)

T	**T**hiazides calcium carbonate and lithium → alters PTH set-point for inhibition of hormone secretion by circulating Ca
R	**R**habdomyolysis (PEARL: initially hypocalcemia)
A	***A***ids
P	↑ **P**TH (parathyroid adenoma 80%) **P**aget disease

* Neoplasm: solid tumors are most likely to result in hypercalcemia due to secretion of parathyroid hormone related proteins (PTHrp) from the tumor; PTHrp stimulate osteoclast activity leading to increased bone resorption. The resultant hypercalcemia leads to an osmotic diuresis and dehydration. Production of vitamin D analogues is associated with lymphoma and less common in solid tumors

PEARL: HYPER-Calcemia is associated with HYPO-Kalemia (33% of patients)
PEARL: 90% of cases of hypercalcemia = malignancy and primary hyper-parathyriodoism

PAGET DISEASE

- Disorder of bone remodeling → excessive bone resorption (osteoclastic activity) followed by a compensatory ↑ bone formation (osteoblastic activity) → structurally disorganized mosaic of bone (woven bone), which is weaker, larger, less compact, more vascular and more susceptible to fracture than normal adult lamellar bone
- Etiology is unknown
- ↑ Ca 2+
- ↑ bone vascularity may → high-output CHF; increased likelihood bleeding complications following surgery
- Most common neurological problem is hearing loss → compression of CN VIII
- Vertebral involvement may lead to nerve-root compressions and cauda equina syndrome

SIGNS AND SYMPTOMS OF HYPERCALCEMIA

Mnemonic - Stones, Bones, Psychic Moans, Abdominal groans

Stones	renal calculi
Bones	osteolysis = bone pain
Psychic moans	mental status change, seizures, apathy, stupor, coma
Abdominal groans	N/V/anorexia, constipation, PUD, pancreatitis

TREATMENT OF HYPERCALCEMIA

- Initial and most important: ***rehydration*** (0.9% NS)
- **Glucocorticoids:** hydrocortisone 200mg/day → inhibits activation of Vitamin D → inhibits bone resorption and GI absorption of calcium; used in chronic granulomatous diseases
- **Bisphosphates**: inhibit calcium release from bone
  Pamidronate (Aredia) 60 to 90 mg over 2 hours
  Zometa (Zoledronic Acid - ZA) 4 mg IV over 15 minutes; considered agent of choice for malignancy-associated hypercalcemia because it is more potent and effective then Pamidronate
- **Calcitonin:** 4 international units (IU)/kg SC or IM every 12 hours; reduces serum calcium by increasing renal calcium excretion inhibits bone resorption
- **Dialysis**
  - Emergent hemodialysis is indicated for patients with:
  - Calcium > 18
  - Neurologic symptoms
  - Patients who can't get fluids (congestive heart failure or renal failure)
- **Correction of underlying condition**
- **Parathyroidectomy:** for hyperparathyroidism

HYPOCALCEMIA CAUSES

- Renal failure, hypoparathyroidism (↓PTH), hypomagnesemia (↓Mg), massive transfusions, shock or sepsis, pancreatitis, rhabdomyolysis, Vitamin D deficiency, alcoholism and drugs

Causes of Hypocalcemia - Medications

- Drugs: cimetidine, phenytoin, phenobarbital, gentamycin, tobramycin, heparin, protamine, theophylline, nipride, phosphate enemas/laxatives, cisplatin, norepinephrine, loop diuretics, steroids and magnesium sulfate

Causes of Hypocalcemia - Tox

- Valproic acid overdose
- Ethylene glycol toxicity
- Burns from military white phosphorous munitions (also causes hyperphosphatemia & hepatotoxicity)

- **PEARL:** Most common cause of hypocalcemia = hypoparathyroidism (low PTH)
- **PEARL:** Most common cause hypoparathyroidism (low PTH) = partial or total thyroidectomy (parathyroid gland)
- **PEARL:** Parathyroid gland: located immediately behind and is partially or totally attached to the thyroid gland
- Other causes of hypoparathyroidism: infiltration of the parathyroid glands: metastatic carcinoma, hemochromatosis (autoimmune), or Wilson disease (rare genetic disorder characterized by excess copper storage)
- **PEARL:** DiGeorge syndrome = congenital syndrome results in hypocalcemia due to absence of the parathyroid glands

HYPOCALCEMIA SIGNS / SYMPTOMS

- Depends on serum level and rapidity of decline
- Chvostek and Trousseau signs, tetany, seizures, psychosis, and prolonged QT; reduced myocardial contractility → hypotension, and CHF; perioral and distal extremity paresthesias
- **PEARL:** most symptoms = neuromuscular → progressive neuromuscular hyperexcitability
- **Chvostek sign:** a twitch at the corner of the mouth when the examiner taps over the facial nerve (CN VII) in front to the ear
- **Trousseau sign:** more reliable indicator of hypocalcemia: BP cuff maintains a pressure above systolic for 3 minutes → positive if carpal spasm produced

HYPOCALCEMIA TREATMENT

- Ca Chloride: 360 mg elemental / 14 meq calcium
- Ca Gluconate 90 mg elemental / 4 meq calcium
- 1 amp = 10 cc of 10% solution (either CaCl or Ca Gluconate)
- The ionized calcium will increase for only 1 to 2 hours → follow by repeated doses or an infusion at a rate of 0.5 to 2 mg/kg/hr

RHABDOMYOLYSIS

- CPK: 5x normal
- Urine: Hematuria with 0 RBCs
- Most common metabolic abnormality in rhabdomyolysis = hypocalcemia (↓$Ca2+$)
  Early in rhabdo you get calcium deposition in injured muscle. Later, hypercalcemia (↑ $Ca2+$) secondary to mobilization of deposited calcium and secondary hyperparathyroidism
- Other lab findings: ↑ $K+$, metabolic acidosis, acute renal failure, DIC
- **PEARL:** ↓$K+$ or ↓Phos: contribute to development of rhabdomyolysis
- **Causes:** traumatic, exercise induced, toxicologic (CO, toluene, statins, ASA, caffeine, ETOH, neuroleptics/ antipsycotics, cocaine/sympathomimetics), environmental (hypo or hyper-thermia, metabolic (↓$K+$, ↓Phos, ↑ or ↓$Na+$, hypo or hyper-thyroidism, DKA or HHS), infectious (influenza most common), snake bites, black widow spider bites, immunologic and inherited
- Treatment: fluid (isotonic crystalloid 500 mL/h and titrate to maintain a urine output of 200 mL/h), urinary alkalinization, mannitol and loop diuretics
- Hemodialysis: persistent hyperkalemia despite therapy, severe acid-base disturbances, refractory pulmonary edema and progressive renal failure

ELECTROLYTE PEARLS

- **Categories of Hyponatremia**
  - **Hypervolemic** (CHF, cirrhosis, nephrotic syndrome)
  - **Euvolemic** (SIADH, psychogenic polydipsisa)
  - **Hypovolemic** (Addison's, renal-GI-third space losses
  - **Pseudohyponatremia** (hyperlipidemia, hyperproteinemia)
  - **Redistributive** (hyperglycemia) – water drawn from cell dilutes $Na+$

- **MEDICATIONS / TOX CAUSES OF HYPONATREMIA**
  - Trileptal (Oxcarbazepine) - 2.5%, mechanism unknown
  - Carbamzepime (Tegretol) - SIADH
  - SSRIs - SIADH
  - Antipsychotics - SIADH
  - COX-2 inhibitor - Celebrex (Celecoxib) - SIADH
  - Chemotherapeutic agents
  - MDMA (Ecstasy)

INFECTIONS ASSOCIATED WITH HYPONATREMIA

MNEMONIC – LDL WR

L	**L**egionella
D	**D**engue hemorrhagic fever
L	**L**eptospirosis
W	**W**NV
R	**R**MSF

- Correct acute hyponatremia: 1 to 2 mEq/L/hr
- Correct chronic hyponatremia: 0.5 mEq/L/hr
- Do not increase serum sodium more than 10 meq/L during the first 24 hours
- **Required dose of hypertonic saline to correct hyponatremia:** (desired Na+ – measured Na+) x 0.6 (weight in kg) = mEq Na+ administered
- In patients who require **emergency therapy:** hypertonic saline 100 mL bolus given over 10 minutes; should raise the serum sodium by 2 meq/L. If seizure persist or worsen repeat bolus one or two more times at 10 minute intervals
- Overaggressive correction of hyponatremia can lead to Central Pontine Myelinolysis (CPM) → destruction of myelin in Pons → CN palsies, quadriplegia or coma. More likely to occur in patients with chronic hyponatremia
- Most common causes of **hypomagnesemia** = malabsorption and chronic alcoholism
- Most likely **ECG findings in severe hypomagnesemia**: PVCs and ventricular dysrhythmias (VT, torsades); other ECG findings = AFIB, MAT, PSVT, ↑QT
- Magnesium is essential cofactor for the **Na+-K+-ATPase pump**
  - Refractory hypokalemia (↓K+) if hypomagnesemia is not corrected along with hypokalemia correction
  - **H**ypomagnesemia will worsen digoxin toxicity induced dysrhythmias
- **Chronic alcohol use: multiple electrolyte abnormalities** = hypomagnesemia, hypokalemia and hypophosphatemia; hypocalcemia (parathyroid hormone resistance from low magnesium)
- Most common cause of **hyperphosphatemia** and **hypermagnesemia** = renal failure
- 50% of alcoholics = **hypophosphatemia** (↓Phos)
- Prominent muscle weakness consider = **hypokalemia** (↓K+); paralysis may occur with serum levels < 2.0 mEq/L; also **hypophosphatemia** (↓Phos)
- Consider *hyperthyroidism* in patients with **hypokalemic periodic paralysis**
- Decrease in the serum K+ of 1.0 mEqL = 370 mEq deficit of total potassium (in the absence of acute shifts caused by acid-base disturbances
- **Pathophysiology of Hypokalemia from vomiting:**
  Alkalosis: K+→ into cells in exchange for H+
  Volume loss → hypovolemia → aldosterone secretion → preserve Na+ & Bicarb in exchange for K+

- **High levels of blood urea nitrogen (BUN) can cause:**
  - Pericarditis
  - Platelet dysfunction
  - AMS
  - Anemia
  - Nausea / vomiting

PEARL: ESRD patients that miss hemodialysis may experience significant bleeding secondary to uremia-induced platelet dysfunction; Treatment: Desmopressin + Cryoprecipitate

- Most important blood protein buffer = hemoglobin
- ↑ or ↓ in pH of 0.10 causes a ↓ or ↑ (opposite change) in PaO2 of about 10%
  PaO2 = partial pressure of oxygen dissolved in blood
  ↑ acidosis → Hgb gives up O2 more readily → ↑ PaO2 for a particular oxy-Hgb saturation → rightward shift of oxygen-hemoglobin dissociation curve
- pH < 7.35 = Acidosis pH > 7.45 = Alkalosis
- Normal values: pH 7.35 to 7.45 PaCO2 35 to 45
- PaCO2 and pH move in the opposite direction = Respiratory process PaCO2 and pH move in the same direction = Metabolic process
- Acute: for every change of 10 in PaCO2 → the pH moves in the opposite direction (↓ or ↑) by 0.08 + 0.02
- Chronic: for every change of 10 in PaCO2 → the pH moves in the opposite direction (↓ or ↑) by 0.03
- Anion Gap = Na – [HCO3 + Cl] Normal range = 5 to 12
- Most common acid-base disorder in seizing patient = respiratory acidosis

CAUSES OF ANION GAP ACIDOSIS

Mnemonic: (CAT MUDPILES)

C	CO, CN (inhibit cytochrome oxidase a-a3 → ↑ lactate)
A	**A**lcoholic ketoacidosis
T	**T**oluene (secondary) to acidic metabolites
M	**M**ethanol, Metformin
U	**U**remia
D	**D**KA
P	**P**araldehyde
I	**I**NH (Isoniazid, inhibits lactate ↔ pyruvate, therefore → ↑ lactate) **I**ron (hypovolemia and anemia → tissue hypoperfusion → ↑ lactate)
L	**L**actic acidosis
E	**E**thylene glycol
S	**S**alicylates

CAUSES OF NON-ANION GAP ACIDOSIS

Mnemonic: (A HARD CUP)

A	**A**ddison's Disease

H	**H**yperalimentation
A	**A**cetazolamide (Diamox)
R	**R**enal Tubular Acidosis (proximal)
D	**D**iarrhea

C	**C**holestyramine
U	**U**terosigmoidostomy
P	**P**ancreatic fistulas

NORMAL ADRENAL PHYSIOLOGY

1. Stress → corticotropin-releasing hormone (CRH) (hypothalamus) →
   Adrenocorticotropic hormone (ACTH) (anterior pituitary) → stimulates the →
   Adrenal cortex (zona fasciculata, middle layer of adrenal cortex) →
   ↑ cortisol

   PEARL: ACTH is produced from a large precursor protein → in the process, other hormones are generated → ↑ MSH

2. ↓ renal blood flow →
   Renin secretion → angiotensin II production → aldosterone secretion from adrenal cortex (zona glomerulosa /outer layer of adrenal cortex) → ↑ reabsorption of Na+ / water and ↑ secretion of K+ →
   ↑ BP

   PEARL: Aldosterone is also produced to a lesser extent by ACTH
   PEARL: ACTH deficiency doesn't cause mineralocorticoid deficiency, but ACTH excess does cause mineralocorticoid excess

3. Then inner most layer of adrenal cortex = zona reticularis → androgens (DHEA)
4. Adrenal Medulla = core of adrenal gland → catecholamines (epinephrine and norepinephrine)

ADRENAL GLAND - 2 REGIONS

1. Adrenal Cortex
2. Adrenal Medulla

ADRENAL CORTEX

Mnemonic: (GFR)

G	Zona Glomerulosa (outer layer) - s**A**lt
F	Zona Fasciculata (middle) - s**T**ress
R	Zona Reticularis (inner) - s**E**x

ADRENAL INSUFFICIENCY (AI)

- Most common cause of Adrenal insufficiency = **autoimmune**
- Most common infectious cause of Adrenal insufficiency worldwide = TB
- Most common infectious cause of Adrenal insufficiency in US = HIV
- ↓Na+ most common about 80%
  a) Sodium loss and volume depletion (**aldosterone deficiency**)
  b) **Increased vasopressin / antidiuretic hormone (ADH) secretion** and subsequent water retention and reduction in plasma Na concentration, caused by cortisol deficiency (lose negative feed back loop to Corticotropin-releasing hormone (CRH) in hypothalamus

- ↑ K+ (40%) aldosterone production failure (see hyperkalemia mnemonic)
- Normocytic Anemia 15%
- ↑ Ca2+ is seen in 6 to 33%
- ↓ Glucose - Sensitivity to exogenous insulin is increased because of loss of the gluconeogenic effect of cortisol
- ↓ BP Postural dizziness or syncope; hypotension (volume depletion - aldosterone deficiency)
- Weakness, weight loss, abdominal pain myalgia and arthralgia
- Severe or longstanding untreated AI have psychiatric symptoms (depression, psychosis, hallucinations, delusions catatonic posturing, mania, anxiety disorientation, delirium, memory impairment, confusion, stupor)
- **PEARL:** Cushing Disease: caused by adrenocorticotropic hormone (ACTH) secreting pituitary gland adenoma

MAJOR DIFFERENCES BETWEEN PRIMARY & SECONDARY ADRENAL INSUFFICIENCY

- Oral mucous membrane **hyperpigmentation is pathognomonic primary AI** (Addison's Disease) → result of compensatory adrenocorticotropic hormone (ACTH) and melanocyte-stimulating hormone (MSH) secretion
- **Secondary adrenal insufficiency:** adrenal insufficiency is from pituitary infarction (Sheehan's syndrome) or hypothalamic insufficiency; secondary adrenal insufficiency = lack of ACTH production
  - Hyperpigmentation is not present, because corticotropin (ACTH) secretion is not increased
  - Dehydration is not present, and hypotension is less prominent
  - Hyponatremia and volume expansion may be present (reflecting increased vasopressin secretion) but hyperkalemia is not (reflecting the presence of aldosterone)
  - Gastrointestinal symptoms are less common, suggesting that electrolyte disturbances may be involved in their etiology
  - Hypoglycemia is more common in secondary adrenal insufficiency
  - Draw blood for serum electrolytes, glucose and measurement of plasma cortisol and ACTH
  - **Treatment in confirmed cases of adrenal insufficiency**: Hydrocortisone 100 mg IVP and D5W 0.9% NS IV to prevent hypoglycemia; pressors are ineffective
  - **Treatment in non-confirmed /suspected cases of AI:** Dexamthasone 4mg IV
  - Dexamthasone will not affect the serum cortisol level → not interfere with the diagnosis of AI using the cosyntropin stimulation test
  - Measure cortisol levels → administer cosyntropin (Cortrosyn), a synthetic form of ACTH, → measure serum cortisol levels at 60 min → AI excluded if basal or post-stimulation level > 550 nmol/L

ADRENAL CRISIS

- Predominant manifestation of adrenal crisis = shock
- 90% of each adrenal gland must be non-functioning for clinically significant AI to manifest
- Patients often have **nonspecific symptoms** = anorexia, nausea, vomiting, abdominal pain, weakness, fatigue, lethargy, fever, confusion, or coma
- **Causes:** Adrenal hemorrhage, sepsis, intensification of chronic insufficiency and rapid steroid withdrawl; Incidence with septic shock = 60%

PRIMARY ADRENAL INSUFFICIENCY

- **Invasive meningococcemia** (Waterhouse-Freidrichsen syndrome) = primary adrenal insufficiency; disseminated meningococcemia results in hemorrhage and thrombosis of the adrenal gland, leading to life-threatening hemodynamic instability; other infectious causes = *Strep pneumoniae, Haemophilus influenzae* or *Pseudomonas*
- **Non-infectious causes of adrenal hemorrhage** = trauma, burns, anticoagulant use, coagulopathy, thromboembolism, or other severe illness (cardiac disease)

THYROID NORMAL PHYSIOLOGY

- Thyrotropin-Releasing Hormone (TRH) (hypothalamus) → Thyroid Stimulating Hormone (TSH) or Thyrotropin (anterior pituitary gland) → thyroid gland → capture iodine from blood to synthesize, store & release thyroxine (T4)

PRIMARY HYPERTHYROIDISM - CAUSES

- Grave's = most common cause; nodular toxic goiter; thyroid CA; thyroiditis; apathetic hyperthyroidism

SECONDARY HYPERTHYROIDISM - CAUSES

- Pituitary Adenoma; stuma ovarii' HCG tumors and factitious

THYROID STORM FINDINGS

- High fever, disproportionate tachycardia, dehydration, psychosis, seizures, restlessness, sweating, muscle weakness, high output CHF, atrial fibrillation, edema, N / V / D, abdominal pain

TREATMENT OF THYROID STORM

Give medications in this order

1) **Block peripheral effects of thyroid hormone**
   a.Propranolol 1 to 2 mg IV q 5 min prn (If COPD or CHF - consider esmolol)
   b.Guanethidine (inhibits NE release from post-ganglionic adrenergic nerve endings)
   c.Reserpine (depletes stored catecholamines both centrally and peripherally → inhibits release)

2) **Inhibit hormone synthesis (Thionamides)**
   a.Propylthiouracil (PTU) 600 to 1,000 mg po, followed by 250 mg po q 4-6h
   b.Methimazole

3) **Block hormone release**
   a.Lugol solution or potassium iodide (SSKI) (give one hour after PTU)
   b.Lithium carbonate – difficult to titrate and toxic effects common

4) **Prevent peripheral conversion of T4 → T3**
   a. Propranolol
   b. PTU
   c. Glucocorticoids (may also be useful in preventing relative adrenal insufficiency due to hyperthyroidism); Hydrocortisone 100mg IV q 8 hours

- Provide general support: airway, monitor, fluids, cooling blanket, Tylenol Low threshold for starting broad-spectrum antibiotics as infections commonly cause thyroid storm
- **PEARL:** Avoid ASA, will result in → ↑ Free T4
- **PEARL:** Avoid Amiodarone - iodine-rich antidysrhythmic with poorly-defined effects on thyroid function that has been associated with both hyperthyroidism and hypothyroidism
- **PEARL:** Give beta-blocker first = *blocking peripheral adrenergic hyperactivity of thyroid crisis may be the most important factor in reducing mortality and morbidity*
- **PEARL:** If asthma, COPD or CHF substitute for B1 selective medication = Esmolol, Guanethidine or Reserpine = alternatives

SIGNS / SYMPTOMS OF HYPOTHYROIDISM

- Puffy face, dry skin, hoarse voice, myxedema, bradycardia, galactorrhea, HTN, yellow-tinged skin, erythema nodosum, absent lateral 1/3 eyebrows, prolonged relaxation phase DTR's, pericardial, pleural and /or peritoneal effusions; bilateral carpal tunnel syndrome, AMS, constipation, pareshtesias, cold intolerance, weight gain, myalgias menorrhagia and sluggishness
- **Treatment:** Levothyroxine daily

MYXEDEMA COMA

Remember - HYPO's

- **Hypo**tenson - edema
- **Hypo**natremia - common
- **Hypo**glycemia
- **Hypo**ventilation → respiratory acidosis
- **Hypo**thermia – virtually all cases; correlates with survival (worst if < 90 degrees F)
- **Hypo**chloremia

- ↓ HR (Bradycardia) Sinus bradycardia most common rhythm
- ↓ Hct (Normochromic, normocytic anemia)
- ↑ Cholesterol > 250 mg/dL
- ↑ Transaminases, CPK, LDH

- Pericarditis → cardiac tamponade
- Mental status changes, lethargy, seizures
- Erythema nodosum, dry coarse hair, alopecia (lateral 1/3 of eyebrow), hoarse voice, bilateral carpal tunnel syndrome
- High SGOT, LDH, CPK

Myxedema Diagnosis ↓ T4 and ↑TSH

- Most common precipitating factor for Myxedema Coma = infection; others = cold exposure, CVA, CHF, drugs, anesthetics, GI bleed, metabolic disturbances, trauma, surgery, noncompliance with medication, MI, narcotics, sedatives and anesthetics
- **PEARL**: Amiodarone has been associated with both hyperthyroidism and hypothyroidism
  Hypothyroidism = blocks conversion of T4 → T3
  Hyperthyroidism = due to iodine content of Amiodarone

- **PEARL**: Amiodarone can cause chemical epididymitis, hypothyroidism / hyperthyroidism, interstitial lung disease (pulmonary fibrosis), blue-grey skin discoloration, corneal microdeposits, radycardia, heart blocks, dysrhythmias, prolonged QT, hypotension
- **Myxedema - Treatment**
  Levothyroxine IV + hydrocortisone 300 mg IV followed by 100 mg IV q 6 to 8 hrs

DIABETES INSIPIDUS (DI)

- Lose large amounts of dilute urine because of the loss of concentrating ability of distal nephron
- Central = lack of ADH secretion from Posterior Pituitary
- Nephrogenic = lack of responsiveness to circulating ADH

Normal Physiology

- ↑ Plasma osmolarity or
- ↓ BP or
- ↑ Angiotensin II

  ↓
- → Arginine Vasopressin (AVP) or antidiuretichormone (ADH) hormone formed in the hypothalamus → Transported via axons to, and released from posterior pituitary → Collecting ducts of kidney → Reabsorption of water back into the circulation →↑ blood volume
- **PEARL:** Vasopressin also → vasoconstrictor → ↑ MAP

Causes of DI

- Central = idiopathic, infection, tumor, bleed, granulomatous disorders, head trauma
- Nephrogenic = Obstructive uropathy, PKD, renal dysplasia, congenital disorders
- Systemic with renal involvement = Sickle cell, sarcoid, amyloid
- Drugs = Lithium, amphotercin, phenytoin, aminoglycosides

Lab

- ↓ Urine specific gravity
- ↓ Urine osmolality
- ↑ Na+

Treatment of Central DI

- Parenteral or IN vasopressin

ANTERIOR PITUITARY HORMONE RELEASE

Mnemonic: (FLAT PEG)

F	**F**ollicle Stimulating Hormone (FSH)
L	**L**uteinising Hormone (LH)
A	**A**renocorticotrophic Hormone (ACTH)
T	**T**hyroid Stimulating Hormone (TSH)

P	**P**rolactin (PRL)
E	**E**ndorphin
G	**G**rowth hormone (GH)

VITAMIN DEFICIENCIES

THIAMINE (B1) DEFICIENCY

- Alcoholics
- Anorexia, malaise, skin anesthesia, palpitations, calf tenderness, leg heaviness
- Wet Beriberi = edema, JVD, CHF, ↑HR, ↑BP, ↓UO; dilated cardiomyopathy (DCM)
  Dry Beriberi = nervous system pathology such as **Wernicke's**
- Polyneuritis

WERNICKE'S ENCEPHALOPATHY TRIAD = (AOA)

1. **A** = Ataxia
2. **O** = Ophthalmoplegia (most frequently seen oculomotor sign = lateral nystagmus)
   Other signs = lateral rectus (CN VI) palsy and conjugate gaze palsy
3. **A** = AMS

- **PEARL:** Give Thiamine 100mg IV BEFORE glucose in the treatment of Wernicke's
- **PEARL:** Thiamine (B1) is used with Pyridoxine (B6) and Fomepizole in the treatment of Ethylene Glycol Toxicity
- **PEARL:** Thiamine (B1) is used used with Pyridoxine (B6) in the treat of Hyperemesis Gravidarum

RIBOFLAVIN (B2) DEFICIENCY

- Sore mouth/tongue, stomatitis, glossitis, purple swollen tongue (seen in other B deficiencies)
- Photophobia, loss of VA, corneal ulcers
- Seborrheic dermatitis

NIACIN (B3) DEFICIENCY

- Constituent of NAD+ and NADP+
- Pellagra = 3 D's and 3 G's
- 3 D's of Pellagra = **D**iarrhea, **D**ermatitis and **D**ementia;
- 3 G's of Pellagra = **G**lossitis, **G**ingivitis and **G**eneralized stomatitis;

- Two main types of pellagra
  - **Primary:** due to a diet that does not contain enough niacin
  - **Secondary:** due to a poor ability to use the niacin within the diet (alcoholism, long-term diarrhea, carcinoid syndrome, and a number of medications (ie, isoniazid (INH)

PYRIDOXINE (B6) DEFICIENCY

- Peripheral neuritis
- Refractory seizures in neonates = Pyridoxine Deficiency = autosomal recessive

PYRIDOXINE (B6) PEARLS

- Used with Thiamine (B1) and Fomepizole in the treatment of Ethylene Glycol Toxicity
- Used to treat Hyperemesis Gravidarum
- Used to treat seizures in Isoniazid (INH) Toxicity
- Refractory seizures in neonates = Pyridoxine Deficiency = autosomal recessive
- Used with INH in the treatment of Latent TB infection in malnourished patients, pregnant or breastfeeding women, or those prone to neuropathy
- High dose B6 = used in the management of Gyromitra mushroom toxicity

FOLATE (B9) DEFICIENCY

- Folate is required for RBC production and fetal development
- Present in alcoholics
- Malnutrition
- Macrocytic anemia
- **PEARL:** Used in the treatment of methanol toxicity

COBALAMIN (B12) DEFICIENCY

- Megaloblastic and pernicious anemias
- Depression
- Optic Neuritis
- Glossitis, hypospermia, GI disorders (can't absorb B12 = colorectal surgery, pernicious anemia, strict vegetarians)
- **PEARL:** Used in treatment of cyanide toxicity

VITAMIN A DEFICIENCY

- Night blindness
- Loss of mucous membrane integrity →↑host susceptibility → infection

ASCORBIC ACID (C) DEFICIENCY

- Cofactor in collagen synthesis
- Scurvy; swollen/inflamed gums, loosening of teeth, follicular hyperkeratosis
- Impaired wound healing
- **PEARL:** IV Vitamin C = Used in mushroom (Amanita) toxicity

VITAMIN D DEFICIENCY

- Rickets

VITAMIN E DEFICIENCY

- Peripheral neuropathy, anemia

ENDOCRINE PEARLS

- Most common cause of coma in patient with diabetes = hypoglycemia
- Hypoglycemia: usually glucose < 60

Symptoms of hypoglycemia

- Tachycardia, diaphoresis, tremulous, paresthesias, HA, confusion, agitation, irritability, anxiety, blurred vision, seizures, coma; focal neurologic deficits possible, however usually symmetrical (non-focal) neurological deficits

Hypoglycemia treatment

- D50 amp
- If no IV → glucagon 1.0 mg IM
- Meal (long acting carbohydrates, recheck glucose)
- If long-acting oral agent = need continued treatment/observation 12-24 hours

Sulfonylureas - prolonged hypoglycemia

- Glimepiride (Amaryl), Glipizide (Glucotrol), Glyburide (Diabeta, Glynase)
- Prolonged half-life = risk of recurrent hypoglycemic episodes (up to 24 hours post ingestion)
- Sulfonylureas act by stimulating pancreatic beta cells to secrete more insulin
- Additionally, they increase the sensitivity of peripheral tissues to insulin
- **Treatment** = Octreotide (somatostatin analog) → inhibits glucose stimulated insulin release → prevents recurrent hypoglycemia

PEARL: Patients on metformin who require a CT scan with intravenous contrast = hold metformin for 48 hours to reduce the risk of lactic acidosis

PEARL: Strategy to determine if a patient is surreptitiously self-administering insulin:
A low C-peptide level + high insulin level → diagnostic for factitious hypoglycemia
Pancreatic beta cells make → Pro-insulin → Insulin + C-peptide (inactive peptide)

PEARL: Pancreatic alpha cells make → Glucagon → glycogenolysis, gluconeogenesis

Effects of Insulin

- Inhibition of glycogenolysis
- Inhibition of gluconeogenesis
- Increased glucose transport into fat and muscle
- Increased glycolysis in fat and muscle
- Stimulation of glycogen synthesis

- Primary reason for mental status changes in DKA = elevated osmolarity

- Urine dipstick for ketones uses a nitroprusside reaction which measures = acetoacetate ... not beta-hydroxybutyrate; usual ratio in DKA 1:3 acetoacetate / beta-hydroxybutyrate (may be as high as 1:30), therefore urine dip stick does not reflect true level of ketosis

- Average adult fluid deficit in DKA = 5 to 10 liters
- Average adult fluid deficit in HHS = 8 to 12 liters
- Correct Na+ in DKA = add 1.6 for every 100 mg/dl over the norm

DIABETIC KETOACIDOSIS (DKA)

- Begin Insulin 0.1 units/kg/hr if K+ is at least 4.0; add dextrose when blood glucose < 250
- Fluid: give a lot see above
- Add 20-40 mEq K to each liter after renal function evaluated
- Phosphorous shifts intracellularly as DKA treated
- Do not need bicarb unless pH < 6

HYPEROSMOLAR HYPERGLYCEMIC STATE

Diagnostic Features of **Hyperosmolar Hyperglycemic State** (HHS) per American Diabetic Association

- Plasma glucose > 600 mg/dL
- Serum osmolarity > 320 mOsm/kg
- Serum pH > 7.30
- Bicarbonate > 15 mEq/L
- Small ketonuria and absent-to-low ketonemia
- Profound dehydration up to an average of 9L
- Some alteration in consciousness
- Most common precipitating factor for Hyperosmolar Hyperglycemic State (HHS) = infection (UTI and pneumonia most common; others = uremia, viral illness, ACS, drugs, metabolic, iatrogenic and GI bleed
- HHS → Start fluid resuscitation first with isotonic saline (0.9% NaCl)
- Insulin can precipitate vascular collapse if given prior to volume expansion in HHS
- HHS mortality = 50%
- **Initial treatment of alcoholic ketoacidosis** = intravenous D5NS; also, correct K+, add thiamine to regenerate NAD; Glucose is the most critical component of treatment; takes about 12 to 24 hours to reverse alcoholic ketoacidosis; Vomiting = significant chloride losses. 0.9% NS is a better fluid choice (higher concentration of chloride, 155 mEq/L vs 109 mEq/L for Lactated Ringers

HYPEPARATHYROIDISM

- Most common cause of Hyperparathyroidism = adenoma 80%; hyperplasia 15-20%, carcinoma < 1%; ↑PTH → ↑Ca
- The most common presentation of primary hyperparathyroidism = asymptomatic hypercalcemia

SHEEHAN SYNDROME

- Ischemic necrosis of the pituitary gland following maternal hemorrhage and hypotension in the peripartum period

HYPOPITUITARISM

- Hypothyroidism - cold intolerance, fatigue, constipation, weight gain, hair loss, slow thinking, bradycardia, hypotension, decrease free water clearance (hyponatremia)
- Adrenal insufficiency - hyponatremia, hypoglycemia, hyperkalemia, anemia
- Amenorrhea
- Initially asymptomatic; difficulty breastfeeding (agalactorrhea) or amenorrhea

CUSHING SYNDROME

- The most common overall cause of Cushing syndrome = iatrogenic (due to exogenous glucocorticoid medication use)
- The most common cause of Cushing syndrome (not taking steroids) = Cushing disease = caused by an adrenocorticotropic hormone (ACTH) secreting pituitary gland adenoma
- If cause is pituitary tumor then it's called Cushing's disease
- Tumors of the adrenal cortex account for 5–10% of Cushing syndrome cases

PHEOCHROMOCYTOMA

Vascular tumor of the adrenal medulla Secretion of epinephrine and norepinephrine

Clinical findings 7 P's

- **P**ounding Pain (severe headaches)
- **P**erspiration (excessive sweating)
- **P**alpitations (tachycardia)
- **P**anic (anxiety/nervousness)
- **P**ain (lower chest / upper abdomen / SOB)
- **P**ressure (elevated BP)
- **P**allor

- Classic Triad: HA's, palpitations and sweating = 40%

Rule of 10's:

- 10% familial
- 10% bilateral
- 10% malignant
- 10% calcify
- 10% located outside the medulla

PEARL: Common site = bladder. Consider in patient with episodic HTN with urination

Labs: Urinary VMA (breakdown of NE) and plasma catecholamines

ENVIRONMENTAL

HYPOTHERMIA

- **Chilblains (Pernio):** inflammatory erythematous to violaceous acral lesions after exposure to cold; pruritic and/or painful; treatment: rewarming, gently bandage, elevate; consider Nifedipine (Procardia)
- **Hypothermia**: temperature of less than 95 °F (35 °C)
- **Severe Hypothermia:** temperature < 90°F (32 °C)
- **Shivering** ceases at 88 °F (31 °C)
- Move the hypothermic patient as little as possible – irritable myocardium → VF
- The amplitude of the **J-wave (Osborne wave)** is proportional to the degree of hypothermia; does not relate to pH and is not prognostic; may appear when temperature falls to < 32 °C (89.6 °F)
- **J-wave other causes:** Hypercalcemia; brain injury; pericarditis; ventricular fibrillation (VF)
- Hypothermia: **sequence of cardiac deterioration:** sinus bradycardia → AF (30 °C / 86 °F) → VF (28 °C / 82 °F) → Asytole (< 18 °C / 64 °F)
- **Cerebral metabolism** ↓ decreases 6% for each 1 °C ↓ decline in temperature
- **Treatment for severe hypothermia (temperature** < 39 °C (90 °F): active core re-warming (warmed humidified oxygen, IV fluids heated to (40 – 42 °C) (104 –107 °F), possibly heated peritoneal dialysis and cardiopulmonary bypass)
- Lactated Ringer solution is not recommended because hypothermic liver cannot metabolize lactate
- **DKA /hypothermia:** insulin is not effective at core temp < 30 °C (86 °F)
- **Defibrillation /hypothermia:** rarely effective < 30 °C (86 °F)
- **Core-temperature afterdrop:** further ↓ in core temperature & clinical deterioration after rewarming; peripheral tissues are warmed → vasodilation → sudden return of cooler, acidotic, hyperkalemic blood from the extremities → central circulation → core-temperature afterdrop → dysrhthmogenic

FROSTBITE

Most common presenting symptom of frostbite = numbness 75%

Treatment options

- Rewarming by immersing the affected area in a water bath heated to 37 to 39 °C (98.6 to 102.2 °F) Previous recommendation was 40 – 42 °C (104 –107 °F), however temps > 40 °C found to not warm tissue faster and cause the process to be more painful
- Splint the affected frostbite area to minimize injury
- Early debridement is contraindicated in frostbite
- tPA (intra-arterial) for severe frostbite injury **presenting within 24 hours**, ASAP after initial management + UFH or enoxaparin
- Technetium (Tc)-99m scintigraphy (bone scan) can be used to predict long-term viability of affected tissue and help guide decisions about thrombolytic therapy
- **Present within 48 hours of the initial insult, treatment**: iloprost, a synthetic form of prostacyclin

HYPERTHERMIA

HEAT EXHAUSTION

- Core body temperature is usually 101 to 104°F (38.3 to 40.0°C) at the time of collapse
- Clinical syndrome
- HA / fatigue / malaise / agitation / N/ V / D/ tachycardia / muscle & abdominal cramps, ataxia, light-headedness, but normal mental status
- **Treatment**: rest, cool environment and rehydration

HEAT STROKE

- Core body temperature > 105°F
- CNS involvement - confusion, ataxia, AMS, seizures or coma
- Treatment: rapid cooling; best option for rapid cooling = evaporative cooling - spray the body
- with fine mist and place near fans to increase evaporative loss; supportive
- **PEARL:** Tylenol/ASA not recommended in heat stroke, may be deleterious

OTHER HEAT RELATED ILLNESSES

- Heat Cramps
- Heat Edema
- Heat Syncope
- Heat Tetany

PEARL: Heat cramps: related to Na+ (salt) deficiency; lab findings: ↓Na+, ↓Cl , ↓UNa+ and ↓UCl levels; salt your beer!

SPIDERS

Black Widow bites

60% erythematous macule; other findings: target lesions, tiny dual fang marks
Pathognomonic bite: patch of sweat and a little red dot

- **Black Widow Pathophysiology**
  Neurotoxin → ↑ Ach and NE release → SLUDGE BAM + HTN (severe abdominal pain).
- **Treatment:** supportive, observe 4 hours → if no symptoms discharge home; if HTN and tachycardia do not respond to supportive measures → Equine derived Antivenin available

Brown recluse spider

Venom causes local necrotic skin lesion surrounded by an erythematous ring

Management

- Supportive care: ice application, clean, irrigate and elevate wound, tetanus prophylaxis as indicated analgesics for pain
- There have been no medications (including dapsone, steroids or antibiotics) that demonstrate any improved outcome over supportive care

Tarantula

Irritating venomous barbed abdominal hairs, which can be ejected several feet like a javelin → allergic reactions; more painful than damaging (only serious if hairs get into eyes)

VENEMOUS SNAKES

Rattlesnake
The most common poisonous snake in the US
Triangular shaped head, elliptical pupils, heat sensing notril pits

Water moccasins (cottonmouths)
Copperheads are members of the family Viperidae, subfamily Crotalinae (formerly Crotalidae)
They are also commonly called pit vipers, (refers to the heat sensing pit located behind the nostrils)

- **Local effects:** severe pain at the site of the bite, edema, erythema, rhabdomyolysis and compartment syndrome.
- **Systemic effects:** paresthesias, generalized weakness, and CP, SOB, metallic taste
- **Labs:** coagulopathy, thrombocytopenia, hypofibrinogenemia and bleeding complications
- Admit patients to the hospital for 24 to 48 hours → serial determinations of platelets, prothrombin time, and urinalysis to check for myoglobin and hemoglobin
- **Treatment:** Crotalidae Polyvalent Immune Fab (Ovine) (CroFab; FabAV)
- **"Dry" bites:** no venom is injected, patient is asymptomatic, 25% of bites; Management: careful observation for at least 8 hours

CORAL SNAKES

- *Red on yellow, kill a fellow*
  Red on black, venom lack
- **Toxicity:** competitive inhibition of the muscarinic acetylcholine receptors at the neuromuscular junction → neurotoxicity = descending muscle weakness, paresthesias, ptosis dysarthria, dysphagia and respiratory failure (measure NIF)
- **Coral Snakes Management:** admit patients for 24 to 48 hours for observation (delayed signs and symptoms may occur); anyone bitten by Eastern Coral Snake should be given antivenin IV → 3 to 5 vials in 500cc NS
- **PEARL:** Adjunctive therapy for coral snake envenomation = Anticholinesterases (neostigmine)
- **PEARL: Gila Monster**: One of only 2 venomous lizards in the world; Mild Neurotoxin; crazy painful bites
- **PEARL: Box Scorpion:** do not treat with narcotic and barbiturates → ↑toxic effects of venom; Antivenin available

HYMENOPTERA STINGS

- Most dangerous venom from **hymenoptera** family = honey bee → venom causes greater histamine release per gram than any other hymenopteran venom
- After stinging a victim honey bees release a pheromone that attracts other bees

PEARL: These bees are only capable of stinging once
- Honeybees
- Africanized bees
- Bumblebees

PEARL: These Vespids are capable of stinging multiple times
- Wasps
- Hornets
- Yellow jackets

Africanized “killer” bees and North American honybees venom potencies are equivalent; **Africanized “killer” bees** have lower threshold for provocation, heightened response and resulting increased number of bees that will attack; hybrids of African honeybees that escaped labs in Brazil, now in southern regions of US and are more aggressive then North American honeybees

MARINE ENVENOMATIONS

- **Jellyfish /man-o-war treatment:** wash off with salt water; 5% acetic acid (vinegar) neutralizes Nematocyte; Use credit card & scrap skin to get nematocyts off skin
- **PEARL:** Freshwater rinsing stimulates nematocyst discharge and make jellyfish stings worse
- **PEARL:** Most jellyfish stings are minor; however, Box Jellyfish stings may present with life-threatening systemic effects: severe pain and spasms, paralysis, respiratory weakness, cardiac arrest

Sting ray, Starfish, Sea Urchin, Sea Cucumbers and Lion Fish

- **Treatment:** immersion in hot water up to a temperature of 45 °C (113 °F) for 30 to 60 minutes

Hemorrhagic bullous lesions with history of sea water-contaminated abrasions or eating raw seafood: consider ***Vibrio vulnificus;*** Treatment: Ciprofloxacin 750mg po bid

ELECTRICAL PEARLS

- Most common cause of death in electrical injury = cardiac
- Most common arrest arrhythmia after electrical injury = ventricular fibrillation
- *Low* voltage alternating current (**AC**) → ventricular fibrillation
- *High* voltage alternating current (**AC**) → Asystole
- Low voltage **AC** example = Electric outlet
- **AC** 3x more dangerous then DC; longer duration = worse the injury
- Most common shoulder dislocation with AC electrical injury = posterior should dislocation
- **Other injuries:** cataracts, compartment syndrome, AKI (myoglobinuria)
- **AC** 3x more dangerous then DC; longer duration = worse the injury
- Direct current (**DC**) → Asystole
- **DC** examples = battery, lightning
- **Injuries** associated with DC electrical injuries = fractures
- **Low-voltage exposures** < 240 V and are rarely associated with significant injury
- **High-voltage exposures** > 1,000 V; Regardless of exam or symptoms → admit / observe for at least 12 hours, even if asymptomatic

Injury associated with:

1. Increased **voltage**
2. Length of exposure **time**

- **Labs:** check for renal injury, electrolyte disturbances, rhabdomyolysis, and cardiac dysrhythmias
- Electrical burns rarely require skin grafting but should be evaluated closely for compartment syndrome given the significant internal muscle destruction that can occur

- All electrical burns should be transferred to a burn center once stabilized
- **PEARL:** Arc burns are flash electrical burns that do not penetrate deeper than the skin
- **PEARL:** Oral commissure burn (kid biting electrical cord) are associated with labial artery bleed 7 to 10 days post injury; discharge home with plastics consult

Resistance of Body Tissues

- (MOST) Bone > Fat > Tendon > Dry skin > Mucous Membranes > Blood > Nerves (LEAST)
- Skin is a good resistor of electrical flow, although moisture decreases skin's resistance; Ohm's Law: Current = Voltage / Resistance

LIGHTNING INJURIES

- Lightning strike: high voltage DC depolarization; current pathway = "**flashover**", not horizontal (hand to hand) or vertical (hand to foot) seen with low or high-voltage AC
- **Lightning injury findings:** Confused and amnestic after event; TM rupture 50%; bilateral cataracts; asystole; **Lichtneberg figures**
- ***Lichtenberg figures:*** superficial ferning pattern are pathognomonic for lightning strike
- **Keraunoparalysis ("Lightning paralysis"):** Transient paralysis following lightning strike; associated with cold, mottled skin and and sensory disturbances (extreme vasoconstriction)

ACUTE MOUNTAIN SICKNESS (AMS)

- Benign
- Self-limited
- Onset 4-12 hours after ascent
- HA / anorexia / N / V/ dizziness / weakness/ exertional dyspnea
- Difficulty sleeping due to periodic breathing
- Ataxia is useful sign of progression of AMS to HACE

Management

- Halt ascent until symptoms resolve; don't necessarily need to descend
- Can be avoided by gradual ascent
- *Climb high - sleep low*
- Oxygen
- Acetazolamide: used in prevention and treatment of AMS
- Dexamethasone: used in treatment of AMS

HIGH ALTITUDE PULMONARY EDEMA (HAPE)

- Most commonly at altitudes > 8,000 feet in unacclimatized patients
- Fatigue, dyspnea at rest, cough dry → productive copious clear secretions, rales
- Decreased exercise tolerance/dyspnea at rest is an early symptom of HAPE

Chest X-ray

a) Non-cardiogenic pulmonary edema
   Results from hypoxia induced pulmonary artery HTN → elevated hydrostatic pressures and capillary leak
b) Patchy alveolar infiltrates, most commonly right middle lobe (RML)

Management

- Cornerstone of **HAPE** Treatment: oxygen (intubation/NIV if needed) and descent
- Nifedipine: prevention and treatment
- Sildenafil (Viagra) and tadlafil (Cialis): blunt hypoxia induced vasoconstriction and have benefit in prevention and treatment of HAPE
- Acetazolamide NOT effective in treatment

HIGH ALTITUDE CEREBRAL EDEMA (HACE)

- Decreased partial pressure of oxygen leads to cerebral edema
- Most common fatal manifestation of high-altitude illness
- Life threatening
- Ataxia
- Severe HA
- N/V/Seizure
- Retinal hemorrhages

Management

- Immediate descent
- Dexamethasone
- Elevate head
- Oxygen
- Hyperbaric therapy (HBOT)
- Gamow Bag: a unique, portable hyperbaric chamber

Acetazolamide is a Carbonic anhydrase inhibitor

- Causes HCO3 (bicarbonate) diuresis → non-AG Acidosis → to maintain serum pH the body increases ventilation to decrease PCO2 → as a result serum PO2 is increased

DECOMPRESSION SICKNESS

- Clinical diagnosis; symptoms begin within 6 hours of diving; may be delayed up to 12-24 hours after surfacing
- Decompression sickness is a form of dysbarism that occurs due to the reformation of dissolved nitrogen into gas bubbles in various tissues

Neurologic manifestations

- "The staggers": profound vertigo, hearing loss, and nausea due to inner ear involvement
- Spinal cord involvement: paresthesias, paralysis
- Cerebral involvement: HA and vision disturbances, stroke (cerebral embolism)

Musculoskeletal manifestations

- "The bends": arthragias & myalgias

Pulmonary manifestations

- "The chokes": SOB / CP & cough

Cutaneous involvement

- "Skin bends": pruritus or burning of the skin or mottling (purpura marmorata), erysipelas-like rash over fatty areas

Cardiac
- MI (coronary embolism)

Risk factors for Decompression Sickness
- Depth of dive
- Rapidity of ascent
- Multiple dives within the same day
- Air travel within 24 hours of dive
- Obesity as nitrogen is fat soluble
- Fatigue
- Alcohol use
- Dehydration
- Heavy exertion
- Respiratory infections
- Older age
- Strenuous exertion underwater

Management
- **Initial mangement:** administration of 100% oxygen via nonrebreather, IV fluids, lying supine and ASA
- **Definitive management:** recompression in a hyperbaric chamber
- This should be done for all but the mildest of symptoms
- Prevention of decompression sickness is via slow ascent with frequent "stops," limiting depth or time of dives, and abstaining from air travel for at least 24 hours

ARTERIAL GAS EMBOLISM

Divers: most common cause of stroke, LOC, ACS

- Expanding gas → ruptures pulmonary alveoli → air enters into the pulmonary venous system → left heart → leading to systemic micro-gas emboli
- This is possible due to bypassing filtration of the lungs and moving directly back to the left heart and out to the systemic circulation
- Most frequently occurs when divers hold their breath on ascent

Classic presentation: a diver who surfaces and loses consciousness within 20 minutes of ascent due to embolus to the cerebral vasculature
- Arterial gas embolism may also affect other systems:
  - Lung: PE like symptoms: dyspnea, hemoptysis and CP
  - Brain: stroke-like symptoms (weakness, dysarthria)
  - Heart/coronary arteries: MI like symptoms: CP, diaphoresis and dysrhthmia

Treatment
- Initial Treatment: keep patient ***supine***, oxygen
- Definitive management: recompression in a hyperbaric chamber. This places the diver back under high pressure, which will force the gases in the embolism to dissolve into the blood
- Primary prevention of arterial gas embolism is by frequent exhalation on ascent from dives

DROWNING

Leading cause of death in children 1 to 14 years old worldwide; cervical spine injuries rare

- **Wet drowning:** 85-90% of cases; laryngospasm relaxes due to hypoxia → aspirate water → loss of surfactant → hypoxia → brain death after 3 minutes
- **Dry drowning:** 10-15% of cases; aspiration of small amount of fluid → laryngospasm → severe hypoxia → seizure or death

RADIATION

- **Alpha particles:** penetrate only the epidermis
- **Beta particles:** penetrate skin to about 8mm (may decay to more dangerous gamma rays)
- **Gamma rays:** deep penetration with deep tissue injury
- **Tissues that are *most* radiosensitive** = fastest rate of cellular division: spermatogonia, epidermal, GI and hematopoietic
- **Tissues that are *least* radiosensitive** = nerve cells and muscle fibers

Protection from radiation exposure

1. Maximizing distance from source
2. Minimizing exposure time
3. Shielding from exposure

- **Mean lethal dose (LD50)** = dose required to kill half the members of a tested population after a specified test duration
- The **mean lethal dose (LD50)** of acute radiation exposure = 3.5 Gray (Gy) or 350 rads
- **Absolute lymphocyte count 24 hours after radiation exposure** is a good indicator of patients clinical course → > 1,200 → no lethal dose.
- If lymphocyte count 300-1,200 at 48hrs → lethal dose of radiation expected

DERMATOLOGY / ALLERGY

Success in Medical School and Beyond / Mnemonics and Pearls

DERMATOLOGY PEARLS

NIKOLSKY'S SIGN

- The outer epidermis separates easily from the basal layer on exertion of firm sliding manual pressure
- **Conditions with positive (+) Nikolsky's Sign:** Pemphigus vulgaris (autoimmune), TEN and Staph Scalded Skin Syndrome, Steven-Johnson Syndrome (SJS) & Bullous Impetigo
- **PEARL:** Nikolsky's Sign may be present even in unaffected skin

BULLOUS PEMPHIGOID

- Autoimmune Vesiculobullous Disease
- Auto-antibodies against basement membrane
- Mucous membranes almost never involved
- Older patients (> 65 years)
- Begins as pruritic papules → large tense blisters

PEMPHIGUS VULGARIS

- Autoimmune Vesiculobullous Disease
- More common to have mucosal involvement
- IgG autoantibodies to desmosomes (transmembrane adhesion moleculess) which results in the loss of cohesion between keratinocytes in the epidermis.
- + Nikolsky sign
- **Treatment:** steroids & immunosuppressants

TOXIC EPIDERMAL NECROLYSIS (TEN) / LYELL DISEASE

- Involves > 30% of the body surface; first affects eyes and spreads caudad; + Nikolsky's sign
- Stevens-Johnson Syndrome (SJS) involves < 30%; MR 10%; 70% mucosal involvement
- AIDS patients on Sulfa prophylaxis 10,000-fold higher risk of getting TEN

ERYTHEMA MULTIFORME (EM)

- Acute immune-mediated reaction
- **Erythema Multiforme Major:** EM with mucosal involvement (and may have associated systemic symptoms, such as fever and arthralgias)
- **Erythema Multiforme Minor:** EM without (or with only mild) mucosal disease and without associated systemic symptoms
- Target lesions palm/sole involvement; 70% mucosal involvement
- Steroids provide symptomatic relief, but unproven benefit in duration and outcome
- Causes: drugs, bugs, immunizations, malignancy (leukemia), idiopathic
- Most common cause: infection; most common infection: Herpes Simplex Virus (HSV 1); Other causes: *Mycoplasma, Strep. pyogenes* as well as drugs: sulfa, phenytoin Penicillin and APAP

STEVEN-JOHNSON SYDROME (SJS)

- Involves skin and mucous membranes. Starts with viral syndrome picture, followed by a painful rash that spreads and blisters. Causes: Cytotoxic immune reaction; most common drugs: sulfamethoxazole/trimethoprim (Bactrim) and lamotrigine (Lamictal)

ERYTHEMA NODOSUM

- Vasculitis that presents with tender, erythematous nodules on the pretibial area, torso or other extensor surface of the body
- **Causes:** Ulcerative colitis, Yersinia enterocolitica, Srep., Chlamydia, TB, sarcoid, histoplasmosis, coccidiomycosis, hypothyroidism, pregnancy, idiopathic, drugs: Phenytoin, PCN, OCP's, Sulfonamides
- Most common drug-induced cause of erythema nodosum = oral contraceptives
- **Treatment:** NSAIDs, rest and elevation & treat underlying condition

IMPETIGO

- Most common cause of **impetigo** = Staph. aureus
- Group A, beta-hemolytic streptococci (Strep pyogenes) #2, distant second
- Most common location = face and extremities
- Children ages 2 to 5 years
- Classically presents as papules that progress → to form vesicles on an erythematous base; Vesicles turn to → pustules that rupture to form thick "honey-colored" golden crust classic for impetigo; pruritic; non-painful; fever is rare
- **Treatment** of localized impetigo: topical antibiotics mupirocin (Bactroban) or Retapamulin (Altabax) being first-line treatments
- More extensive impetigo may require systemic antibiotics
- **Complication:** post-streptococcal glomerulonephritis

TINEA VERSICOLOR

- Yeast infection, *Pityrosporum ovale or P. orbiculare* are synonyms for Malassezia furfur; variety of colors (tan, pink white), hypopigmented scaly macules or patches on chest or back. Usually seek medical attention because spots do not tan; lesions resolve in 1-2 months without permanent scar. Common fungal infection of the skin. The fungus interferes with the normal pigmentation of the skin, resulting in small, discolored patches.
- Recurrence in common.
- **Treatement:** oral Ketoconazole (Nizoral) 400mg x1 or 200mg q24 hr x 7days or 2% cream 1x q24 hr x 2 weeks; rule-out erythrasma

ERYTHRASMA

- Chronic superficial infection intertriginous areas of skin; ***Corynebacterium minutissimum***; well-demarcated brown-red macular patches; Treatment: Erythromycin 250mg q 6hr x 14 d

PORPHYRIA CUTANEA TARDA

- Erosions and bullae to sun-exposed areas exposed to trauma; Painful blisters; Avoid sunlight

WOOD'S LIGHT

Organism → fluorescent pattern
Porphyria cutanea tarda → urine color change to orange or yellow
Erythrasma → coral red or pink
Tinea versicolor → green or yellow
Pseudomonas → yellow or green

PITYRIASIS ROSEA

- Pink or pigmented maculopapular rash over the trunk following Langers' lines.
- Eruption is classically preceded by a week by the appearance of a "herald patch" (2 to 6 cm plaque) and follows a dermatomal, "Christmas-tree pattern" distribution on the trunk
- Usually children and young adults; asymptomatic or pruritis; self-limiting, resolves in 8 to 12 weeks without treatment; etiology unclear, possibly viral

LICHEN PLANUS

- Autoimmune; violaceous papules; most commonly affects individuals between 30 and 60 years of age; 4 Ps" = 1) purple 2) pruritic 3) polygonal 4) papules

LUPUS PERNIO

- Pathognomonic for sarcoidosis
- Chronic, violaceous, raised plaques and nodules commonly found on the cheeks, nose, and around the eyes

DERMATOMYOSITIS

- Dermatomyositis: often associated with malignancy
- Gottron papules: symmetric erythematous papules on the extensor surface of the hands
- Heliotrope rash: erythematous eruption around the eyes and the nasolabial fold

ACANTHOSIS NIGRANS

- Velvety hyper-pigmented patch of skin = marker for underlying malignancy or DM

MIGRATORY THROMBOPHLEBITIS (TROUSSEAU SYNDROME)

- Rare; suspicion for an underlying pancreatic malignancy

ICHTHYOSIS

- Fish-like scales on the skin

PYODERMA GANGRENOSUM

- Not an infection; associated with systemic disorders: TB, Cancer, UC, RA may respond to Dapsone

- **PEARL:** SLE = facial "butterfly rash"
- **PEARL:** Amiodarone can cause chemical **corneal micro-deposits**
- **PEARL:** Lead lines = bluish lines along gumline

VASCULITIS

- Presents with tender, erythematous nodules on the pretibial area, torso or other extensor surface of the body; Treatment = NSAIDs, rest and elevation and treat underlying condition

ERYTHRODERMA / EXFOLIATIVE DERMATITIS

- "Red skin"; severe and potentially life-threatening condition that presents with diffuse erythema and scaling involving all or most of the skin surface area (≥ 90%)

- Most common cause of erythroderma = exacerbation of a preexisting inflammatory dermatosis, most often psoriasis or atopic dermatitis
- Other causes: idiopathic (30%), hypersensitivity drug reaction, hematologic or systemic malignancies

- **Sezary syndrome** is an aggressive form of cutaneous T-cell lymphoma and affect the skin - Erythroderma
- It is characterized by a widespread red rash he presence of cancerous T cells (called Sezary cells) in the blood, and abnormally enlarged lymph nodes
- Other signs and symptoms may include intense itchiness, scaling and peeling of the skin
- May see high output cardiac failure

BEHÇET'S SYNDROME

- Recurring genital ulcerations
- Recurring oral ulcerations
- Relapsing uveitis
- Ulcerations, painful; necrotic center with surrounding red rim

Treatment

- Corticosteroids: palliative
- Cytotoxic medications indicated in ocular, CNS, and vascular disease

MOLLUSCUM CONTAGIOSUM

- Infection on the face should raise concern for underlying HIV/AIDS infection
- The severity of immunosuppression correlates with the number of lesions found on the face
- There is an inverse relationship between the number of lesions and the patient's CD4 count
- The infection is caused by a DNA poxvirus
- Lesions: flesh-colored, dome-shaped and have a pearly appearance, papular and have dimpled center. Most commonly found on the trunk, axillae, extremities, face and genitalia
- Spreads via autoinoculation, scratching, contact with lesions, and fomites
- Immunocompetent patients: condition is generally self-limited and resolves spontaneously in 6 to 9 months; Immunocompetent patients can be referred to a dermatologist for removal
- **Genital molluscum contagiosum** in a child should raise concern for = SEXUAL ASSAULT

POISON IVY

- Allergic contact dermatitis
- Delayed immunologic response (type IV hypersensitivity)
- Allergen not in bullae of vesicles, so after washing of the involved site, contact with rash does not cause it to spread; Treatment: antihistamines, oatmeal baths and topical steroids; IvyBlock

Steroids in Poison Ivy

- If widespread oral steroids: 30 to 80 mg/day tapered over 21 days

PEARL: Steroids in Zoster

- Treatment: if within 3 days of onset of rash; ↓ discomfort during acute phase of zoster; does not ↓ incidence of post-herpetic neuralgia or lessen rate of the healing of lesions
- 21 day steroid taper: 30mg bid (days 1-7), 15mg bid (days 8-14) 7.5mg bid (days 15-21)

PEARL: Hutchinson's sign - with HZ infection V1 distribution = vesicle at the tip of the nose

EVALUATION OF PIGMENTED LESION

A = Asymmetry (a line drawn down the middle of the lesion does not create 2 equal halves
B = Border irregularity
C = Color (lesion may look jet black or contain shades of red, white, blue or gray)
D = Diameter (lesion > 6mm, the size of a pencil eraser = suspicious
E = Elevation (lesion the elevates rapidly over a short period of time = nodular melanoma)

BASAL CELL CARCINOMA

- Central ulcer, with raised pearly-white border
- 90% of skin cancers in the US
- Most common of all cancers

SQUAMOUS CELL CARCINOMA

- Firm, red nodule or papules or plaques
- Usually seen in sun exposed areas

MELANOMA

- Not good

NEUROFIBROMATOSIS

- Genetic disorder that causes tumors to form on nerve tissue (brain, spinal cord, acoustic neuromas (vestibular schwannoma), meningiomas and peripheral nerves)
- Three (3) major clinically and genetically distinct forms: neurofibromatosis types 1 and 2 (NF1 and NF2) and schwannomatosis; NF1 (von Recklinghausen disease) is the most common type
- Hallmarks of NF1 = multiple café-au-lait macules and cutaneous neurofibromas

ALLERGY

HYPERSENSITIVITY REACTIONS

Type I hypersensitivity reaction

- Immediate hypersensitivity
- IgE-mediated hypersensitivity. Binding of antigens to IgE on mast cells and basophils leads to derganulation of mediators
- Examples: anaphylaxis, urticaria and angioedema
- **PEARL:** Dermographism may be seen in patients with urticaria

Type II hypersensitivity reaction (cytotoxic)

- Involves cell lysis resulting from antibody binding to membrane-bound antigens
- IgG-mediated cytotoxic hypersensitivity with resultant complement activation
- Examples: Goodpasture syndrome, erythoblastalis fetalis blood transfusions and autoimmune hemolytic anemia

Type III hypersensitivity reaction (immune complex-mediated reactions)

- Antibodies bind to antigens to form immune complexes
- Immune complexes are deposited on vessel walls leading to complement activation and resultant local inflammation
- Examples: serum sickness, Lupus (SLE), RA, post-strep GN, PAN, reactive arthrits, serum sickness, arthus reaction, HSP, "Farmers's lung")
- Serum sickness presents with rash, fever / flu-like symptoms, polyarthralgias and usually begins 1-2 weeks after exposure to a causative agent

Type IV reactions (Delayed)

- T-cell mediated (other are antibody mediated) inflammation against cell surface bound antigens. Contact dermatitis (poison ivy), Stevens-Johnson syndrome (SJS), toxic epidermal necrolysis (TEN), TB skin test, transplant rejection, sarcoid, Crohn's, MS, metals (nickel); scabies
- **PEARL:** Nickel is the most common cause of metal dermatitis and a common cause of allergic contact dermatitis

TREATMENT OPTION FOR ANAPHYLAXIS

- Diphenhydramine 50mgIV
- Solumederol 125 mg IV
- H2 Blocker
- Fluids
- Epinephrine 1:1000, 0.3 mg IM lateral thigh

If patient is crashing/anaphylactic shock

- Epinephrine IV over 10 minutes
- Take Epi off crash cart, draw up 1 mL
- Dilute this in 9 mL 0.9%NS
- Give slowly over 10 minutes
- **PEARL:** Epinephrine acts by binding to adrenergic receptors (beta-receptor)
- Patients taking beta-blockers may exhibit refractory hypotension despite being administered fluids and epinephrine
- To circumvent the beta-receptor, glucagon can be administered, which will bypass the beta-adrenergic second messenger system, potentiate the circulating epinephrine, and help restore vasomotor tone

RED MAN SYNDROME

- ***Anaphylactoid reaction*** to vancomycin
- **Clinically**: pruritus and erythematous rash to face, neck, and upper torso (upper body > lower); less common symptoms = fever, dizziness, burning sensation, myalgia and hypotension
- ***Anaphylactoid reactions*** directly activate mast cells → histamine release, independent of IgE (as opposed to anaphylaxis, which is mediated by IgE)
- **Treatment:** antihistamine and removal of the offending agent (vancomycin) Vancomycin can be restarted at a slower rate of infusion only AFTER symptoms have resolved and there is no evidence of true anaphylaxis

INFECTIOUS DISEASE

Success in Medical School and Beyond | Mnemonics and Pearls

SEPSIS DEFINITIONS

Multiple definitions create confusion

CMS and the Third International Consensus (Sepsis-3) definitions are currently used in clinical practice, with distinct terminology and different identification criteria, including blood pressure and lactate cutoff points

- The CMS definition continues to recommend SIRS for sepsis identification.
- Sepsis-3 disregards the concept of SIRS and uses the sequential organ failure assessment (SOFA) or the quick version (qSOFA) to define sepsis
- Sepsis-3 removes severe sepsis from official nomenclature and this has led to confusion and challenges in protocol development

QUICK SEQUENTIAL ORGAN FAILURE ASSESSMENT

1. Respiratory rate at least 22 breaths/minute
2. Systolic blood pressure 100 mm Hg or lower
3. Altered mental status (Glasgow Coma Scale score < 15)

Problem: Sepsis-3 relies on clinician's ability to identify infection as the cause of organ dysfunction, which may not be apparent early on, making it less sensitive than SIRS for diagnosing early sepsis

CMS DEFINITIONS

These definitions are widespread and easily understood

SYSTEMIC INFLAMMATORY RESPONSE SYNDROME (SIRS)

2 or More Criteria Must be Met

1. Temperature
   a. > 38° C (100.4° F) or
   b. < 36° C (96.8° F)
2. Heart Rate > 90 beats/min
3. Respiratory Rate (respiratory alkalosis is often the first sign of SIRS)
   a. > 20 breaths/min or
   b. P_aCO_2 < 32 mmHg
4. WBC
   a. > 12,000 or
   b. < 4,000 cells or
   c. > 10 % bands

SEPSIS

SIRS + suspected or documented source of infection

SEVERE SEPSIS

Sepsis + infection induced organ dysfunction, hypoperfusion or hypotension
Organ dysfunction includes but not limited to: oliguria; lactic acidosis; AMS changes; hypotension, AKI, bilirubin > 2.0; platelets < 100,000; INR > 1.5 or PTT > 60 seconds

SEPTIC SHOCK

Severe Sepsis + refractory ↓ BP despite adequate fluid resuscitation
OR
Lactate ≥ 4

PEARL: Most common source of infection in septic patient = respiratory system
PEARL: Overwhelming **P**ost-**S**plenectomy **I**nfection **(OPSI):** septic shock, DIC and adrenal hemorrhage; may be post surgery or inadequate splenic function (sickle cell)

HIV/AIDS

HIV REPLICATION

The genetic material of HIV is RNA; the virus uses enzymes to attack host with final goal to convert HIV RNA into DNA and then insert this HIV DNA into host CD4 cell
Virally encoded enzymes include: reverserse transcriptase, integrase and protease

1. Reverse transcriptase: used to to convert HIV RNA into DNA → after reverse transcription → the viral DNA migrates to the nucleus of the cell → Nucleoside analog Reverse Transcriptase Inhibitors (NRTIs) and non-NRTIs bind to HIV reverse transcriptase → block DNA polymerase → preventing the production of a DNA copy of viral RNA (think of NRTIs and non-NRTIs as agents that are "unzipping" a zipper)
2. Integrase: used to integrate (insert) viral DNA into the DNA of the host CD4 cell → INtegrase Strand Transfer Inhibitors (INSTIs) inhibit the process of integration
3. Protease: used to cut the long HIV polyprotein chains into smaller functional HIV proteins to make a mature, infectious viral particles
   Protease inhibitors inhibit activation of HIV proteins and therefore, prevent this final step in the replication cycle

- Sexual transmission = most common means of **transmission** of HIV
- Worldwide, the most common epidemiological pattern is heterosexual transmission
- In the US male-to-male sexual transmission is more common, representing 67% of new cases.
- In the US, population groups disproportionately affected by HIV = African Americans and Hispanics
- Risk of seroconversion after needlestick from HIV + patient = 0.3%
- Risk of HIV from blood transfusion = 1/600,000 to 2,000,000
- Primary HIV occurs 2 to 4 weeks after exposure **(Acute Retroviral Syndrome)**
- **Presentation** = mono-like syndrome; Fever, fatigue, sore throat, lymphadenopathy (cervical most common), weight loss, myalgias, HA, N/V/D/, and maculopapular erythematous rash (most commonly on trunk) and leukopenia
- Develops in 40-90% patients; Diagnosis: HIV RNA assay

DIAGNOSIS

- HIV antigen/antibody test that detects HIV antibody as well as the p24 antigen Adding the p24 antigen shortens the "window period" where HIV could go undetected previously
- CD4 Count: predictor of susceptibility to opportunistic infections
- Viral Load: most important predictor of disease progression to AIDS and death

ACQUIRED IMMUNODEFICIENCY SYNDROME (AIDS)

HIV + AIDS defining condition OR CD4 count < 200 cells/mm3
< 200 cells/mm3 = development of opportunistic infections

AIDS PEARLS

- Most common GI symptom = Diarrhea
- Most common cause of diarrhea = Cryptosporidium (parasite) & CMV
- Most common cause of chronic diarrhea = Cryptosporidium & Isospora belli (parasite)
- Most common GI infection = Oral Candidiasis
- Most common cause of blindness in AIDS patient = CMV
- Most common cause of focal encephalitis = Toxoplasmosis (parasite)
- Most common neurologic problem = AIDS Dementia
- Most common opportunistic infection = Pneumocystis jiroveci pneumonia (fungus)
- Most common infectious cause of Adrenal Insufficiency in the US = HIV,
- worldwide TB; Most common cause of AI overall in US is autoimmune
- TB is 200-550x higher then general population; sputum AFB smears and cultures
- PPD + in early HIV often negative in late HIV
- PPD > 5mm = clinical TB infection
- Most common bacterial infection = Mycobacterium avium complex (MAC)
- Most common malignancy in AIDS patients = Kaposi's sarcoma (KS)
- KS associated with = Human herpesvirus 8 (HHV-8)

AIDS – GI PEARLS

- Oral/esophageal candidiasis: affects 80% of AIDS patients; white plaques are easily scraped off
- HSV Esophagitis
- Oral Kaposi Sarcoma (KS)
- Hairy Leukoplakia - EBV, white material on the tongue and palate in an HIV-positive patient that CANNOT be scraped off
- Viral Hepatitis: HBV / HCV
- Pancreatitis (medication side effects, viral injury, gall bladder disease)
- Proctitis (HSV, GC, Chlamydia, HPV, Enterobius vermicularis, trauma)
- Diarrhea - most frequent GI symptom /complaint = 50-90%; Causes: Salmonella, Shigella, Campylobacter, CMV, Cryptosporidium and Isospora

4 MALIGNANCIES THAT ARE CONSIDERED AIDS-DEFINING ILLNESSES:

1. Kaposi's sarcoma (most common)
2. Cervical cancer
3. Burkitt's lymphoma
4. Primary CNS lymphoma

PNEUMOCYSTIS

- Most common opportunistic infection in AIDS patients: *Pneumocystis jiroveci*
- Pneumocystis jiroveci formerly called "carinii"
- Still called PCP pneumonia ("Pneumocystis pneumonia")
- Ascomycetous fungus
- **Presentation:** Gradual onset of symptoms over weeks over 2-3 weeks; fever, non-productive cough and DOE which → dyspnea at rest
- **Labs:** LDH often elevated; CD4 count < 200
- **CXR:** bilateral interstitial infiltrates ("Bat wing" appearance), pneumothorax (bilateral) and pneumatoceles are common
- **Treatment:** Bactrim; if sulfa allergic: clindamycin + primaquine or pentamadine
- Steroids if PaO2 < 70 mmHg or Aa gradient > 35; steroids 15-30min before medications reduces respiratory failure and death

- **PEARL:** If **TB is suspected:** steroids are contraindicated
- **PEARL: PCP prophylaxis:** if history of PCP or CD4 count is < 200: TMP/ SMX 1 DS Q day or 3 times / week

- Most common cause of serious opportunistic viral infection in HIV patient = **CMV**
  - **CMV retinitis** is the most common cause of retinitis and blindness in AIDS patients
  - **Ophthalmic examination:** Cotton wool spots; yellow patches with or without hemorrhage ('cottage cheese and ketchup" appearance)
  - **Treatment:** Ganciclovir

- Most common bacterial infection with CD4 count < 50 patient
  - ***Mycobacterium avium complex (MAC)***
  - Diagnosis AFB in stool or other body fluids
  - **Treatment:** Rifabutin + Clarithromycin + Ethambutol

Most common cause of pneumonia in HIV / AIDS patients = still *Streptococcus pneumoniae*

HIGHLY ACTIVE ANTIRETROVIRAL THERAPY (HAART)

- HAART decreases the patient's total burden of HIV
- Treatment is now recommended for all HIV + positive patients as it reduces mortality as well as AIDS and non-AIDS related (cancer, cardiovascular disease, liver/renal disease) complications

ANTIRETROVIRAL THERAPY (ART)

- For most individuals, an ART regimen consists of a dual nucleoside combination (2 NRTIs) + a third agent from a different class

HIV MEDICATIONS

NON-NRTIS

Most commonly used non-NRTIs: Efavirenz (Sustiva) and Nevirapine (Virmaume)

Efavirenz, EFV (Sustiva)

- Side effects: Vivid dreams, HA, severe rash, anxiety, insomnia, dizziness, and lightheadedness.

Nevirapine, NVP (Virmaume)

- Side effects: Hepatotoxicity, TENS, SJS

PROTEASE INHIBITORS

Indinavir, IDV (Crixivan): protease inhibitor (inhibit activation of HIV proteins)

- Side effects: kidney stones, hyperbilirubinemia, and hepatitis

Lopinavir / Ritonavir, LPV/r (Kaletra): combination protease inhibitor

- Side effects: Hepatitis, N / V /D

INTEGRASE STRAND TRANSFER INHIBITORS (INSTIS)

Dolutegravir, DTG (Tivicay)

- Not prescribed to any person of childbearing age

Elvitegravir EVG (Vitekta)

- Not prescribed to any person of childbearing age

HIV MEDICATIONS - SIDE EFFECTS

NRTI medications the cause pancreatitis

Mnemonic (Z - LSD)

Drug, abbreviations (Brand Name in the US)

Z	**z**alcitabine (ddC); also 30% neuropathy
L	**L**amivudine, 3TC (Epivir)
S	**S**tavudine, d4T (Zerit); also 30% neuropathy
D	**D**idanosine, ddI (Videx); also 15% neuropathy

Zidovudine, AZT, ZDV (Retrovir)
NRTI associated with bone marrow suppression, anemia, and macrocytosis

NRTIs are also associated with lactic acidosis, if lactate > 2.5 NRTI should be stopped

TB 200 to 550x greater in AIDS patients
CXR: nonspecific; PPD may be nonreactive

TREATMENT OF TB IN HIV

Mnemonic - **(RIPE)**

R	**R**ifampin
I	**I**soniazid (INH)
P	**P**yrazinamide
E	**E**thambutol

OCCUPATIONAL POST-EXPOSURE PROPHYLAXIS (PEP)

Highest risk for transmission of blood borne disease = percutaneous exposure

HIV

- PEP given with mucous membrane exposure or skin compromise
- Tenofovir (Viread) Nucleoside reverse-transcriptase inhibitor (NRTI) + Emtricitabine (FTC) (Emtriva) Nucleoside reverse-transcriptase inhibitor (NRTI) + Raltegravir (RAL) (Isentress) Integrase inhibitor

- **PEARL:** Combo drug = emtricitabine/tenofovir (Truvada)
- **PEARL:** PEP reduces risk of HIV seroconversion by 80% if treated within 36 hours; no efficacy > 72 hours

HBV

- Prior vaccination: PEP not needed
- No prior immunization: HBIG + HBV vaccine

HCV: no PEP available

TOXOPLASMOSIS

Toxoplasma gondii

- Obligate intracellular parasite transmitted by cats or undercooked meat
- **Diagnosis:** Contrast Head CT: ring-enhancing lesions with surrounding edema
- CSF non-specific or normal
- Immunocompetent infected hosts are asymptomatic
- Latent infection can persist for lifetime
- Immunocompromised, HIV patient < CD4 100 = reactivate disease
- **Symptoms:** Fever, headache, AMS, seizures are common; 80% have focal neurological deficits
- **Treatment:** Pyrimethamine + Folinic acid (Leucovorin) (prevents heme toxicity from pyrimethamine) + Sulfadiazine or trimethoprim/sulfamethoxazole IV
- Life-time prophylaxis with trimethoprim/sulfamethoxazole

CRYPTOCOCCUS

Cryptococcus neoformans

- Most common opportunistic CNS fungal infection in AIDS patients:
- ↑↑ ICP; seizures uncommon
- **Presentation:** meningismus is uncommon F/HA/N/AMS/focal neuro deficits; photophobia
- CD4 count usually < 100; India Ink staining of CSF = 60-80% Sn
- CSF cryptococcal antigen = 100 % Sn & Sp
- **Imaging:** frequently shows no abnormality or cerebral atrophy without obstruction or other pathology; less commonly, hydrocephalus. Mass lesions (cryptococcomas) are seen in about 10%
- **Treatment:** 14-day course of Amphotericin + Flucytosine (both are fungicidal); followed by 8 weeks of Fluconazole (fungistatic) to clear the CSF of pathogen
- Life-time prophylaxis with Fluconazole

WEST NILE ENCEPHALITIS (WNE)

- Arthropod-borne virus (arbovirus) endemic to the Middle East and throughout US
- Transmitted by Aedes mosquito
- Birds serve as host
- Most patients remain asymptomatic or have a mild viral syndrome
- Maculopapular rash
- Meningoencephalitis < 1%
- Headache, fever, psychiatric symptoms, cognitive deficits, seizures, flaccid paralysis, and tremors;
- Bladder/bowel dysfunction; no sensory abnormalities
- Less common: mild hepatitis, rhabdomyolysis, hyponatremia, pancreatitis, myocarditis, myositis, orchitis
- Chorioretinitis: chorioretinal lesions multifocal with a "target-like" appearance
- **Serology / CSF:** pleocytosis - mostly lymphocytes, normal to elevated glucose, and increased protein
- Immunoglobulin M (IgM) antibodies in serum or CSF: the cornerstone of diagnosis
- Leukopenia with a pronounced and prolonged lymphopenia, which can aid in distinguishing it from other causes of encephalitis
- **Imaging:** MRI if needed
- **Treatment:** supportive

PEARL: Most women infected with WNV during pregnancy have delivered infants without evidence of infection; some evidence that transplacental transmission of WNV can occur

INFECTIOUS MONONUCLEOSIS

Most commonly caused by Epstein-Barr virus

- **Presentation / Exam:** low-grade fever, headache, malaise, severe fatigue, mildly tender lymphadenopathy), posterior cervical chain), hepatosplenomegaly (> 50%); Atypical lymphocytes on peripheral smear, > 50% lymphocytosis; transmitted via salivary secretions ("kissing disease")
- **Diagnosis:** heterophile antibody test (monospot test), or a generalized maculopapular rash following administration of amoxicillin
- **Treatment:** self-limiting, refrain from contact sports for 4 weeks post-infection
- **PEARL:** Antibiotics associated with morbilliform rash in a patient with infectious mononucleosis: Ampicillin and Amoxicillin

EPSTEIN-BARR VIRUS (EBV)

- Infectious mononucleosis
- B-cell lymphoma
- Hodgkin disease
- Burkitt lymphoma
- Nasopharyngeal carcinoma
- EBV can affect nearly all organ systems.
- Neurologic complications: encephalitis, meningitis, and Guillain-Barré (GBS)

LYME DISEASE

- *Borrelia burgdorferi* = spirochete
- Vector = Ixodes dammini / Ixodes scapularis – deer tick
- Zoonotic reservoirs = white-tail deer and white footed mouse
- Most prevalent in Northeast, mid-Atlantic states and upper Midwest
- Most common vector-borne disease in the US;
- Tick needs to be attached > 48 hours for transmission to occur;
- Only 50% remember tick bite

3 STAGES OF LYME DISEASE INFECTION

Stage 1
Early Localized Phase

- Erythema Chronicum Migrans (ECM): pathognomonic; 2 to 20 days after tick bite;
- Viral syndrome + ECM: sharply demarcated borders, blanching, large, flat or raised, central clearing, "bulls eye" appearance

Stage 2
Early Disseminated Phase

- Around 4 weeks after tick bite; fever, adenopathy arthralgias, 50% get multiple annular lesions which are the most characteristic component of Stage 2. Hematogenous spread leads to Diffuse Erythema Migrans' spares palms/soles
- Carditis: 8%; 1st degree AVB, Wenkebach, CHB
- CNS: unilateral or bilateral CN VII palsies (most common neuro symptom); peripheral neuropathy; memingoencephalitis

Stage 3
Late Phase

- > 1 year after infection; chronic arthritis (knee most common), myocarditis, chronic encephalopathy, peripheral neuropathy.

INITIAL SCREENING

- Two-Step testing of blood for specific antibodies; it takes 4 to 6 weeks to develop antibodies (antibody testing often negative in early LD)
- Enzyme immunoassay (EIA) or immunofluorescence assay (IFA) —> followed by Western Blot (WB) to confirm diagnosis
- CSF: detect using PCR

MANAGEMENT APPROACH

- Post-Exposure Prophylaxis: Recommended if deer tick is attached at least
- 36 hours: Doxycycline 200mg po x1
- Treatment for Early or Mild Disseminated Infection: Doxycycline or Amoxicillin 14-21 days
- Patients with neurologic or cardiac manifestations should be admitted and treated with IV Ceftriaxone

BABESIOSIS

- ***Babesia microti*** (NE US) and ***Babesia gibsoni*** (NW US) and ***B. divergens*** (Europe) = protozoan
- Vector = Ixodes dammini – deer tick (same vector as Lyme disease)
- Zoonotic reservoirs = deer, rodents and domesticated mammals (cattle, horses, dogs and cats)
- Malaria-like disease; protozoan similar in structure and life-cycle to plasmodia
- Blood transfusions have been implicated in transmission of babesiosis
- 20% have concurrent Lyme disease
- Viral syndrome presentation with ↑ spiking fevers; hepatosplenomegaly; emotional lability
- ↓thrombocytopenia, ↓leukopenia, ↑LFTs, renal failure (dark urine)
- Hemolytic anemia = ↑IBIL, ↑reticulocyte count, ↑LDH, ↓haptoglobin
- Diagnosis = intra-erythrocytic parasite on Giemsa stained peripheral blood smear
    - (“Maltese Cross” formation)
- Treatment = Clindamycin + Quinine or Atovaquone + Zithro [12, 6th ed., pg 973] and [10, 5th ed., pg 1869]

RELAPSING FEVER

Borrelia recurrentis = spirochete [12, 6th ed., pg 1256]

- Vector = lice (singular: louse) or ticks
- Zoonotic reservoirs = humans and wild rodents [12, 6th ed. pg 973]
- Viral syndrome presentation
- ↑LFTs,↓thrombocytopenia, ↓BP; severe cases → meningoencephalitis, DIC, liver failure, myocarditis
- Relapsing fevers
- Diagnosis = thick smear (similar to Malaria)
- Treatment = Tetracycline 200 mg po or Erythromycin 1gm po x one dose

EHRLICHOSIS

- *Ehrlichia chaffeensis;* Gram-negative coccobacilli
- *Anaplasma phagocytophilum* Gram-negative
- South Central, South Atlantic and upper Midwest United States
- 90% of patients recall tick bite; June-August
- **Vector:** Ixodes scapularis (deer tick); Amblyomma americanum (Lone star tick)
- **Zoonotic reservoirs:** White-tailed deer; white-footed mouse
- dogs and other mammals
- Infects circulating leukocytes → maculopapular rash 20%
- Abrupt onset of fever, HA, myalgias and shaking chills; jaundice, vomiting and diarrhea rare (Pearl: Lyme does not present abruptly)
- **Labs:** 50 to 90% of patients have ↓leukopenia ↓thrombocytopenia, ↑LFTs; rarely encephalitis and renal failure
- **Diagnosis:** suspected if clinical features + exposure
  - Confirmed
  - 1. Antibody titers
  - 2. PCR assay for organism-specific DNA
  - 3. Identification of morulae in leukocytes
  - 4. Immunostaining on biopsy
  - 5. Culture
- **Treatment:** Doxycycline 100mg po bid x 7 to 14 days

Q-FEVER

- ***Coxiella burnetii;*** intracellular, small Gram-negative
- **Vector**: tick; more common route of infection = inhalation of organisms from air that contains airborne barnyard dust contaminated by dried placental material, birth fluids, and excreta of infected herd animals
- **Zoonotic reservoirs:** livestock (cattle, sheep, goats), cats
- 50% infected with C. burnetii show signs of clinical illness. ↑ Chills /Fever (104-105° F), fever with relative bradycardia severe HA, myalgias, non-productive cough, N/V/D, abdominal pain, and CP. 30-50% of symptomatic infection will develop pneumonia.
- Atypical pneumonia, meningitis, endocarditis, granulomatous hepatitis
- **Treatment:** Doxycycline , Azithromycin or Quinolone

ROCKY MOUNTAIN SPOTTED FEVER

- Despite the name, most cases occur along the eastern coastline, Northeast, Southeast, and South
- Rickettsia rickettsii; intracellular, Gram negative
- **Vector:** Dermacentor tick
- **Zoonotic reservoirs:** deer, horses, cattle, cats, dogs or rodents

- **Classic triad:** fever, rash, and history of tick exposure (20%)
- **Rash**: Blanching maculopapular rash; starts on palms/soles, wrists/ankles
- Rash spreads centripetally (from ankles/wrists —> trunk)
- Evolves into purpura, petechiae, or red lesions with a purplish core
- **PEARL: Rumpel-Leede Phenomenon** = petechiae formation after BP cuff inflation
- Fever with relative bradycardia; lymphadenopathy, jaundice, hepatomegaly, splenomegaly, HA, myalgias, abdominal pain, N /V/D, AKI, photophobia; myocarditis, meningitis or encephalitis
- Myalgias; Calf pain COMMON

- **PEARL:** calf pain also with Leptospirosis
- **Diagnosis:** Clinical; Skin Biopsy
- **Labs:** hyponatremia, neutropenia, thrombocytopenia, and elevated liver enzymes
- CSF: pleocytosis, no organism
- Treatment: Doxycycline (even children)

TULAREMIA

- *Francisella tularensis,* small, Gram Neg, aerobic, rod
- Forms of *F. tularensis* infection recognized in humans include: Ulceroglandular (80%, chancer- like ulcer - with raised margins), Glandular, Oculoglandular, Oropharyngeal, Typhoidal/Septicemic and Pneumonic
- Transmission:
  - Direct penetration of the skin (hair follicles, or cuts/abrasions or contaminated by exposure of an infected animal)
  - Indirectly from bites of deerflies, ticks or mosquitoes (bacterium not isolated in saliva; scratch after bite → introduce infected feces)
  - Exposure of mucous membranes with blood or tissue of infected animals
  - (rabbits, squirrels, foxes, skunks, mice, rats)
  - Ingestion of contaminated food or water
- Inhalation
  - Regardless of presenting form of tularemia systemic symptoms of *fever with relative bradycardia in 42%,* chills and rigors, myalgias (often prominent in low back), weakness, malaise and headache
  - Treatment: Streptomycin; alternative = Gentamicin

TRAVEL CHEMOPROPHYLAXIS

- http://www.cdc.gov/travel

DENGUE FEVER

- Arbovirus; Most common serious febrile tropical disease after malaria
- Mosquito transmission = *Aedes aegypti* (day biting mosquito)
- Incubation period = 4 to 7 days
- Asymptomatic or viral syndrome presentation with rash:
- Acute onset of severe HA, myalgias and arthralgias *("Break-Bone Fever")*
- Facial flushing, conjunctival injection, retro-orbital pain and facial edema *("Dengue Facies")*
- Rash = macular or maculopapular on trunk spreads → extremities and face
- Note: West Nile virus (transmitted by *Culex* mosquito) = lymphadenopathy → **absent** in Dengue

DENGUE HEMORRHAGIC FEVER (DHF)

- A small percentage of previously infected patients develop → DHF
- Begins as classic Dengue Fever followed by→
- Hemorrhagic pleural effusions, purpura, petechiae, bleeding diathesis
- Diagnosis = ELISA IgM; lab = ↓leukopenia, ↓thrombocytopenia, false ↑Hct, ↑LFTs; ↓Na (most common electrolyte abnormality); ↑PT/PTT, ↓fibrinogen and ↑fibrin degradation products
- Supportive care; Treat fever with Tylenol not NSAIDs due anticoagulant properties.

DENGUE SHOCK SYNDROME

- Circulatory failure (↓BP, Altered mental status, ↑ HR, Altered MS, cool/clammy, narrow pulse pressure with ↑ peripheral vascular resistance

HANTAVIRUSES

- Inhale material contaminated with mouse urine/feces → hemorrhagic fever + renal failure *or*
- Syndrome of severe respiratory failure and shock

- ↑leukocytosis with atypical lymphs, ↓thrombocytopenia
- CXR = bilateral interstitial infiltrates in dependent areas
- Death from CV collapse; Mortality rate 6%, if respiratory syndrome mortality much higher

MALARIA

Most deadly vector-borne disease in the world

5 species of malaria are known to infect humans:

- ***Plasmodium falciparum*** (most common), ***vivax, malariae, ovale*** and ***knowlesi*** = protozoa
- Over 90% of malaria seen in he US is due to *P. falciparum or P. vivax*
- Mosquito transmission = Female Anopheles (bite at dusk and dawn)
- Also direct transmission → blood transfusion & mother → fetus

- Viral syndrome presentation: Paroxysm shivering and chills → followed by ↑fever → when ↓ fever → patient diaphoretic /exhausted → paroxysms of malaria (correspond to length of asexual erythrocytic cycles; merozoites invade RBC's → cells lyse → new merozoites further invade uninfected RBCs); less common symptoms = N/V/D/HA and jaundice

- ***P. falciparum*** = most deadly form of malaria; complications = cerebral malaria, ↓hypoglycemia (parasites metabolize glucose from RBCs; especially children), metabolic acidosis, severe ↓anemia, renal failure, pulmonary edema, DIC and death

- Blackwater fever = dark urine secondary to RBC hemolysis from high parasitemia

Malaria Diagnosis

- Giemsa or Wright's - stained thin and thick blood smears

Malaria Treatment

- Treatment of adults and children with uncomplicated *P. falciparum* malaria (except pregnant women in first trimester)
- 3-day treatment with artemisinin combination therapy (ACT) using any of the following:
  - Artemether/lumefantrine
  - Artesunate/amodiaquine
  - Artesunate/mefloquine
  - Dihydroartemisinin/piperaquine
  - Artesunate plus sulfadoxine/pyrimethamine

Treatment of uncomplicated *P. falciparum* malaria in special risk patients

- Treat women in first trimester of pregnancy with 7 days of quinine plus clindamycin
- Treat infants weighing < 5 kg with an ACT at same mg/kg target dose as children weighing 5 kg

Treatment of Severe Malaria

- Aretesunate IV followed by either artemether/lumefantrine, atovaquone/proguanil, doxycycline, clindamycin (if pregnant), or mefloquine (if other options not available)
- Aretesunate only available from CDC 770-488-7788

Do not use Primaquine if glucose-6-phosphate dehydrogenase deficiency → hemolysis of RBCs

- Quinine given po or IV; if rapid infusion → ↓ profound hypoglycemia
- Other side effects = ↓BP and cardiac dysrhythmias

LEPTOSPIROSIS

World's most widespread zoonotic infection; common in tropical climates

- Leptospira interrogans = spirochete
- Fresh water contaminated by bovine, pig, canine or rat urine; 2 to 20 days incubation
- Leptospires multiply in the small blood vessel endothelium
- Two syndromes: anicteric (which is self-limiting) 90% of cases and icteric leptospirosis (Weil's disease) which is more severe form characterized by multi-organ failure
- Two distinct phases of illness observed in the mild anicteric form → septicemic (acute) phase and the immune (delayed) phase. In icteric leptospirosis, the 2 phases of illness are often continuous and indistinguishable
- Viral syndrome presentation with severe ↑HA, petechial rash which may involve the palate, conjunctival injection, myalgias (calf, low back) and **fever with relative bradycardia**

  → Symptoms resolve after 4 to 7 days, followed by → asymptomatic period or progress directly→more severe disease
- Aseptic meningitis, hepatitis/liver failure, nephritis/RF, uveitis, rash (jaundice and purpura), TTP, HUS, DIC, pneumonitis/consolidation due to alveolar hemorrhage, acalculous cholecystitis, pancreatitis, myocarditis → CHF, Afib and rarely CV collapse
- → May last up to 4 weeks
- Mortality rate in icteric leptospirosis (Weil's disease) = 5 to 40%
- **Diagnosis:** isolate leptospires from blood or CSF
- Oral Doxycycline or Amoxicillin if treated within first 3 days
- Penicillin or Ampicillin IV for severe cases

LEISHMANIASIS

- Leishmania: intracellular protozoan
- Transmission: Lutzomyia or Phlebotomus → sandflies
- (Rural Africa, Asia, Mediterranean basin, Central/South America, Brazil, India and Sudan
- ↑ Leishmaniasis in returning U.S. military personnel and their dependents from the Middle East, especially from Iraq (mainly cutaneous)

Clinical Syndromes

1. Cutaneous = most common
2. Mucocutaneous = chronic and relentless disease complicated by secondary infections and pneumonia
3. Diffuse Cutaneous = chronic, difficult to treat, few resulting deaths
4. Visceral (Kala-azar or Black fever) = most fatal form caused by Leishmania donovani

- Darkening of skin is characteristic = Kala-azar or black fever; lymphadenopathy
- "Kala-azar" comes from India → Hindi for black fever
- Infiltration of the hematopoietic system → pancytopenia

- ↑ mortality due to secondary infections (pneumonia, TB, dysentery); hemorrhage or severe anemia
- Pentad: fever, weight loss, ↑ hepatosplenomegaly, ↓pancytopenia and hypergammaglobulinemia

- **Diagnosis:** aspirate bone marrow, spleen, lymph nodes or punch biopsy from ulcer edge
- Stained smears: Leishman-Donovan bodies = stained amastigotes in macrophages
- Treatment of cutaneous leishmaniasis where the potential for mucosal spread is low, topical Paromycin
- **Treatment: Pentavalent Antimonial compounds;** injection only; call CDC for this one
- If failure/resistance, use Amphotercin

BACTERIAL FOLLICULITIS

- *Staphylococcus aureus* most common cause of bacterial folliculitis
- Mild *S. aureus* folliculitis with a few pustules may resolve without medical treatment
- *S. aureus* folliculitis that persists; topical antibiotic therapy
- **Treatment:** topical mupirocin or topical clindamycin
- More extensive *S. aureus* folliculitis or *S. aureus* folliculitis that fails to resolve or recurs after topical treament - treatment options include: dicloxacillin and cephalexin If MRSA suspected: trimethoprim/ sulfamethoxazole, Clindamycin, or Doxycycline

- **PEARL**: **Pseudofolliculitis barbae (PFB)** or shaving bumps - no antibiotics
- More common in African Americans

- Hot tub folliculits: **Pseudomonas follicultits** generally self-limited; no antibiotics
- Etiology: exposure to inadequately chlorinated swimming pools and hot tubs; Oral ciprofloxacin 500 mg twice daily can be used for severe cases or immunocompromised patients

CELLULITIS (INCLUDING ERYSIPELAS)

- Bacterial infection underneath the skin surface characterized by redness, warmth, swelling, and pain
- Most common cause: β-hemolytic streptococci Groups A, B, C, G and F
- Most common group = group *A Streptococcus (Strep pyogenes*)
- *S. aureus* (including MRSA) is less common cause

CELLULITIS

- Involves the deeper dermis and subcutaneous fat
- More common in middle-aged and older adults

ERYSIPELAS

- Involves the upper dermis and superficial lymphatics
- More common in young children and older adults
- Acute onset of symptoms
- Systemic manifestations, including F / C / HA, severe malaise
- There is clear demarcation between involved and uninvolved tissue
- Classic descriptions: "butterfly" involvement of the face
- Vast majority of erysipelas cases are caused by Strep pyogenes
- Involvement of the ear (Milian's ear sign) is a distinguishing feature for erysipelas, since this region does not contain deeper dermis tissue

IMPETIGO

Group A Strep (Strep Pyogenes)
Staph aureus

BULLOUS IMPETIGO

Staph aureus

NECROTIZING FASCIITIS

- Hallmark: Pain out of proportion to exam
- Toxic appearing
- Crepitus (Type I) may precede skin findings of erythema and blistering
- Late: pain may subside as nerves become damaged from necrosis and gangrene
- Most common risk factor = DM

CLASSIFICATION

- **Polymicrobial (Type I)**
  - Anaerobic species: Most commonly Bacteroides, Clostridium, or Peptostreptococcus
  - Aerobic enterobacteriaceae: E. coli, Enterobacter, Klebsiella, Proteus
  - Pseudomonas aeruginosa (Obligate aerobe) - rarely component of such mixed infections

- **Monomicrobial (Type II)**
  - GAS or other beta-hemolytic streptococci
  - Infection may also occur as a result of Staphylococcus aureus

- Presence of gas in soft tissue on radiographic imaging (CT with IV contrast preferred)
  - Type I = gas present
  - Type II = gas absent

TREATMENT

- Empiric antibiotic treatment: Piperacillin-tazobactam + Vancomycin + Clindamycin
- Surgical consult for debridement

CELLULITIS AFTER WOUND IN FRESH WATER LAKE: CONSIDER AEROMONAS HYDROPHILIA

- **Treatment:** Quinolone; alternate: Bactrim
- **PEARL:** If mild Aeromonas hydrophilia folliculits: no treatment

MENINGITIS PEARLS

- > 1st year of life, you can assess nuchal rigidity. Two signs of meningeal irritation: **Kernig's** and **Brudzinski's**
- **Kernig's sign:** with patient lying supine, hip and knee flexed to about 90°, knee extension → in meningeal irritation → neck pain (Kernig's - Knee)
- **Brudzinski's sign:** with the patient supine, passive flexion of the neck → involuntary flexion in the hips, if there is meningeal irritation (meningitis, SAH or encephalitis); Brudzinski's - Bend the brain
- Sensorineural hearing loss is a complication of herpes and *Haemophilus influenzae* meningitis and less common with meningococcal meningitis

COMMON CAUSES OF NEONATAL SEPSIS / MENINGITIS (< 1 MONTH)

Mnemonic: GEL

G	Group B Strep. (Strep. agalactiae) Most common cause 49%
E	E. coli 18%
L	Listeria 7%

TREATMENT OF NEONATAL MENINGITIS

- Ampicillin (will cover Listeria) 50 mg/kg q 6 hrs (max dose 2 grams) + Cefotaxime (Claforan) 200 mg/kg/day divided q 6-8 hrs (max dose 2 grams) or Gentamycin
- If CSF pleocytosis and negative gram stain consider adding Acyclovir empirically for HSV

MOST COMMON CAUSES OF BACTERIAL MENINGITIS > 1 MONTH TO 50 YEARS

- *Streptococcus pneumoniae* and *Neisseria meningitidis*. Less common cause *H. Influenzae*
- *N. meningitidis* : the most common cause of meningitis in young adults age 16 to 21
- **PEARL:** If > 50 years or alcoholism or other debilitating associated diseases or impaired cellular immunity consider Listeria
- **PEARL:** *Listeria monocytogenes* risk > 60x ↑ in AIDS patients and 3/4 present with meningitis
- **PEARL**: Most common cause of **focal encephalitis** in patients with AIDS: ***Toxoplasma gondii***

TREATMENT OF MENINGITIS > 1 MONTH TO 50 YEARS

- Dexamethasone + Ceftriaxone or Cefotaxime + Vancomycin
- Ceftriaxone: 100 mg/kg (2 gm IV max) q 12 hrs
- Dexamethasone: 0.15 mg/kg IV q 6 hrs x 2 to 4 days; give 15 min prior or con-comitant with first dose of antibiotic to prevent neurologic complications
- Vancomycin:15 mg/kg IV q 6 hours; Adults max dose of 2-3 gm/day is suggested: 500 to 750mg IV q 6 hours
- If > 50 years or alcoholism or other debilitating associated diseases or impaired cellular immunity add, Amplicillin 2gm IV q4h to regimen above cover possible *Listeria*
- Regimens are most effective in started as early as possible

- **PEARL: Encephalitis:** presence of abnormal brain function (AMS, focal neurologic deficits, altered behavior, and speech or movement)
- **PEARL: Sensorineural hearing loss** is a complication of herpes and *Haemophilus Influenzae* meningitis and less common with meningococcal meningitis

LP may be performed without Head CT in some patient groups during evaluation for meningitis

- Age less than 60
- Immunocompetent
- No history of CNS disease
- No recent seizure
- Alert and oriented
- No papilledema
- No focal neurologic deficits
- Signs suspicious for **space-occupying lesions:** papilledema and focal neurologic deficits

RING-ENHANCING BRAIN LESIONS ON CT

- Bacterial abscess
- Toxoplasmosis
- Cryptococcosis
- Neoplasm (e.g., glioma, lymphoma)
- Cysticercosis
- Vascular malformations
- Granulomatous disease
- Multiple sclerosis
- Infarction
- Tuberculoma
- Cerebral contusion

LUMBAR PUNCTURE (LP) PEARLS

- Conus Medullaris ends at
  - Infants = L2-L3
  - Adults = L1-L2
- Interspace level for LP
  - Infant = L4-L5 and L5-S1
  - Children and adults
  - L3-L4
  - L4-L5
- **PEARL:** The decision to perform a head CT before lumbar puncture should not prevent the immediate administration of antibiotics

Although the yield of CSF cultures and CSF Gram stain may be diminished by antimicrobial therapy given prior to LP, pretreatment blood cultures and CSF findings (i.e., elevated WBC count, diminished glucose concentration, and elevated protein concentration) will likely provide evidence for or against the diagnosis of bacterial meningitis

TYPICAL CSF CHARACTERISTIC OF NORMAL & INFECTED HOSTS

Case	Color	Opening Pressure	WBC	Glucose	Protein
Normal Infant	Clear	< 180 mm	< 10mm3	> 40 mg/dL	90 mg/dL
Normal child or Adult	Clear	< 180 mm	0	> 40	< 40
Bacterial Meningitis	Cloudy	> 200 mm	200-10,000 (> 80% PMN)	< 40	100 – 150
Viral Meningitis	Clear	< 180 mm	25-1,000 (< 50% PMN)	> 40	50-100
Cryptococcal Meningitis	Clear	> 200 mm	50-1,000 (< 50% PMN)	< 40	50-300

NEISSERIA MENINGITIDIS PROPHYLAXIS - CLOSE CONTACTS

- Close contacts should be treated with prophylactic antibiotics to prevent meningitis
- A close contact includes:
  - Anyone that was within 3 feet of the patient for > 8 hours in the week prior to their illness (housemates, intimate partners)
  - Anyone with direct exposure to oral secretions (e.g. kissing, endotracheal intubation, suctioning)

- Droplet precautions at least until 24 hours after antibiotics started
- Prophylactic regimens include:
  - Ceftriaxone
  - Ciprofloxacin
  - Rifampin

SPINAL EPIDURAL ABSCESS

Classic triad:
1. Localized severe back pain
2. Fever
3. Neurologic deficits (motor/sensory deficits, loss of bowel or bladder function)

- The triad is rare; back pain in 85-90%, fever 35-60%;
- Most common cause = hematogenous spread
- Risk factors: DM, IVDA, CRF, endocarditis, recent back surgery, epidural puncture, alcoholism, and immunosuppression
- Most common organism = Staphylococcus aureus: Other: streptococci, anaerobes, gram-negative bacilli, and Pseudomonas aeruginosa
- MRI is the diagnostic modality of choice; Lumbar 60% > thoracic 30% > cervical 10%;
- Erythrocyte sedimentation rate (ESR) is a sensitive screening marker; ESR will always be elevated; order blood cultures
- **Treatment:** Cefepime 2gm IV q 8 hours + Vancomycin 15-20 mg/kg IV q 8-12 hours; Neurosurgical consult

TRICHINOSIS

- Parasitic disease caused by roundworms of the Trichinella type
- Undercooked pork
- N / V / D / crampy abdominal pain, elevated CPK
- Diagnosis: Muscle biopsy; ELISA
- Treatment: mebendazole + steroids (reduce muscle inflammation)

CYSTICERCOSIS

- Infection caused by the eggs of Taenia solium, or pork tapeworm
- Most common parasitic infestation affecting the central nervous system (CNS)
- Approximately 90% of patients with cysticercosis have CNS involvement
- Cerebral cysticercosis: patient will present with new onset seizures and a history of eating undercooked pork

- **Head CT:** cystic lesions, ring enhancing lesions, and calcifications
- Viable cysts are round, nonenhancing hypodense lesions usually 5 to 20 mm in diameter; As the cyst begins to degenerate, the cyst wall increases in density and is often accompanied by edema or contrast enhancement. Following collapse of the cyst, a residual calcified granuloma may be present
- Calcifications are solid, nodular lesions 2 to 4 mm in diameter (range 1 to 10 mm)
- Calcified lesions are usually non-enhancing but may be associated with perilesional edema in some cases
- Treatment is not always indicated but if started is usually albendazole + steroids +/- praziquantal +/- antiseizure medication

ENCAPSULATED ORGANISMS

Mneumonic: Some Nasty Killers Have Some Capsule Protection

Some	**S**treptococcus pneumonia
Nasty	**N**eisseria meningitides
Killers	**K**lebsiella pneumonia
Have	**H**aemophilus influenzae
Some	**S**almonella
Capsule	**C**ryptococcus neoformans (yes a fungus with a capsule)
Protection	**P**seudomonas aeruginosa

AMPC BETA-LACTAMASE (AMPC) PRODUCING ORGANISMS

(Enzymes which convey resistance to penicillins, second and third generation cephalosporins)

Mneumonic: SPICE

S	**S**erratia
P	**P**rvovidencia
I	**I** "Indole-positive" Proteus sp (does not include Proteus Mirabilis)
C	**C**itrobacter
E	**E**nterobacter

Also, Cronobacter, Edwardsiella, Hagnia, Morganella, Aeromonas, Pseudomonas and Acinetobacter

TETANUS

- Inhibits release of inhibitory (GABA) neurotransmitter → continuous stimulation by excitatory neurotransmitter
- Initial symptoms: trismus ("lock jaw" = risus saronicus - think of the Joker from Batman), dysphagia → and then progressing in a descending fashion to the the muscles of the neck, trunk, and extremities; rigidity of muscles (opisthotonos); diaphoresis, HTN and tachycardia

Tetanus Treatment

- Supportive, opioids and Benzodiazepines
- Tetanus immune globulin (TIG) near the site of the wound
- Metronidazole (Flagyl)
- Muscle relaxant
- Neuromuscular blockade

RABIES - RABIES PEP REGIMEN

Product	Recommended time of administration
HRIG	Day 0 (if not administered on day 0 can be given up to and including day 7 of the first dose of vaccine)
Administration details 20 IU/kg If anatomically feasible, infiltrate the bite wound with the full dose. Any remaining volume should be given IM at a site distant from vaccine administration. The deltoid, (opposite arm from where vaccine is given) is recommended. If a non-bite exposure occurred, HRIG can be given IM at a site distant from vaccine administration (deltoid opposite arm from where vaccine is given). Not needed for patient previously given full series of rabies PEP or patient pre-exposure vaccinated for rabies.	

Product	Recommended time of administration
Rabies VACCINE dose 1	Day 0
Administration details Administered IM. In deltoid for adults. For small children, anterolateral aspect of the thigh is also acceptable The gluteal area should NEVER be used because it results in lower titers. **Rabies vaccine dose 2** Day 3 See vaccine dose 1 information **Rabies vaccine dose 3** Day 7 See vaccine dose 1 information **Rabies vaccine dose 4** Day 14 See vaccine dose 1 information **Rabies vaccine dose 5** (for immunocompromised patients only) Day 28 See vaccine dose 1 information	

RABIES PEARLS

- **Major carriers:** raccoons (30%) > bats (29%) > skunks (26%); others = cats, dogs, cattle, coyotes, foxes, mongooses and beavers
- **The gold standard for diagnosis:** histological evaluation of the grey matter - visualization of Negri Bodies (eosinophilic intracellular lesions in which viral replication takes place within in the CNS) is pathognomonic for infection with the rabies virus.

PEDICULOSIS CAPITIS (HEAD LICE)

- Nits (eggs) are attached to the host's hair and are difficult to remove (unlike dandruff)
- Nit (egg) → hatches in 8 days → Nymphs → Nymphs become adults
- Itching develops secondary to patient's hypersensitivity reaction to saliva and fecal material of louse; itching that gets worse at night
- Posterior cervical and occipital lymphadenopathy; excoriation, and secondary bacterial infection from scratching
- Transmitted by close personal contact and contact with infected objects (direct contact, lice do NOT jump, fly or use vectors)
- Infection outbreaks: schools, daycare facilities, nursing homes, and families
- **Treatment:** Permethrin (safe in pregnancy and children < 2 years old);
- 95% cure rate
- Permethrin causes respiratory paralysis of adult louse, however, it is NOT effective on recently laid eggs
- Applied to dry hair and requires REPEAT treatment in 2 weeks to remove any eggs that were present during the first application
- Available as over-the-counter medication and in a prescription strength formula
- **PEARL:** Avoid Lindane anyone weighing < 50 kg and children < 2 years old, associated with seizure activity
- **PEARL:** Mayonnaise will kill adult lice in < 10 minutes

BIOLOGICAL TERRORISM

ANTHRAX

Bacillus anthracis

- Gram-positive (+), spore-forming, rod with capsule
- Exists in environment as a spore
- Spore persists in soil for decades
- Germinates into virulent form upon ingestion or inoculation into animal host

Four (4) syndromes defined by route of exposure

- Cutaneous anthrax
- Inhalational anthrax
- Gastrointestinal anthrax
- Injectional anthrax

PLAGUE

Yersinia pestis

- Gram-negative (-) coccobacilli, capsule
- Resembles a safety pin
- Facultative intracellular anaerobe

Three (3) syndromes

- Bubonic plague
- Pneumonic plague
- Septicemic plague

TULAREMIA

Francisella tularensis

- Small, non-motile, aerobic, gram-negative (-) coccobacillus
- One of the most infectious pathogenic bacteria known. It requires inoculation or inhalation of as few as 10 organisms to cause disease
- Several Types
  - Pulmonary – bioterrorism option
  - Ulceroglandular (accounts for about 75%-80% of cases)
  - Oculoglandular: eye becomes painful, swollen, and red, and pus
  - Oropharyngeal
  - Typhoidal
    - Accounts for about 20%-25% of cases
    - Characterized by fever, abdominal pain, hepatosplenomegaly

CUTANEOUS MANIFESTATIONS OF BIOWEAPONS

CUTANEOUS ANTHRAX

- Painless, depressed, black necrotic eschar (anthrax = Greek for "coal")
- Begins as a papule → vesicle → painful lymphadenopathy -> after about a week → black necrotic eschar
- After next 2-3 weeks eschar sloughs off and illness is over or you become bacteremic and die
- Mortality without antibiotic treatment =20%
- Mortality with antibiotic treatment = 1%
- Investigation by CDC of 2001 U.S. bioterrorism anthrax attacks, 11 cases, none fatal

BUBONIC PLAGUE

- Most common form of plague
- Incubation period for 2 to 8 days
- Viral syndrome
- Fever + regional lymph node infection (buboes)
- Femoral lymph nodes most common > inguinal > axillary > cervical
- Erythemetous, warm, very painful, tender, swollen lymph nodes (buboes) with considerable surrounding edema
- Buboes usually non-fluctuant and rarely, suppurate
- Mortality rate 5-15% with treatment

SEPTICEMIC PLAGUE

- Primary Septicemic Plague – no detectable buboes
- Septicemia can occur secondarily to pneumonic or bubonic plague
- About 10-20% of cases
- Begins with GI symptoms -> progresses to systemic symptoms
- Fever + hypotension, ARDS
- Acral gangrene ("black death")
- Mortality rate = 20-90%

ULCEROGLANDULAR TULAREMIA

- Viral syndrome
- Erythematous, tender papule at inoculation site → becomes pustular → ulcerates within days; painful open sores (ulcers)
- The local ulcer is raised with sharply demarcated margins with depressed center (chancriform)
- Painful, swollen lymphadenopathy at site of inoculation

TRICHOTHECENE MYCOTOXINS ("YELLOW RAIN")

- Protein synthesis inhibitors and inhibit mitochondrial respiration and cause bone marrow suppression; 400x more potent than mustard in producing skin injury/ ↑blisters
- Charcoal binds mycotoxins

SMALLPOX

- Smallpox rash has a **centrifugal** distribution and spread.Rash begins on the face and upper extremities, spreads to lower extremities and finally the trunk over 7 days. All lesions are **synchronous** (in the same phase of development at a given time), umbilicated, deeply embedded in the dermis, are painful and non-pruritic; rash may involve the palm and soles
- Patients are infectious from the time the rash first appears until all scabs fall off. (1-2 weeks)
- Smallpox vaccine can lessen the severity/prevent illness if given within 3 days of exposure
- Vaccination within 4-7 days may modify severity of illness
- **PEARL:** Chickenpox rash is pruritic, starts on the trunk does not involve palms/soles and the rash is **asynchronous**
- **PEARL:** Chickenpox illness usually lasts 4 to 7 days vs Smallpox which lasts 14 to 21 days

PULMONARY MANIFESTATIONS OF BIOWEAPONS

INHALATIONAL ANTHRAX

- Viral syndrome with non-productive cough; rhinorrhea ***uncommon***
- Patient may improve before acute deterioration within 24 to 48 hours → diaphoresis, dyspnea, stridor, cyanosis, hemorrhagic mediastinitis, septic shock, death; 50% hemorrhagic meningitis
- **CXR**: Wide mediastinum, hemorrhagic pleural effusions. Results from U.S. anthrax attacks 2001 from first 10 patients = 7 had infiltrates, multilobar in 3 patients

PNEUMONIC PLAGUE

- Pneumonia and hemoptysis
- Viral syndrome: fever, chest pain and dyspnea
- **CXR**: bilateral infiltrates or lobar consolidation; any pattern possible, including ARDS
- Within 24 hours without treatment → fulminant pneumonia associated with hemoptysis, septic shock, DIC, respiratory failure, circulatory collapse and death; 6-10% get meningitis
- Mortality rate nears 100%

PULMONARY TULAREMIA

- Initial picture of systemic illness without prominent signs of respiratory disease: abrupt onset of high fever with relative bradycardia in 42%, chills, rigors, malaise, sore throat, headache and pleuritic CP, myalgias (often prominent in low back) and non-productive cough
- **CXR**
  - Earliest radiographic finding = peribronchial infiltrates
  - Advancing to bronchopneumonia in one or more lobes
  - Hilar lymphadenopathy and effusions are common

BIOTERROISM AGENTS - TREATMENT

https://www.uptodate.com/contents/treatment-of-anthrax

CUTANEOUS ANTHRAX WITHOUT SYSTEMIC INVOLVEMENT

NON-PREGNANT ADULTS:

- Ciprofloxacin 500 mg every 12 hours or
- Doxycycline 100 mg every 12 hours or
- Levofloxacin 750 mg every 24 hours or
- Moxifloxacin 400 mg every 24 hours

PREGNANT, LACTATING, AND POSTPARTUM WOMEN:

- Ciprofloxacin 500 mg every 12 hours

CHILDREN

- Ciprofloxacin 30 mg/kg per day divided every 12 hours (not to exceed 500 mg/dose)
  or
  For penicillin-susceptible strains (MIC ≤0.5 mcg/mL), amoxicillin 75 mg/kg per day divided every 8 hours (not to exceed 1 g/dose)

Alternatives include:

- Doxycycline
  <45 kg: 4.4 mg/kg per day divided every 12 hours (not to exceed 100 mg/dose)
  ≥45 kg: 100 mg every 12 hours or
- Clindamycin 30 mg/kg per day divided every 8 hours (not to exceed 600 mg/dose) or Levofloxacin
  <50 kg: 16 mg/kg per day divided every 12 hours (not to exceed 250 mg/dose)
  ≥50 kg: 500 mg every 24 hours

ANTHRAX WITH SYSTEMIC INVOLVEMENT

Systemic anthrax is defined as anthrax meningitis; inhalation, injection, and gastrointestinal anthrax. Patients with cutaneous anthrax with extensive edema or lesions of the head or neck should also be treated according to the recommendations for systemic anthrax

- Ciprofloxacin 400 mg IV every 8 (eight) hours ***PLUS*** Clindamycin 900 mg every 8 hours or Linezolid 600 mg every 12 hours

- PEDS: Ciprofloxacin 30mg/kg per day divided every 8 hours (not to exceed 400m mg per dose ***PLUS*** Clindamycin 40 mg/kg per day divided every 8 hours (not to exceed 900 mg per dose

- *PLUS* **Antitoxin Therapy** *PLUS* **Anthrax Immunoglobulin**

SYSTEMIC ANTHRAX WITH SUSPECTED OR PROVEN MENINGITIS

- Ciprofloxacin – In adults: 400 mg intravenously (IV) every 8 hours; in children: 30 mg/kg per day divided every 8 hours, not to exceed 400 mg per dose **PLUS**

- Meropenem – In adults: 2 g IV every 8 hours; in children: 120 mg/kg per day divided every 8 hours, not to exceed 2 g per dose **PLUS**

- Linezolid – In adults: 600 mg IV every 12 hours; in children <12 years of age: 30 mg/kg per day divided every 8 hours, not to exceed 600 mg per dose; in children ≥12 years of age: 30 mg/kg per day divided every 12 hours, not to exceed 600 mg/dose

- PLUS **Antitoxin Therapy** *PLUS* **Anthrax Immunoglobulin**

ANTHRAX ANTITOXINS

Included as soon as possible in the treatment regimen for any patient suspected to have systemic anthrax; greatest benefit when used early in the course of disease
Raxibacumab (ABthrax) or Anthim (obiltoxaximab)

ANTHRAX IMMUNOGLOBULIN

Anthrax immunoglobulin derived from the plasma of Anthrax Vaccine Adsorbed (AVA)-immunized persons is available from the CDC or through state and local health departments for the treatment of inhalation anthrax, in patients with cutaneous anthrax with extensive edema or lesions of the head or neck or anthrax meningitis in combination with antimicrobial therapy. Anthrax immunoglobulin neutralizes toxins produced by *B. anthracis*

ANTHRAX TREATMENT - GLUCOCORTICOIDS / DURATION OF TREATMENT

- **Glucocorticoids** — Glucocorticoids should be considered as adjunctive therapy for patients with anthrax meningitis, cutaneous anthrax with extensive edema involving the head and neck, anthrax in the setting of recent glucocorticoid therapy, or anthrax with vasopressor-resistant shock
- Begin IV treatment initially before switching to oral antimicrobial therapy
- Continue oral and IV treatment for 60 days

ANTHRAX POST-EXPOSURE PROPHYLAXIS (PEP)

Antimicrobial drug prophylaxis for 60 days

Non-pregnant adults:
- Ciprofloxacin 500 mg every 12 hours or
- Doxycycline 100 mg every 12 hours

Pregnant, lactating, and postpartum women:
- Ciprofloxacin 500 mg every 12 hours

Children
- Ciprofloxacin 30 mg/kg per day divided every 12 hours (not to exceed 500 mg/dose)
  or
  Doxycycline
  <45 kg: 4.4 mg/kg per day divided every 12 hours (not to exceed 100 mg/dose)
  ≥45 kg: 100 mg every 12 hours

PLUS
A three-dose series of anthrax vaccine adsorbed

PNEUMONIC PLAGUE

- **Treatment**
  - Preferred choices: Streptomycin
    - 1 g intramuscularly twice daily (30 mg/kg/day) in adults
    - 15 mg/kg intramuscularly twice daily (maximum daily dose 2 g) in children
  - Gentamicin
    - 5 mg/kg/day intramuscularly or IV (or 2 mg/kg loading dose followed by 1.7 mg/kg every 8 hours) in adults
    - 2.5 mg/kg intramuscularly or IV every 8 hours in children
  - Alternative choices: Doxycycline or Ciprofloxacin or Chloramphenicol
  - Treatment for 10 days
- **Post-exposure prophylaxis**
  - Doxycycline 100 mg po bid x7 days
  - Levofloxacin 500mg po daily x10 days

PULMONARY TULAREMIA

TREATMENT

- Treatment with Streptomycin, Gentamicin, or Ciprofloxacin should be continued for 10 days
- Treatment with Doxycycline or Chloramphenicol should be continued for 14-21 days

Adults	**Preferred choices:** Streptomycin, 1g IM twice daily Gentamicin, 5 mg/kg IM or IV once daily **Alternative choices:** Doxycycline, 100 mg IV twice daily Chloramphenicol, 15 mg/kg IV 4 times daily Ciprofloxacin, 400 mg IV twice daily
Children	**Preferred choices:** Streptomycin, 15 mg/kg IM twice daily (should not exceed 2 gm/d) Gentamicin, 2.5 mg/kg IM or IV 3 times daily **Alternative choices:** Doxycycline If weight >= 45 kg, 100 mg IV If weight < 45 kg, give 2.2 mg/kg IV twice daily Chloramphenicol, 15 mg/kg IV 4 times daily Ciprofloxacin, 15 mg/kg IV twice daily
Pregnant Women	**Preferred choices:** Gentamicin, 5 mg/kg IM or IV once daily Streptomycin, 1 g IM twice daily **Alternative choices:** Doxycycline, 100 mg IV twice daily Ciprofloxacin, 400 mg IV twice daily

POST-EXPOSURE PROPHYLAXIS

Adults	**Preferred choices:** Doxycycline, 100 mg orally twice daily Ciprofloxacin, 500 mg orally twice daily
Children	**Preferred choices:** Doxycycline, and If >=45kg give 100 mg orally twice daily If <45 kg then give 2.2 mg/kg orally twice daily Ciprofloxacin, 15 mg/kg orally twice daily
Pregnant Women	**Preferred choices:** Ciprofloxacin, 500 mg orally twice daily Doxycycline, 100 mg orally twice daily

Exposed persons should be prophylactically treated for 14 days
Postexposure prophylactic treatment of close contacts of tularemia patients is not recommended because person-to-person transmission is not known to occur

BOTULISM

7 types of botulism neurotoxins known as types A-G
Exotoxin (botulinus toxin) → descending symmetrical paralysis

PATHOGENESIS

- Inhale / digest neurotoxin → circulation → nerve synapses → blocks the release of acetylcholine → Symmetrical descending flaccid paralysis with prominent bulbar palsies →
- Dysarthria (difficulty speaking)
- Dysphagia (difficulty swallowing)
- Dry mouth
- Diplopia (double vision)
- Dilated or non-reactive pupil (blurred vision)
- Dsysphonia
- Droopy eye (Ptosis)
- Respiratory Failure
- Absence of fever and no sensory deficits

TREATMENT

- Equine Serum Heptavalent Botulism Antitoxin; Antitoxin does not reverse paralysis but arrests its progression 2-8 weeks ventilatory support may be required; Antibiotics are not indicated
- **PEARL:** Guillain-Barré Syndrome (GBS) → ascending paralysis

CHOLERA

- Enterotoxin →↑ cAMP → secretion of water and chloride ions → massive "rice-water" stool; fluid losses may exceed 5 to 10liters per day
- Treatment
  - Fluid and electrolyte replacement
  - Ciprofloxacin 1.0 gm po x once OR
  - Doxycycline 300 mg po x once
  - For children and in pregnancy: erythromycin or trimethoprim-sulfamethoxazole

BIOTERRORISM PEARLS

- Abdominal symptoms are seen with: inhalational anthrax, pneumonic plague, Q-fever, Ebola
- Person to person transmission has ***not*** been reported in: inhalational anthrax, bubonic and septicemic plague, pulmonary tularemia, Q-fever pneumonia
- Person to person transmission ***has been*** reported in: pneumonic plague, viral hemorrhagic fevers (not yellow-fever), and smallpox
- Decontamination, bleach effective: anthrax, plague, tularemia, Q-fever, cholera, ricin, VHFs, nerve agents, blister agents
- Hypochlorite solution does ***not*** inactivate Trichothecene Mycotoxins
- Common characteristic features of VHFs & plague: petechiae, purpura, ecchymosis, DIC
- Hemoptysis is present in both VHFs and plague, however other pulmonary findings are uncommon with VHFs

CHEMICAL TERRORISM

BLOOD AGENT - CYANIDE

- Is a tissue toxin - the military incorrectly categorizes with blood agent
- Binds cytochrome oxidase and disrupts oxidative phosphorylation →↑ anaerobic metabolism
- Symptoms: HA/N/V/confusion/combativeness/seizures and coma
  - Reddish lips (blue in dark skinned patient)
  - Odor = almonds
- Signs: initially ↑ HR and BP followed by → ↓ HR and BP and profound metabolic acidosis; respiratory, CNS and myocardial depression (bradycardia → asystole) within minutes of significant exposure

Treatment

- Preferred Treatment Options
  - Na-Thiosulfate
  - Hydroxocobalamin (Vitamin B12), is bright red and causes reddish discoloration of skin, urine and plasma
- Alternative Treatment Option: Cyanided Antidote Kit

  #1 Amyl Nitrite - inhaled by the patient (held under the patient's nose or via ETT) for 30 seconds of each minute x 3 minutes

  #2 Na-Nitrite → converts RBC hemoglobin (Hgb) → to Methemoglobin
    - Methemoglobin → combines with cyanide to form → cyanometh-Hgb
    - Cyanometh-Hgb and free cyanide are detoxified by sulfur transferase (rhodanese) → to thiocyanate
    - Thiocyanate is → eliminated in urine
    - Rhodanese function ↑s with the availability of sulfur donor
    - **Na-Thiosulfate is a sulfur-containing compound**

  #3 Na-Thiosulfate + cyanometh-Hgb, via rhodanese enzyme → Na-thiocyanate
  Na-thiocyanate → eliminated in urine

- **PEARL:** If simultaneous **carbon monoxide** and **cyanide poisoning** - Na-Thiosulfate should be used ALONE
- Adjunctive therapy: sodium bicarbonate to correct metabolic acidosis & benzodiazepines for seizures

BLISTER AGENTS

- Lewisite
- Nitrogen and sulfur mustards
- Phosgene oxime
- Most sensitive are warm, moist thin areas → perineum, genitalia, axilla, neck & antecubital fossa (thicker skin of hands may be spared)
- On the skin mustard causes no immediate pain sensation (delayed symptoms, hours after exposure)
- Lewisite and phosgene oxime cause immediate pain
- Lewisite antidote: Dimercaprol (British Anti-Lewisite - BAL)

CHEMICAL TERRORISM

NERVE AGENTS

- Sarin, Soman, Tabun, GF & VX
- Inhibitors of acetylcholinestease → cholinergic excess → SLUDGE BAM Syndrome
- Treatment
  - Atropine: large amounts, (10-20 mg), may be needed over 24 hours
  - Pralidoxime chloride (2-PAM, Protopam) reverses the cholinergic nicotinic effects

CHOKING AGENTS

- Phosgene and Chlorine = non-cardiogenic-pulmonary edema
- Delayed symptoms with phosgene; immediate symptoms are noted with chlorine
- Nebulized 3.75% sodium bicarbonate symptomatic improvement to treat chlorine exposures

INDUCTION AGENTS

DRUG	DOSE	ONSET / DURATION PEARLS	SIDE EFFECTS
Etomidate (Amidate)	0.3 mg/kg	Onset < 15 seconds Duration: 5-15 minutes Minimal BP effects	Potential adrenal suppression in septic patients
Propofol (Diprivan)	1.5-3mg/kg	Onset 10-20 seconds Duration: 10-15 minutes Bronchodilation	Hypotension
Midazolam (Versed)	0.2 mg/kg	Onset 1-5 minutes Duration: 30-60 minutes Amnesia	Hypotension
Ketamine (Ketalar)	1-2 mg/kg	Onset < 2 minutes Duration:10-15 minutes Status asthmaticus (bronchodilation); beneficial in hypotension; amnesia; analgesia	Bronchorrhea Laryngospasm HTN
Fentanyl (Sublimaze)	2 mcg/kg	Onset 1-2 minutes Duration: 30 minutes Use if concern for increased ICP attenuates the increase in BP (20 mm Hg on average) that occurs with laryngoscopy	Hypotension

PARALYTIC AGENTS

DRUG	DOSE	ONSET / DURATION PEARLS	SIDE EFFECTS
Succinylcholine (Anectine)	1 .5 mg/kg (adults) 2.0 mg/kg (children)	Depolarizing agent Onset < 1 minute Duration: 4-6 minutes	Hyperkalemia
Vecuronium (Norcuron)	0.2 mg/kg	Non-depolarizing agent Onset 1.5-3 minutes Duration: 20-60 minutes	Long duration of action
Rocuronium (Zemuron)	1.0 mg/kg	Non-depolarizing Onset < 1 minute Duration: 45 minutes	Long duration of action

SUCCINLYCHOLINE CONTRAINDICATIONS

- Rhabdomyloysis
- Crush injuries > 5 days old
- Burns > 1-5 days old involving > 10% BSA
- Denervation injuries (CVA, spinal cord) > 5 days old until
- 6 months post-injury
- Neuromuscular diseases indefinitely (muscular dystrophies)
- Guillian Barre Syndrome (GBS)
- Intra-abdominal sepsis > 5 days until resolution
- Malignant hyperexia

8 P'S OF RAPID SEQUENCE INTUBATION (RSI)

P 1.	**P**erform H & P (MAPLE), consider indications, risks, alternatives, Mallampati score
P 2.	**P**reparation: personal, drugs & equipment
P 3.	**P**ulse oximetry, monitor, good IV access, automated BP device, end-tidal CO2
P 4.	**P**reoxygenate
P 5.	**P**rime (induction): Etomidate, Propofol, Midazolam, Ketamine or Fentanyl
P 6.	**P**aralyze: Succinylcholine, Vecuronium, or Rocuronium
P 7.	**P**lacement of ETT
P 8.	**P**ost-intubation: verify tube placement and assure adequate sedation

ENDOTRACHEAL TUBE (ETT) SIZE

- ETT size = the inner diameter in mm
- ETT size adult males = 8.0-8.5 advance tube to 23cm (from carina to corner of mouth)
- ETT size adult females = 7.5-8.0 advance tube to 21 cm (from carina to corner of mouth)

- After intubation, order PCXR, ETT should be 2 cm above the carina; check end-tidal CO2
- PEARL: If end-tidal CO2 = yellow → good ETT placement (*yellow = mellow*)

END-TIDAL CO2 PEARLS

High ETCO2 reading

- Altered mental status
- Severe difficulty breathing
- Hypoventilation
- Patient may need to be intubated

Low ETCO2

- Hyperventilation

PRE-INTUBATION ASSESSMENT FOR DIFFICULT AIRWAY

Mnemonic: (LEMON)

L	**L**ook externally
E	**E**valuate (3:3:2 rule) = 3 fingers between incisors; mandible length 3 fingers from tip of chin to hyoid bone and distance of the hyoid to the thyroid – 2 fingers distance
M	**M**allampati classification (I-IV); I fully visible tonsils; IV only hard palate visible)
O	**O**bstruction
N	**N**eck

POST-INTUBATION PROBLEMS

Mnemonic: (DOPE)

D	**D**islodged ETT
O	**O**bstructed ETT
P	**P**neumothorax
E	**E**quipment failure

POST-INTUBATION HYPOTENSION

Mnemonic: (AAHH SHITE)

https://rebelem.com/post-intubation-hypotension-the-ah-shite-mnemonic/Reference provided by Dr. Adam Madej

A	**A**cidosis
A	**A**naphylaxis
H	**H**eart (cardiac tamponade)
H	**H**eart (pulmonary hypertension)
S	**S**tacked breathing
H	**H**ypovolemia
I	**I**nduction agent
T	**T**ension pneumothorax
E	**E**lectrolytes (hyperkalemia)

PEDIATRIC AIRWAY PEARLS

Airway Differences vs Adults

- Large tongue
- Floppy epiglottis
- Anterior and cephalad cords
- Narrowest diameter = cricoid ring (below the cords)
- Head and occiput proportionally larger
- Neck is shorter (trachea shorter)
- Adenoids larger
- Risk of mainstem intubation is higher in pediatrics due to short trachea and bronchus

ESTIMATING ETT SIZE

- Uncuffed = (Age / 4) + 4
- Cuffed = (Age / 4) + 3.5

- ETTs should be cuffed for all pediatric intubations except neonates and newborns
- ETTs cuff pressures should be kept to < 20 cm H2O

- ETT x 2 = NG and Urinary Catheter size
- ETT x 3 = Depth of ETT insertion (position of ETT at the lips (in cm;s)
- ETT x 4 = Chest tube size

- Weight in kilograms = (Age x 2) + 8

Weight estimates

- Newborn = 3 kg
- 1 y/o = 10 kg
- 5 y/o = 20 kg
- 10 y/o = 30 kg

Upper limit of SBP = (Age x 2) + 80

IMPORTANT NUMBERS

Success in Medical School and Beyond I Mnemonics and Pearls

THE #3 IS AN IMPORTANT NUMBER

INFECTIOUS DISEASE

3 Stages of Lyme Disease: Early localized, Early disseminated (around 4 weeks) and Late (> 1 year)

3 Phases of Pertussis: Catarrhal phase, Paroxysmal phase and Convalescent phase

Most common complication of Pertussis: seizures **3**%

3 Forms of Plague: Bubonic, Pneumonic and Septicemic plague

3 steps (important virally encoded enzymes) in HIV Replication: reverse transcriptase, integrase and protease (anti-virals work against each step)

3 important Spirochetes (spiral-shaped bacteria): Treponema (syphilis & yaws); Borrelia (Lyme disease & relapsing fever) and Leptospira

Triad Rocky Mountain spotted fever (RMSF): Fever, Rash and Tick exposure

TOXICOLOGY

3 phases of Ethylene Glycol Toxicity: CNS (1 to 12 hours), Cardiopulmonary (12 to 24 hours) and Nephrotoxic (24 to 72 hours)

3 phases of Amanita mushroom illness: Gastrointestinal, Quiescent and Hepatic Failure

Stage with the highest mortality in Acetaminophen (APAP) toxicity = Stage **3**

Stage with the highest mortality in Iron (Fe) toxicity = Stage **3**

Triad of sublethal arsine (gas form of arsenic) exposure: abdominal pain, jaundice and hematuria

NEUROLOGY

3 Types of neurofibromatosis: Types 1 and 2 (NF1 and NF2) and schwannomatosis; NF1 (von Recklinghausen disease) = most common type

3 Components of uvea (uveal tract): from inner to outer = iris, ciliary body, and choroid

Triad Menier's Disease (Idiopathic endolymphatic hydrops): Sensorineural hearing loss, tinnitus and episodic vertigo

Triad Wernicke's Encephalopathy: AMS, ophthalmoplegia and ataxia

Triad Spinal epidural abscess: fever, back pain and neurological deficits (rare)

3 Step treatment approach in status epilepticus: 1) benzodiazepines 2) Fosphenytoin *or* Levetiracetam 3) phenobarbital *or* Pentobarbital *or* Propofol

Triad normal pressure hydrocephalus: urinary incontinence, mental confusion and ataxia ("wet, wacky, and wobbly")

CARDIOLOGY / PULMONARY

Aorta consists of **3** layers: intima, media, and adventitia

Aortic dissection, Male:Female ratio **3:1**

Aortic diameter > **3** cm is considered aneurysmal (AAA)

Triad Ruptured AAA: Hypotension, pulsatile abdominal mass and flank/back pain; May be incomplete in as many as 50%

Triad Aortoenteric Fistula: GI bleeding (massive or simple sentinel bleed), abdominal pain, palpable mass

Triad Aortic Stenosis: Syncope, Angina and Dyspnea (SAD)

Multifocal Atrial Tachycardia (MAT): **> 3** differently shaped P's; irregular rhythm

Triad EKG Findings in WPW: Wide QRS complex (QRS > 120 msec), short PR interval (PR < 120 msec) and slurred upstroke of QRS complex ("Delta wave")

Virchow's **triad**: hypercoagulable state, venous stasis, venous injury

Triad pulmonary embolism (PE): Dyspnea, CP, hemoptysis < 20%

Chronic bronchitis definition: mucous-producing cough most day of the month, **3 months** of a year, for 4 years in a row without other explanation for cough

3 D's of Beck's Triad: Distant (muffled) heart sounds, Drop in BP (hypotension), Distended jugular veins (increased CVP)

GI / SURGERY

US finding consistent with appendicitis: **3 mm** wall thickness (diameter > 6mm, target sign, not compressible appendix)

US findings consistent with cholecystitis: **> 3 mm** GB wall thickening; the most sensitive US finding = sonographic Murphy's

US aortic diameter **> 3 cm** is considered aneurysmal (AAA)

Diagnosing pancreatitis: lipase needs to be **> 3x** upper limit with history consistent with pancreatitis

Charcot's **triad**: Fever, RUQ abdominal pain and jaundice

Plummer-Vinson **triad**: dysphagia, esophageal webs and iron-deficiency anemia

Boerhaave syndrome, Mackler's **triad**: CP, vomiting, and subcutaneous emphysema, < 50%

3 common sites for esophageal FBs to lodge: Cricopharyngeus (level of C6, most common), Aortic arch (level of T4) and GE junction (level of the diaphragmatic hiatus)

3 meds, "triple therapy", for H. pylori: proton pump inhibitor, clarithromycin, and amoxicillin or metronidazole; most common cause of PUD

3 D's of Pellagra: Diarrhea, Dermatitis and Dementia; Niacin (B3) deficiency

3 G's of Pellagra: Glossitis, Gingivitis and Generalized stomatitis; Niacin (B3) deficiency

PEDIATRICS

3 kg = Weight of a newborn; (1 year-old = 10 kg; 5 year-old = 20 kg and a 10 year-old = 30 kg)

3 x ETT size = Depth of ETT insertion; (ETT x2 = NG/Foley catheter size; ETT x3 = depth of ETT insertion; 4 ETT size = Chest tube size; pediatrics)

3% = Incidence of febrile seizures; recurrence rate = 30%

2-**3%** = Chance of developing epilepsy after simple febrile seizure > compared with 1% rate of epilepsy in general population

3rd Most common childhood cancer = neuroblastoma (most common site = adrenal glands): Leukemia and brain tumors most common childhood cancers

Colic definition: crying for > **3 hours**/day, for > **3 days**/week in an infant < **3** months of age

Triad Hemolytic Uremic Syndrome: MAHA (schistocytes on peripheral smear), Thrombocytopenia & AKI

Triad Pediatric Intussusception: abdominal pain, vomiting & bloody stools (hematochezia) = 33%

OTHER

3 causes Acute tubular necrosis (ATN): renal ischemia, nephrotoxic and sepsis

Triad Glomerulonephritis: Hematuria, HTN and periorbital edema

Triad Granulomatosis with PolyAngiitis (GPA), formerly known as Wegener's granulomatosis (WG) = sinusitis, pulmonary infiltrates and nephritis

3 Basic requirements of EMTALA: Medical Screening Exam (MSE), stabilization and transfer

3 D's of Endometriosis: Dysmenorrhea (painful menstruation), Dyspareunia (painful sexual intercourse), Dyschezia (painful bowel movement)

3 D's of Colles Fracture: Distal radius fracture, Dorsal displacement of radial fragment, Dinner fork deformity

THE #4 IS AN IMPORTANT NUMBER

4 Stages of acetaminophen (APAP) Toxicity: Stage 1 (First day); Stage 2 (days 1 to 3); Stage 3 = (days 3 to 4 fulminant hepatic failure = bad) and Stage 4 = (> 4 days), resolution, HF or death

4 King's College Prognostic Criteria to consider during APAP toxicity and need for liver transplantation: pH < 7.3 after fluid resuscitation, PT > 100 seconds or > 1.8x control or INR > 6.5, creatinine > 3.4 mg/dL and Grade III or IV hepatic encephalopathy

4 hours after ingestion = time to draw Acetaminophen (APAP) level to determine toxicity

4 to 8 hours = time after ingestion to draw serum iron (Fe) concentrations; if
< 500 µg/dL = low risk of significant toxicity; Concentrations of > 500 µg/dL at 6 hours = significant toxicity

3.5 to **4** mEq/L = indication for dialysis in Lithium (Li) toxicity

4 minutes = time to perform perimortem Caesarean delivery; (remember 24 & 4 = > 24 weeks gestation and start with **4** minutes of arrest; 1 min for procedure)

4 Phases of Pericarditis on EKG

4:1 Male:Female ratio in AAA

4:1 Male:Female ratio in Legg-Calve-Perthes disease

4:1 Male:Female ratio in Pyloric Stenosis

> **4mm** thickened pylorus = US findings in pyloric stenosis; elongated > 14mm (most common 2 weeks to 2 months of life)

4 to 6 **hours** = testicular salvage rate is greatest in testicular torsion (96%); drops to 20% after 12 hours

< **4mm** = size of kidney stones with greatest chance to pass (90%), 4 to 6 mm (50%) and > 6mm (10%)

4 to 6 **hours** = observation time for post-obstructive diuresis in patients with chronic urinary retention

Diagnostic Criteria + fever for 5 days to make diagnosis of Kawasaki syndrome = **4** out 5; (Five criteria = CREAM = conjunctivitis, rash, edema, adenopathy and mucosal involvement)

4 Leg muscle compartments: anterior, lateral, superficial posterior, deep posterior; anterior compartment of the leg = most common site for compartment syndrome

4 Grades of hyphema injuries: Grade I = < 1/3 of AC; Grade II = 1/3 to 1/2 of AC; Grade III = Slightly less then total AC; Grade V = "Eight ball" = blood fills entire AC

4 Anatomical locations of metacarpal fractures: metacarpal head, neck, shaft, or base

Treating hypoglycemia in infants: D25 at 2 to **4 mL/kg**
(Neonates = D10 5 to 10 mL/kg)

4 P's in the treatment of Tet Spell: P = position (knee-chest position), Pain control (morphine), Propranolol, Phenylephrine

Estimating ETT Size
Uncuffed = (Age / **4**) + **4**
Cuffed = (Age / **4**) + 3.5

0. **4** to 0.**44** seconds (**4**00 to 440ms) = normal QT interval

4 Classes of Antiarrhythmics: SOme BLOCK, Potassium, Channels = Class I = SOdium channel blockers, Class II = Beta BLOCKers, Class III = Potassium channel blockers and Class IV Calcium Channel blockers

4 Personality disorders in Cluster B: Narcissistic, Antisocial, Borderline and Histrionic

4 Types of consent: Express consent, implied consent, emergent consent and informed consent

4 Elements of negligence: Duty, breach of duty, causation and damage

< **4 mL/kg** = amount of fluid most drowning victims aspirate
(content of water, salt vs fresh, is not clinically relevant)

4 Organisims that cause pneumonia which present with fever + relative bradycardia ("Faget Sign"): Legionella (legionellosis), Coxiella burnetii (Q-fever), Chlamydia psittaci (Psittacosis) & Francisella tularensis (Tularemia)
All **4** organisms also cause transaminitis (Elevated LFTs)

4 Forms of anthrax: Cutaneous, inhalation, gastrointestinal, and the newly designated injection anthrax

4 Clinical stages of Syphilis: Primary, Secondary, Latent and Tertiary

4 drugs in the treatment of TB in HIV:
(RIPE) R = Rifampin, I = Isoniazid (INH), P = Pyrazinamide, E = Ethambutol

Acute HIV infection (Primary HIV infection) or Acute Retroviral Syndrome occurs
2 to **4 weeks** after exposure

THE #20 IS AN IMPORTANT NUMBER

Fluid bolus in pediatric resuscitation = **20 mL/kg**

Pediatric neck masses
20% = branchial cleft cyst (lateral neck, anterior to the border of the sternocleidomastoid near the angle of the mandible; non-tender (unless infected) and fluctuant)

Weight estimates
Newborn = 3 kg
1 y/o = 10 kg
5 y/o = **20 kg**
10 y/o = 30 kg

Intussusception
"Currant jelly" stools (late finding) only present in about **20% of cases**
Siblings of affected patients have a relative risk **20x** > general population

IMPORTANT NUMBERS

Most prevalent parasite in the US
Enterobius vermicularis (pinworm). **20** to 30% kids infected; cause of anal pruritus in kids

20% = elemental iron in ferrous sulfate
Ferrous fumarate = 33% elemental iron
Ferrous sulfate = **20% elemental iron**
Ferrous gluconate = 12% elemental iron

Gyromitra esculenta toxicity
Treat with methylene blue if **methemoglobin level is > 20%** or causing symptoms

Rocky Mountain spotted fever (RMSF)
Triad: Fever, rash, tick exposure, occurs in **20% of cases**

Lyme Disease Stage 1 Early Localized Phase
Erythema Chronicum Migrans (ECM): pathognomonic; 2 to **20 days** after tick bite

Leptospriosis
Leptospira interrogans = spirochete; most widespread zoonotic infection
Fresh water contaminated by bovine, pig, canine or rat urine
2 to **20 days incubation**

Ehrlichiosis
20% present with maculopapular rash

Cysticercosis
Viable cysts are round, non-enhancing hypodense lesions 5 to **20mm** in diameter

Mortality rate of cutaneous anthrax without treatment = **20%**

Hemolytic Uremic Syndrome (HUS): low grade fever in 5 to **20%**

Human rabies immune globulin (HRIG) dose = **20 IU/kg**

Initial Vancomycin dose = **20 mg/kg**

SIRS respiratory rate criteria
a. **> 20 breaths/min** or
b. PaCO2 < 32 mmHg

20% = rate of recurrence herpetic whitlow

20% = sigmoid volvulus mortality rate (if gangrenous > 50%)

Postoperative adhesions are the most common cause of SBOs (60%), followed by **cancer (20%)**, and then incarcerated hernias (10%)

If burns are >**20% BSA** = likely to get an ileus

<20% gallstones seen on KUB

50% of HCV patients develop chronic hepatitis

20% of this group develop cirrhosis within 10 years

20% of patients with Boerhaave syndrome (Mackler Triad) will have Hamman's crunch

20 mL/kg of blood after chest tube insertion = indication for thoracotomy

CXR shows **20** -34% of diaphragmatic injuries

Testicular torsion salvage rate: 4 to 6 hours = 96%; drops to **20%** after 12 hours

Triad pulmonary embolism (PE): dyspnea, CP and hemoptysis seen in **< 20%**

Normal Mean Pulmonary Artery Pressure (MPAP) = 10 – **20 mmHg**

Labetalol dosing in HTN Emergency:
Start with **20 mg** IV over two minutes – repeat or double every 10min to max of 300mg

Procainamide **20** to 50 **mg/minute** IV; monitor every 5 to 10 minutes until the

a) arrhythmia terminates
b) hypotension ensues
c) QRS is prolonged > 50% or
d) Total of 17 mg/kg is given

Adenosine is ultra short acting = **20 seconds**

Lasix, diuretic response = in 10 to **20 minutes**

Strong risk factor for AAA = Family history → patients with 1st degree relative & AAA have a 10-**20 fold ↑risk of developing AAA**

BP difference between upper extremities of > **20 mmHg** suggests aortic dissection
Mortality: 25% at 1 hour, 50% at one week and 90% at one year

Arterial occlusion: arterial embolism most common; second most common cause = thrombosis **(20%)**

AMI + mild CHF, **mortality rate** = 15-**20%**

Most Common Rhythm Disturbance in Digitalis Toxicity
PVC 60% > SVT 25% > **AV block 20%**

AKI, pre-renal azotemia = UNa < **20 mEq/L** and FENa < 1%

AKI, Acute Tubular Necrosis (ATN)
BUN to Cr ratio < **20**
FENa > 2%

Maximal inspiratory pressure (MIP): the maximal negative pressure a patient can generate while inhaling through a blocked mouthpiece after a full exhalation
MIP is also referred to as negative inspiratory force (NIF)
Normal NIF > 60 cm water. If NIF is dropping or nears **20 cm water** = need respiratory support; measure NIF in GBS and MG patients

Most common causes of hyperparathyroidism:
Adenoma 80%
Hyperplasia 15-**20%**
Carcinoma < 1%
↑PTH → ↑Ca

Normal visual acuity (VA) = **20/20** (you can see clearly at 20 feet what should normally be seen at a distance)

Normal IOP < **20 mm Hg**

Normal LP opening pressure: 6 to **20 cmH2O** in the lateral decubitus position

Normal intracranial pressure (ICP) < **20**
CPP = MAP – ICP

20% = mortality rate in status epilepticus

ANTICONVULSANTS IN STATUS EPILEPTICUS

Fosphenytoin (Cerebyx)
Loading dose: 15-**20 mg PE/kg** IV, infuse at 100-150 mg PE/min

Phenytoin (Dilantin)
Loading Dose: 15-**20mg/kg IV**, infuse at 25-60 mg/min

Phenobarbital
Loading dose: 15-**20 mg/kg IV,** infuse at 25-60 mg/min

Levetiracetam (Keppra)
Loading dose: 10-50 mg/kg IV, safe place to start = **20 mg/kg IV**

Diazepam 5 mg IV, or **20 mg PR**

Hunt Hess Grading Scale for Subarachnoid Hemorrhage (SAH)
Classify the severity of a SAH based on clinical condition at presentation (Grade I to V)
20% projected survival for Grade IV = stupor, moderate / severe motor deficit, intermittent posturing (Grade I = 70%; Grade II = 60%; Grade III = 50%, **Grade IV = 20%;** Grade V = 10%)

Seizure > 20 minutes after trauma = worse prognosis; ↑ possibility of internal injury and development of seizures later

Patients with atrial fibrillation are 10 to **20x** more likely to develop stroke, and the majority of these are embolic events

30 day mortality after stoke = **20** – 25%; in-hospital mortality = 15%

Acceptable Metacarpal Angulation in Middle Finger: **< 20°**
(< 10° Index, < 20° Middle < 30° ring and < 40° little finger)

10-**20%** patients with scaphoid fractures will have normal x-ray

Bohler's angle: normal **20** to 40 **degrees**, if less suspect calcaneal fracture

Fat embolism syndrome: mortality rate = **20%**

Achilles tendon rupture: Gravity Equinus Splint: below-the-knee posterior splint with **20** to 30 **degrees** of plantar flexion (equinas position)

Compartment syndrome suspected if pressures > **20 mm Hg**
Diagnosed Compartment Delta Pressure ≤ 30 mm Hg or
Absolute compartment pressure > 30–40 mm Hg

20 weeks = gestational age uterus is palpable at the umbilicus

20% increase in oxygen requirement in pregnancy

20% functional residual capacity (FRC) decrease in pregnancy

FRC and oxygen requirement changes in pregnancy results in → decreased pulmonary reserve → puts pregnant patient at > risk of desaturation during endotracheal intubation

Most common surgical emergency in pregnancy = appendicitis
Higher perforation rate in pregnancy
Fetal loss 20% with perforated appy

Threatened abortion: vaginal bleeding **< 20 weeks** of gestation and a closed internal cervical os; risk of miscarriage in this population is up to 50%

Pseudogestational sac: anechoic fluid collection without a clear double decidual reaction Seen in 10 to **20% of ectopics**

Chlamydia urethritis: **20%** of women will present with dysuria (sterile pyuria)

20% of all psychiatric referrals have organic etiologies

Suicide attempt: after initial attempt, **20%** of patients will retry within one year

Ziprasidone (Geodon) dose for adults = **20 mg IM**

THE #500 IS AN IMPORTANT NUMBER

Postpartum Hemorrhage > **500 mL** of blood in 24 hours

Potentially *lethal dose* of Aspirin (ASA) > **500 mg/kg**

Significant Iron toxicity = concentrations > **500 μg/dL** at 6 hours

IMPORTANT NUMBERS

SOUND ALIKE WORDS

Leriche Syndrome: Aortoiliac Occlusive Disease
Claudication / pain of the buttocks and thighs; Erectile Dysfunction (ED)
Absent /decreased femoral pulses

Lemierre's syndrome: jugular vein suppurative thrombophlebitis
Preceded by pharyngitis, usually in association with tonsil or peritonsillar involvement. Other antecedent conditions include primary dental infection or infectious mononucleosis

Lhermitte sign: electric shock-like sensations down the back and/or limbs upon flexion of the neck of patients with multiple sclerosis (MS)

Fosphenytoin (**Cerebyx**): anti-epileptic medication
Celebrex (Celecoxib): COX-2 inhibitor, NSAID

Opsoclonus-myoclonus syndrome (very rare): involuntary myoclonic muscular contractions and spontaneous conjugate rapid eye movements in all directions of gaze 50% have an underlying neuroblastoma

Opisthotonos: rigidity of muscles in tetanus; PEARL: Initial symptom of tetanus = trismus ("lock jaw"= risus saronicus - think of the Joker from Batman)

Abduction: move "A"way from the "B"ody
Adduction: "Add" to the body (move toward midline of body)

Ilium: bone in pelvis
Ileum: part of small intestine

DysphaSia: difficulty speaking or understanding words ("S" = speaking)
DysphaGia: difficulty swallowing

Berger's disease: Immunoglobulin A (IgA) nephropathy
Buerger's disease: (Thromboangiitis obliterans (TAO) = inflammatory disease that affects the small to medium-sized arteries and veins of the extremities; smokers

Condyloma acuminatum: broad-based, pedunculated, cauliflower-like warts caused by Human papillomavirus (HPV)
Condyloma lata: broad-based, raised, flat, moist papules due to *Treponema pallidum*

SOUND A LIKE WORDS

Hemostasis: controlling/stopping bleeding
Homeostasis: maintaining equilibrium

Trapezius: muscle in back and shoulders
Trapezium: bone in the wrist below thumb

Malleus: small bone in the middle ear
Malleolus: bony protuberance in the ankl

POSTEROLATERAL A KEY WORD IN TEST QUESTIONS

- Most common site of diaphragmatic injury = **Posterolateral**
  (left >> right sided frequency)
- Most common site herniated disks rupture = **Posterolateral**
  Most common site L4-L5 & L5-S1 (95%)
- Almost all spinal hematomas = **Posterolateral**
- Most common site of esophageal tear in Boerhaave's syndrome = left **Posterolateral**
  (distal esophagus), weakest part of esophagus

IV IMMUNOGLOBULIN (IVIG) PEARLS

Primary Immune Thrombocytopenic Purpura
Formerly Idiopathic Thrombocytopenic Purpura (ITP)
Treatment is supportive as the course is self limited with 90% spontaneous remission
• Platelet count < 20,000μL will require treatment: steroids + IV gamma globulin (IVIG) or Anti-D immunoglobulin

Guillain-Barre Syndrome (GBS)
IVIG or Plasmapharesis (not both)
Assess respiratory status: negative inspiratory force (NIF)

Myasthenic Crisis
IVIG + steroids, or Plasmapharesis
Assess respiratory status: negative inspiratory force (NIF)

Kawasaki Syndrome (Mucocutaneous Lymph Node Syndrome)
IVIG + high-dose aspirin (ASA

PATIENT POSITIONING PEARLS

Acute Respiratory Distress Syndrome (ARDS)
Prone positioning (improves gas exchange)

Pulmonary Contusion
Good lung to the Ground

Pulmonary Hemorrhage
Bad side to ground

BONUS PEARLS

Empyema
Bad side to ground

Pregnant patient in transport
Left side down (left lateral decubitus)

Air embolism - positioned to avoid further embolization
Left lateral decubitus = suspected *venous* air embolism
Supine position = *arterial* embolism is suspected

Scuba diver after ascent
Arterial gas embolism
SUPINE

Acute angle closure glaucoma
Supine

Hyphema
Elevate HOB

Elevated ICP
Elevate HOB

Spinal headaches begin within first 24 hours after LP
Worse = upright position
Resolve = SUPINE

Pericarditis
Worse = Supine
Better (less pain) = sitting UP leaning forward

REFERENCES

UpToDate

eMedicine

RoshReview

ICEP Board Review Course 2019

Rogers PT: *The Medical Student's Guide to Top Board Scores.* Chicago: Innovative Publishing and Graphics, Inc. 1992; pgs. 116, 129, 131, 189, 193, 195, 200, 206, 225.

Dr. Antonio Carlino

Dr. Karen Spurgash

Dr. Tajudeen Ogbara

Dr. Eric Farinas, mnemonic provided by Dr. Nancy Bauer

Dr. Dane Nichols

Dr. Thomas R. Scaggs

Author = Dr. Gueyikian, mnemonic provided by Dr. Suzanne Ahn

Dr. Nancy Bauer

Dr. George Hevesy

Dr. Nicole Colucci